THE EMOTIONALLY INTELLIGENT
NURSE LEADER

THE EMOTIONALLY INTELLIGENT NURSE LEADER

Mae Taylor Moss

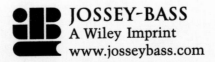

JOSSEY-BASS
A Wiley Imprint
www.josseybass.com

Published by Jossey-Bass
A Wiley Imprint
989 Market Street, San Francisco, CA 94103-1741   www.josseybass.com

Jossey-Bass books and products are available through most bookstores. To contact Jossey-Bass directly call our Customer Care Department within the U.S. at 800-956-7739, outside the U.S. at 317-572-3986 or fax 317-572-4002.

Jossey-Bass also publishes its books in a variety of electronic formats. Some content that appears in print may not be available in electronic books.

Readers should be aware that Internet Web sites used within may have changed or disappeared between when the book was written and when it is read.

Library of Congress Cataloging-in-Publication Data

Moss, Mae Taylor.
The emotionally intelligent nurse leader / Mae Taylor Moss.—1st ed.
p.; cm.
Includes bibliographical references and index.
ISBN 0–7879–5988–X (alk. paper)
1. Nursing services—Administration. 2. Leadership. 3. Emotional intelligence.
4. Nurses—Psychology. 5. Nurse and patient. I. Title.
[DNLM: 1. Nursing, Supervisory. 2. Emotions. 3. Leadership. 4. Nursing
Staff—psychology. 5. Patients—psychology. WY 105 M913e 2005]
RT89.M635 2005
362.17'3'068—dc22
2004014530

Printed in the United States of America
FIRST EDITION
PB Printing   10 9 8 7 6 5 4 3 2 1

CONTENTS

PART FOUR
Changing the Culture of Nursing and the Organization

PREFACE

"KNOW THYSELF" and "To thine own self be true," aphorisms taken from classic literary works and passed down through many generations as standard wisdom, remain popular even today. Centuries ago, when Socrates and Shakespeare penned those now-immortal words, they probably did not know that they were glimpsing a broader, more exact science—that of emotional intelligence. Today, emotional intelligence has blossomed from studies in social behavior to a measurable, predictable pattern of thought and action that influences decision making and success in relationships. References to feelings, emotions, and interpersonal skills abound in management literature, pointing out the relevance of emotional aptitude in our day. The ability to know and understand oneself, as well as to practice integrity in handling one's emotions, is fundamental to emotional expertise.

So relevant is emotional intelligence to leadership that multiple books have been written on the topic. However, nursing leadership presents a special situation: a field in which emotions are inherent in frontline work, leading to a decision structure in which conflicts and ethical dilemmas occur almost daily, and a rapid technological boom and increased financial emphasis that have stripped away the time allowed for pleasant, leisurely conversations.

This book was written to equip the nurse leader with emotional principles for leadership in the twenty-first century. Nurse leaders are responsible not only for patient outcomes but also for the success of those under their leadership. Because nurse leaders lead staff members who deal with the emotional issues of patient care, they also deal with the end result of all of these emotional issues: stress, the need to reflect, the need to be valued, and the need to grow emotionally. In the midst of this leadership challenge, nurse leaders themselves need to grow emotionally, supporting themselves and those around them in healthy, constructive ways.

Over the years, my experience as a staff nurse, educator, leader, and administrator have presented me with specific challenges, all of which presented profoundly emotional themes. There is no doubt that nursing is one of the most emotionally charged professions of our day or that it will continue to be so as this century unfolds. My passion for helping others, especially fellow nurse leaders, to develop their own emotional acuity led me to research the subject of emotional intelligence and provide this information to nurse leaders so that they, too, can understand how critical it is not only to know themselves but also to be true to their colleagues, their department, their organization, and their profession.

This book was made possible through the contributions and influence of many. John Mayer, Peter Salovey, and David Caruso, whose research has led to refinement of the science of emotional intelligence and its application, graciously allowed me to participate in the normalization of their most recent emotional intelligence test, the MSCEIT 2.0. During the research process, I was able to gain valuable insight into how emotional intelligence affects leadership in the health care arena.

I would also like to convey my deep gratitude to Marjorie Byers, PhD, RN, FAAN, former executive director of the American Organization of Nurse Executives, whose outspoken belief that emotional skills are critical to nursing leadership was highly instrumental in making this book a reality.

I would never have been able to write this book without the countless opportunities given to me over the years by nurse leaders—opportunities both to teach them and to learn from them. Today, I work with a team of eighteen nurse leaders who are growing not only in nursing knowledge but also in the ability to relate to and effectively lead their teams. As a result, their teams are leading our organization.

Family members and friends have supported this work and continually encouraged its completion. Many authors conclude that despite the research, the prior knowledge, and the publishing deadlines, it is really the personal support of those closest to them that motivates and makes possible the completion of a work. This work is no exception.

To nurse leaders working everywhere—in hospitals, clinics, disease management organizations, managed care organizations, and government agencies: know thyself, know your colleagues, and know what you can do to make your organization more successful. Please accept my sincere wishes for a lifetime of successful leadership.

MAE TAYLOR MOSS

ABOUT THE AUTHOR

MAE TAYLOR MOSS, RN, MSN, DHA, FAAN, a registered nurse since 1977, holds a master's degree in nursing from the University of Maryland, a master's degree in education from Johns Hopkins University, and a doctorate in health care administration and leadership from the Medical University of South Carolina. She has held educational, administrative, and leadership positions in both hospital and nonhospital health care settings, including vice president of perioperative services and vice president of operations. She has consulted, written, and spoken nationally and internationally on health care leadership and cost containment. Her prior publications include *Re-engineering of Operative and Invasive Services* as well as multiple peer-reviewed articles on leadership in health care. Dr. Moss concentrated her doctoral research on the influence of emotional intelligence in health care leadership and has researched this topic extensively over the past decade, providing a portion of the normalization data for Version 2.0 of the Mayer-Salovey-Caruso Emotional Intelligence Test, which was developed by John Mayer, Peter Salovey, and David Caruso. A native of the Jacksonville, Florida, area, Dr. Moss currently resides in Greensboro, North Carolina, where she is vice president of operations for Accordant Health Services.

To my Mom and Dad, who taught me the foundation for the work that it takes for a team to be successful.

To Donna, whose constant encouragement helped make this book a reality.

INTRODUCTION

"WHY DO YOU WANT TO BE A NURSE?" one might ask a little girl or boy with such aspirations. And the child might reply, "I want to take care of people and make them feel better." There is something quite compelling about that possibility to a young person who has discovered her own ability to affect the well-being and feelings of others, and many nurses can recall a similar drive propelling them into their chosen career.

Where Did the Time Go?

A registered nurse who graduated from nursing school in the early 1990s remembers learning the textbook methods of giving back rubs, making beds, and turning and bathing patients. Accordingly, clinical experiences, at least the fundamental ones, required mastery of these and other skills involved in "taking care of people and making them feel better." But when she emerged onto the cardiac step-down unit for the first time as a registered nurse, she salvaged very little time for these niceties. "I spent almost half of my time documenting," she recalls, "and a good deal of that was done after reporting off to the next shift." Time with patients was confined to the minutes required to do a head-to-toe assessment at the beginning of the shift, medication rounds every two hours, and confirmation that intravenous pumps and other equipment were running smoothly. "If I spent extra time with a patient," she says, "it was because that patient called me. If there was a problem that wasn't quick to solve, it usually meant staying later to chart or being late with someone else's medications." On the anxiety-laden cardiac floor, time was at a premium, and the proverbial squeaky wheels eked out what little remained once the essential tasks were completed.

Gone were the minutes, or even hours, that the nurse once passed by the patient's bedside, conversing and teaching in relaxed, nonstructured ways. Gone was the careful attention to how the patient was really coping with his illness. Gone also was the time to reassure, the time to get acquainted, the time to understand. But certainly the essential nature of reassuring, getting acquainted, and understanding is inherent in any nurse's value structure. Nursing schools tout the emotional element of compassion as fundamental to bedside care.

In reality, there was once more time specifically allocated to compassion in health care than there is today. Nurses who have practiced for thirty to forty years can recall roles and responsibilities much different from those of their younger counterparts. Supporting the patient has taken on a different meaning, a meaning that many older nurses have found difficult to reconcile with the concept of care they learned earlier. Complicated treatment plans, intense drug regimens, and increasingly acute conditions have cornered the nurse between technological accuracy and bedside grace. The hospital is not the world it once was.

What Has Happened to Our Patients?

Not surprisingly, patients have also changed. They are sicker, confined only during the most crucial hours of their recovery. Because patients are sent home so quickly, planning for discharge begins during the admitting process. Patients are expected to independently accomplish in hours what convalescents of the past would have been led through over days or even weeks. They are wheeled in, wheeled through, and wheeled out amid an array of scans, pokes, prods, opinions, discharge instructions, and multiple staff. They are anxious. Their families are anxious. The fact is that patients and their families bring fear, apprehension, anger, and grief to the hospital, just as they did forty years ago. What has changed is nurses' opportunity to deal with these emotions. The environment in which the emotions are experienced has changed as well.

The Emotional Cure

If one were to imagine the scientific advance most immediately needed in nursing, perhaps it would be a way to encapsulate and mete out a cure for the emotions that ail patients entering the health care system, just as we have streamlined and perfected many technical aspects of patient care. However, we could not expect this cure to come in a measured dose or a prescribed protocol. Instead, we would need to be able to

- Identify an emotional state almost instantly
- Understand what the emotion could lead to if unregulated or what it might represent in the patient's recovery process
- Understand the emotion's effect on the family, ourselves, and other caregivers

o Allow our own emotional state to maintain equilibrium in the face
of intense emotions of others

o Help patients, families, and colleagues to manage and regulate
their own emotions (Mayer, Salovey, and Caruso, 2000, 2002)

Why Is the Need So Critical?

Most people would not deny that health care is one of the most emotionally charged of all occupational fields. No one coming into the health
care system is immune from at least some form of vulnerability. Patients
do not always know what is going to happen, despite what their doctors
have told them. Diagnostic tests are foreign to most patients, even if they
know someone else who had one or received detailed descriptions beforehand of what was going to happen. Lack of control pervades the thought
processes of those undergoing medical procedures, as though they were a
passenger flying in a commercial airliner for the first time. No matter how
prepared passengers are for the mechanical sequence of events such as
takeoff and landing, emotions such as anxiety and the feeling of someone
else being in control and responsible for getting them back on the ground
are more difficult to prepare for in advance.

Of course, most nurses would acknowledge that even the best health
care often does not bear the same odds of a favorable outcome as even the
most angst-provoking of airplane trips. The best-case scenario is that an
individual will experience a little discomfort, uncertainty, and unscheduled
disruption on her way to a slightly blemished bill of health. Every flight
into the health care system is prejudiced by the reality that signing up for
the trip means admitting that something is, or may be, or could be going
to go wrong. It is like stepping onto a 747 on which engine trouble is sus-
pected but discovering that the only way to confirm it is to fly about four
hundred miles at twenty thousand feet. Patients may feel a loss of control
in a situation where there is far less cultural reassurance that everything is
perfectly normal and routine than there is on a commercial airliner.

The sense of vulnerability that is eternally typical of the sick has col-
lided head-on with the increasingly technical nature of medicine and
health care. In industries other than health care, increasing use of technology may have mitigated the need for human interaction. With the
advent of automated teller machines (ATMs), for example, consumers
were able to enlist a machine to do a teller's job. These automated systems were initially met with curiosity and sometimes distrust, because
bank customers wondered how the machines actually worked. Was it possible for human interaction to be replaced by a computer that mystically
communicated with unseen stacks of bills and account records?

Our familiarity with and reliance on ATMs has increased steadily over the years. Today, people are able to do their banking twenty-four hours a day, using electronic transfers and commands. The technology is sufficiently user-friendly that any reasonably intelligent individual can competently perform banking transactions once reserved for bank employees. There is less need for human interaction in order to complete the process, although a human being ultimately completes transactions behind the scenes. In short, banking is one industry where we have been minimally affected by the disappearing human element.

Not so in health care, where the rapid advance of technology has outstripped professionals' ability to answer questions concerning its use. Now, health care professionals must cope ever more efficiently with life-and-death decisions, ethical quandaries, heightened expectations, and dashed hopes. Within this environment, nurse managers must balance technological and business knowledge with the emotional footing to support patients, families, and staff.

How This Book Can Help

This book is written for nurse leaders. Wherever a nurse leader practices, he or she is faced with similar issues involving patient care, ethical dilemmas, and the reactions of staff members to the day-to-day impacts of their jobs. With that in mind, the book addresses topics pertinent to nurse leadership, highlights the qualities required of successful nurse leaders, and demonstrates how these leadership qualities can be used to develop and encourage leadership ability in others. The book is divided into four main sections that are best read in sequence: understanding the elements of emotional intelligence; intelligently creating, sharing a vision, and setting an example; intelligent transfer of information; and changing the culture of nursing and the organization.

Understanding the Elements of Emotional Intelligence

Chapters One through Three describe emotional intelligence and how it relates to the world in which we currently live and work—specifically, a world that is ever advancing technologically and thus requires a new type of leadership, especially in health care. From this section, the reader should gain knowledge of what emotional intelligence is and is not, as well as how it influences leadership qualities and characteristics and why it is so important, especially today. Chapter One explains that emotional intelligence is a scientific construct, not one that can be abstractly discussed as a type of social skill, although social skill and emotional intelligence go hand in hand. Chapter Two describes how, in the age of increasing technology, emotions become more and more important, even though the exact opposite might seem true. Chapter Three's focus is specifically on leaders, who must be astute in emotional knowledge and recognition in order to manage the complex issues that these same emotions create.

Intelligently Creating, Sharing a Vision, and Setting an Example

Chapters Four through Six focus on three leadership actions at which emotionally intelligent nurse leaders can be highly successful: creating, sharing a vision, and setting an example for others not only to follow but to become. Creating, described in Chapter Four, requires an innovative leader who is emotionally ready to take an organization or department to the next level, who is ready to change, and who is capable of convincing others of the need to change also. Sharing a vision, the focus of Chapter Five, requires not only that a leader have a vision but that it be a unique picture of the ideal that the leader can transmit to others in such a way that they actually live the vision. And setting an example, explained in Chapter Six, involves not only modeling behavior that others will want to emulate but also giving others the freedom to do exactly what the leader would do.

Intelligent Transfer of Information

Chapters Seven through Nine focus on the transfer of information from the leader to the team, from the team to the leader, and within the team itself. Whenever groups are involved, we can be certain of three things: the leader has knowledge the team needs, the team has knowledge the leader needs, and the collective and individual dynamics of knowledge and opinions will result in conflict. Emotional intelligence is a key determinant in how leaders and teams interact and share knowledge and information. Downloading, discussed in Chapter Seven, involves the leader making knowledge available for the team to tap into at will; the knowledge must be open and available in order to facilitate this process. Uploading, reviewed in Chapter Eight, involves the leader sending individuals and teams exactly the input they require, based on their specific needs. Conflict resolution, a need that grows naturally out of the potential for conflict when two or more opinions collide, is discussed in Chapter Nine, along with emotional competencies that are useful in resolving issues.

Changing the Culture of Nursing and the Organization

The work of this book would be incomplete without a forward-looking review of the culture and structure of nursing as a discipline and its organizations as dynamic, functional units. Chapter Ten discusses what culture means and how it applies to the nursing organization, as well as how much impact nurses can have in changing the culture within an organization. Chapter Eleven focuses on rebuilding the traditional hierarchical pyramid so that group process, not a particular position of management, is at the head and helm of the organization, dictating how it is run and steering it on an effective course. Chapter Twelve, of course, seeks to tie together all the elements of emotional intelligence that were previously discussed and apply them to the future of nursing leadership, to provide the nurse leader with a tool kit of strategies to use in a field that is poised for rapid change.

―――――― o ――――――

Let us begin our exploration of the critical success factor of emotional acuity with an overview of emotional intelligence.

THE EMOTIONALLY INTELLIGENT
NURSE LEADER

PART ONE

UNDERSTANDING EMOTIONAL INTELLIGENCE

AN AGE-OLD, NEW KIND OF NURSING INTELLIGENCE

AT THE FOUNDATION of understanding and applying any new skill is a basic understanding of its core concepts and often its history. Every acquired discipline, from architecture to the practice of law, requires attention to elementary principles. Emotional skill, specifically as it relates to nursing leadership, is no exception. In fact, emotionally intelligent nurse leaders have the opportunity to hone three skills: nursing, leadership, and emotional ability. In the pages that follow, we will explore the foundations of emotional intelligence and set the stage for applying emotional skill to effective leadership in nursing.

The Nurse as Caregiver

Since the dawn of the nursing profession, nurses have been viewed as caretakers or caregivers. A late nineteenth-century description of the nursing role includes the following:

> Every physician recognizes the importance of good nursing. In the treatment of disease medicinal agents are necessary to combat the various symptoms as they arise, but it is equally important that the surroundings of the patient should be so arranged that he may be supported and tided over the critical period of his illness. It is not too much to say that in many illnesses good nursing is more than half the battle. When a man is seriously ill he is practically as helpless as a child, and can neither think nor act for himself. He is fortunate should there be some friend or relative who will take the initiative for him, but there are many people—often men in good social position—who

have no one about them whom they would care to trust. The sick man sends for his doctor, and nurses are provided on whom rests the responsibility of seeing that he is properly cared for, and that no advantage is taken of his helplessness. The trust is a sacred one, and for the honour of the nursing community is rarely or never abused [*Ambulance Work and Nursing,* c. 1898].

Caregiving defines nursing even to the present day. Despite the increasingly technical and knowledge-rich nature of nursing, the expansion of nurses into significant health care leadership positions, and the growing number of nursing professionals who hold master's or doctoral degrees, the patient-nurse relationship still involves giving and receiving care. Highly qualified through certification, advanced learning, and experience, the nurse combines skilled medical administration with the roles of teacher, minister, and friend.

The "sacred trust" formed between nurse and patient is built on more than medical skill. It contains elements that are inevitably social and emotional. As nurses administer metered doses of potent medications, they assess patients for signs of depression and fear. As they explain treatment options to patients, they calm fears and anxieties by means that cannot be ascribed to procedural knowledge. Fundamentally, nursing involves a complex blend of accuracy and intuition, reason and emotion.

Emotion and Reason: The Traditional Dichotomy

The relationship between the rational and the emotional, then, must be explored. Traditionally, the two represent opposite poles of a dichotomy. Most people may be able to recall how emotions were viewed during their childhood, but in order to advance in emotional aptitude, it is helpful to first understand exactly how one was taught to perceive, manage, and express emotion in everyday life. Many people were taught that there was no way for emotion and reason to peacefully coexist and that the two must by nature be at odds with each other. Many were taught the necessity of leaving emotions out of decision making.

Emotion and Reason: Their Interdependency

The emotional and rational realms overlap, interact with, and affect each other. Despite notions of the desirability of separating emotions and reason, both realms must be acknowledged in order to provide quality health care, especially as medicine becomes more technical. Understanding how the two realms overlap is becoming ever more important as medicine presents us with issues such as life support decisions and genetics counseling. Such decisions as opting for elective oophorectomy or mastectomy to avert cancer (Dimond, Calzone, Davis, and Jenkins, 1998) or remaining childless because of genetic test results highlight the impossibility of ignoring the emotional component in rational health care decision making. Nurses especially, as patients' lifelines, need to understand the emotional dimensions in such clinical situations. Recognizing emotions and facilitating the transition from one to another are skills of emotional intelligence that serve nurses in such settings.

Emotion and Nursing Leadership

Increasingly, leaders in all fields acknowledge emotional processing, which was once left to instinct and intuition, as a vital component of executive ability. Without this skill, health care managers in hospitals, home care, outpatient care, nursing facilities, and other settings may face the challenge of rectifying the wrongs that result when emotions are handled ineffectively. Managers may be less able to communicate optimally with clients, families, or other health care professionals than they would be with better emotional skills. Important gains can be made in health care leadership by giving attention to the significant and critical emotional element present in every health care situation and by ensuring that nursing leaders develop their emotional potential, especially now that these competencies are recognized as skills that can be developed rather than less malleable personality traits (Freshman and Rubino, 2002).

Linking Emotional Elements and Leadership Style

For emotional development to occur in leaders, the concepts of emotional intelligence and leadership must be linked in such a way as to demonstrate a relationship between aspects of emotional intelligence and facets of leadership style. Various leadership styles have been described by different theorists (Blake and Mouton, 1978; Kouzes and Posner, 1995; Covey, 1991; Yukl, 1998), and their individual characteristics and actions have been explained (Birrer, 2002; Blake and McCanse, 1997). Because these characteristics are often associated with character traits, intuitive links between types of leaders and specific emotions often derive from experience. For example, one might associate an authoritarian manager with anger or lack of compassion, and a more relaxed or personable managerial style with cheerfulness.

Linking Specific Emotional Abilities to Leadership Style

Beneath these relatively easy-to-identify traits that characterize certain types of leaders lies another aspect of emotion not as readily apparent—the ability to identify, facilitate, understand, and manage emotion (Mayer, Salovey, and Caruso, 2000, 2002). Although we may identify anger with the tyrannical boss, appropriate management of that emotion may net an entirely different leadership style that we would no longer recognize as tyrannical. The personable, cheerful manager may be perceived by colleagues as friendly but may become a more effective leader by better understanding how underlying emotions cause individuals to react to adverse situations and how to help others manage these emotions in times of conflict. One of the first to note that effective leaders tend to have more emotional competencies was David McClelland, and research on this topic continues to this day, especially since the subject was popularized by Goleman (1995) (Freshman and Rubino, 2002).

Mayer and Salovey (1997) defined emotional intelligence as "the ability to perceive accurately, appraise, and express emotion; the ability to access and/or generate feelings when they facilitate thought; the ability to understand emotion and emotional knowledge; and the ability to regulate emotions to promote emotional intellectual growth" (p. 10). Abilities on this scale may be specifically tied to practical aspects of leadership style, and development of these abilities may be tied to professional and personal growth.

It is especially important, then, to explore what it is to be an effective leader in health care and not merely to act like one—intertwining Mayer, Salovey, and Caruso's (1999, 2000, 2002) constructs of emotional ability with specific leadership traits, exploring how these abilities can be learned as part of personality (Mayer, Salovey and Caruso, 2002), and discussing examples from earlier times, before the time went away and during which emotional art was as common at the bedside as medical science. We now have a clearer, more scientific view of what this art was and how it can be applied to other forms of knowledge to synergistically meet the demands placed on nursing leaders today.

Emotionally Intelligent Leaders Create

Leaders who are emotionally literate are more willing to experiment, more willing to make mistakes, and more ready to widen the span of their employees' control. Nursing leaders face a significant challenge in these aspects of leadership. Risk taking in leadership is often associated with liability for the actions of oneself or others, and in the health care setting, this liability involves a significant human life element that is not present in other fields. Policies and procedures abound, and adherence to standards is imperative when quality of care is at stake. How, then, does the nurse leader become one who creates, one who empowers, and one who takes risks within the organization? What abilities beyond a command of clinical and administrative skills give the nurse leader an edge on effectiveness that others may not possess?

Leaders who create take their work beyond duty to inspiration. They shape an enjoyable work culture and encourage employees to shape it as well. They foster a positive emotional climate in order to encourage participation. They are not afraid of failure; instead, they use it to teach success (Farson and Keyes, 2002). Having creative leaders will lead to having creative employees, which will result in more team spirit, more employee loyalty, and better productivity (Kouzes and Posner, 1995).

Emotionally Intelligent Leaders Communicate and Share a Vision

In addition, emotionally literate leaders possess and share a vision of the ideal workplace. They communicate their vision of success, and by doing so, they inspire others to collaborate with them in making the vision a reality. They are planners, developers, and motivational managers (Kouzes and Posner, 1995; Mayer, Salovey, and Caruso, 2000, 2002).

Leaders should be the visionaries of their organizations and should understand what is needed to make them successful; this notion is very much supported in current thought. The Baldrige National Quality Program stipulates visionary leadership as an overarching critical element among performance excellence criteria for health care (Levey, Hill, and Greene, 2002). The Magnet Nursing Services Recognition Program defines and acknowledges features of hospitals that resulted in retention and recruitment of talented staff and improved patient outcomes (Aiken, Havens, and Sloane, 2000), results for which a solid vision is often at the core. Nursing team leaders should be able to communicate the possibilities of the long-term future and how present activities will translate to achieving that vision. In imagining the future, most imagine the ideal. High standards are a consequence of imagining that ideal. Part of being a leader is the ability to communicate persuasively, which includes conveying the conviction that the future will be better, even when the current situation presents a threat or major change (Bardwick, 1996). To achieve this, certain emotional tools are necessary, including the ability to recognize and manage emotions inherent in change (Mayer, Salovey, and Caruso, 2000).

Emotionally Intelligent Leaders Set an Example

Emotionally skilled leaders not only set a high standard but also set an example of excellence for others to follow. Because of their stability, they can encourage others to do as they do as well as to do what they say. They are not afraid of being wrong or admitting it, and they are ready to acknowledge credit for work well done. They operate personally, interpersonally, interdepartmentally, and organizationally in the same way, consistently representing their work and that of others. They balance their lives and expect others to do the same.

What sets these leaders apart is that they challenge the system from within while participating, while making the process better. They are not the managers who stand and criticize, failing to apply to themselves the rules they apply to others. In this way, they encourage others to act and to participate in the ongoing betterment of the work at hand.

Emotions in Organizational Teams

The preceding paragraphs point out that the emotional skills critical to effective patient care actually translate to better leadership ability. In the dual role of caregiver and leader, the nurse manager interfaces laterally with colleagues and vertically with patients, subordinates, and corporate administrators. The interfaces are no longer unilateral but are increasingly collaborative. Nurse managers find themselves not simply giving orders and taking orders but rather engaging themselves and their staff, their superiors, their colleagues, and even their patients, in participative decision making. As shared leadership becomes formalized in many organizations, its collaborative principles already typify even informal interactions in the health care team. It is becoming the norm.

It has to. Without it, patients are patients, doctors are doctors, dietary aides are dietary aides, and administrators are administrators in the senseless world of poking, prodding, and speedy discharge that patients have come to know as "the health care system." Without collaboration and team decision making, patients, nurses, aides, and even doctors may have no idea what the goals are or where they are in relation to their accomplishment.

Admittedly, not all work is done by teams, but the team concept is becoming the norm in many organizations. In health care, diagrams of teams often show interactive, interdisciplinary representation with the client in the center. Because *team* can be misinterpreted to mean "a group of people working on the same thing," it is important to differentiate here between work groups and teams in organizations and to realize that the two are not synonymous. Teams include an interpersonal accountability that work groups do not always have. As such, the development of a team involves an element of risk that the formation of a work group does not (Katzenbach and Smith, 1993). However, despite the risk, analyst Lyle Spencer, Jr., asserts that the synergy of a well-developed team brings "huge leverage" to the organization (Goleman, 1998b, p. 217).

In today's dynamic organizations, and especially in health care, the synergistic contribution of effective teams is critical. While a work group may be sufficient for handling routine or stipulated agendas, such a group may lack the ability to optimally manage the complexities present in health care, with its multimodal emphasis on medicine, ethics, finance, and legal issues. Understanding, not just acknowledging the issues, however, requires emotional literacy (Mayer, Salovey, and Caruso, 2000, 2002).

The Role of Emotional Intelligence in Team Interactions

The ability to work as a team member is especially important in the workplace today, and emotional aptitude can play a considerable role in effective team membership (Goleman, 1998b; Druskat, 2001). A team situation brings together the individual tastes, ideas, opinions, and professional philosophies of everyone at the table. Unlike the revered family dinner table of the 1940s, where individualism was hailed but there was the comfortable assumption that a dad prevailed on anything requiring a decision, today's team setting is likely to yield a variety of opposing and concurring views without ultimate authority for their resolution. In a multidisciplinary team, leadership may shift depending on whose expertise is most critical to the particular decision at hand. Even so, groups of individuals do not automatically become harmonious merely by coming together for the same purpose any more than a string orchestra can play in harmony simply by watching a director. The instrumentalists must listen to one another, listening with an ear that understands when things are going wrong. If they don't listen to one another, they are unable to hear their own notes in a context that affirms their wholeness.

Likewise, team members must listen to each other with an ear that understands when things are not flowing appropriately. This ear must be able to "hear" crushed alliances, foundering certainty, and deflated morale. When problems are recognized, the more team members and leaders can redirect these occurrences by rebuilding alliances, negotiating, and facilitating decision making, in addition to fostering a strong work ethic, the more likely the team is to succeed (Katzenbach and Smith, 1993). Nursing leaders may be team members or team leaders. In many senses, they may be both, acting as care coordinators in a multidisciplinary model while representing the practice of nursing, for example. Whatever his or her role within a team, the nurse's emotional ability can foster a more congruent, effective team environment.

"Primary Greatness" and Emotional Coaching

Further, an emotionally intelligent person, whether a team member or a team leader, can achieve what Covey (1991) calls "primary greatness," which is an alignment of beliefs with behavior. This accomplishment may or may not be rewarded. At this point, having obtained some skills to share, the emotionally intelligent person can coach others in developing their emotional powers. Such coaching fulfills the responsibility of mentoring others. As a parent trains a child or a professor trains a beloved student, the emotional coach not only shares knowledge but also imparts a vision, nurtures a belief in the protégé's abilities for and commitment to the job at hand, and expresses and acts on a dedication to the institution or relationship that shelters both of them.

Emotionally Intelligent Conflict Management

Perhaps one of the most real yet avoided aspects of health care leadership is the need to identify, confront, and resolve conflict. It is nearly enough to say that conflict mediation and resolution rely on three things: communication, communication, and communication. Conflicts are as diverse as the people who experience them, but they can all be moved toward resolution if careful attention is paid to how people are arguing as well as what they are arguing about. Equally important, once these aspects are understood, is an ability to empathize with both sides. Understanding how people are feeling as they argue, including the fears that motivate them, and helping them verbalize those feelings can help bring clarity to what is at stake and determine whether combatants are willing to take the potential losses.

Furthermore, in clinical situations, patients and their families often have to weather bad news—an unfavorable diagnosis, the loss of a loved one, or the prospect of a long battle against disease. Exchanges between caregivers and patients in these situations require careful gauging of the emotional impact of the news and an understanding of the emotional responses of all parties. Think of the physician who demands emotional distance, the patient who needs a hand to hold, and the nurse overextended due to understaffing. In administrative situations, nurse managers have to discover ways to deliver other kinds of bad news—poor job performance reviews, layoffs, or unpopular changes in operations. Managers can be appropriately sensitive in these situations, offer solutions, and be an asset to the organization and the employee by employing the tools of emotional intelligence.

The Concept of Emotional Intelligence

Although the term *emotional intelligence* was used by Salovey and Mayer in 1990 (Salovey and Mayer, 1990), philosophers, researchers, and religious leaders have attempted to focus on monitoring behavior and finding awareness for centuries (Freshman and Rubino, 2002). Here it becomes important to formally define and distinguish emotional intelligence skills from some common misinterpretations of true emotional ability. The information directly following will also distinguish Mayer, Salovey, and Caruso's work in emotional intelligence as the primary basis for this book (Mayer, Salovey, and Caruso, 1999, 2000, 2002).

What Emotional Intelligence Is Not

First, the concept of emotional intelligence, as we know it today, is relatively new, although it has evolved over decades from cognitive and social research (de Beauport, 1996; Goleman, 1995; Sternberg, 1985; Sternberg and Wagner, 1986; Freud, 1960; Gardner, 1983; James, 1963). An attempt to classify genuine concern and compassion as "emotional skill" may be met with a different set of criteria today than it once might have. Despite widespread belief, caring and concern, or even intensity of feeling, are not the equivalents of emotional intelligence, though they may very well coexist. Emotional intelligence does not equate to touchy-feely scenes or sentimental moments. In other words, the most attentive and supportive bedside nurse of twenty years ago might or might not be deemed "emotionally literate" on today's scale, depending solely on specific abilities within the emotional spectrum.

What Emotional Intelligence Is

In 1997, Mayer and Salovey, the academicians whose theory of emotional intelligence was popularized by Daniel Goleman (1995, 1998b), published a definition of emotional intelligence that corrects problems in earlier definitions (Salovey and Mayer, 1990; Mayer and Salovey, 1993): "Emotional intelligence involves the ability to perceive accurately, appraise, and express emotion; the ability to access and/or generate feelings when they facilitate thought; the ability to understand emotion and emotional knowledge; and the ability to regulate emotions to promote emotional intellectual growth" (Mayer and Salovey, 1997). Over the past decade, Mayer, Salovey, and Caruso have created and formalized a structured emotional skill set that delineates basic to advanced skills (Mayer, Salovey, and Caruso, 2000, 2002). This is important now, because psychological research in recent years has been able to demonstrate what has long been accepted as an unproved fact: that those skilled in identifying, using, understanding, and regulating emotions can succeed when those with a high IQ may fail. They can go where intelligence alone cannot take them. Furthermore, unlike IQ, which is believed not to change, emotional intelligence can be taught and its skills refined (Goleman, 1998b).

The History of Emotional Intelligence

It is interesting to note that the modern definitions and concepts of emotional intelligence have their roots in the works of earlier theorists who defined emotion (Fisher, Shaver, and Carnochan, 1990; Fewtrell and O'Connor, 1995; Smith and Lazarus, 1993; Turski, 1994; Vanman and Miller, 1993), "personal intelligence" (Gardner, 1983), and "practical intelligence" (Sternberg and Wagner, 1986). Zeidner, Matthews, and Roberts (2001) referenced a concept by early intelligence theorist Spearman that emotional content was among other aspects of character that were components of will. The work of later theorists (Goleman, 1995; de Beauport, 1996; Cooper and Sawaf, 1997; Greenspan, 1997) elaborates the earlier definition of emotional intelligence proposed by Salovey and Mayer (Salovey and Mayer, 1990, 1994; Mayer and Salovey, 1993), categorizing its functions and proposing various applications for emotional health and success. The definition of Mayer and Salovey (1997) is the culmination of theories equating emotional intelligence with the ability to understand and respond appropriately to feelings.

Much of the research in this emerging field of study can be attributed to dissatisfaction with purely academic measures of intelligence. Theorists who first sought to advance the concept of multifactoral intelligence (Gardner, 1983; Sternberg, 1985) use the self-awareness and relational principles discussed by Freud (1960) to support their theories that intelligence comprises more than just cognitive aspects. Cooper and Sawaf (1997), de Beauport (1996), Goleman (1995, 1998b), and Mayer and

Salovey (1993, 1994) discussed the relationship between emotions and cognitive skills that forms the foundation of modern concepts of emotional intelligence.

Emotional Intelligence as a True Intelligence

Intelligence, in general, refers to an individual's capacity to adapt through information processing and effective cognition. Some define intelligence as mental ability or the ability to absorb complex material. However, intelligence as a general concept does not define all the specific abilities that are components of intelligence (Roberts, Zeidner, and Matthews, 2001).

An intelligence must meet three criteria to be a true intelligence (Mayer, Salovey, and Caruso, 1999): a correlation criterion, which involves defining a set of abilities that can be moderately intercorrelated with one another; a developmental criterion, which requires that tested abilities develop with age and experience; and a conceptual criterion, which involves demonstration of actual mental abilities, not just the desire to possess those abilities. Emotional intelligence does involve this actual demonstration of ability, which is further subdivided by Mayer, Salovey, and Caruso (1999, 2000, 2002) along a continuum from lower, molecular skills to higher, more complex skills. In 1999, Mayer, Salovey, and Caruso presented a new scale for measuring emotional intelligence, known as the Multifactor Emotional Intelligence Scale (MEIS). They argued, based on findings from the use of this scale, that emotional intelligence was much like traditional intelligence. It could be measured with correct or incorrect answers; diverse tasks could be assigned to measure it; and tasks were positively correlated (Mayer, Salovey, and Caruso, 1999, 2002). The Mayer-Salovey-Caruso Emotional Intelligence Test (MSCEIT) measures each of these skills as eight task level scores (such as faces or pictures), which combine to form four branch level scores (such as perceiving emotions in faces and pictures). Branch level scores combine into two area level scores, which represent the two main diagnostic areas of emotional intelligence (experiential and strategic emotional intelligence). These components will be explained more thoroughly in Chapter Three (Mayer, Salovey, and Caruso, 2000, 2002).

Levels of Emotional Intelligence

Emotional identification, the most basic level of emotional aptitude in Mayer, Salovey, and Caruso's model, involves recognizing emotion in artwork or a facial expression (Mayer, Salovey, and Caruso, 1999, 2000,

2002). Facilitation, the next level, requires the ability to contrast emotions with one another and with other thoughts and sensations such as sound, taste, and color. The third level of the model involves emotional understanding. There are unique rules followed by each emotional state—for example, happiness, fear, anger, or sadness. The third level of emotional aptitude involves reasoning about the interactions among these emotional states. The fourth and highest level involves emotion management. This level may include the ability to alleviate the anxiety of another person or to calm oneself after becoming angered. According to Mayer, Salovey, and Caruso (1999, 2000, 2002), proficiency in the fourth stage denotes achievement of the highest level of emotional intelligence.

Stated another way, emotion management is the highest skill attainable on Mayer, Salovey, and Caruso's (1999, 2000, 2002) four stage, or "four-branch" model, whose measurement was briefly described earlier, and must be preceded by understanding emotions. Before emotions are understood they must be facilitated, and before they are facilitated, they must be identified. According to the model, one level cannot be achieved before all lower levels are mastered. For example, understanding cannot precede identification. Mastery of all levels results in true emotional intelligence. Mayer, Salovey, and Caruso's theory is a construct through which it is possible to organize emotion into developmental stages, to perceive a hierarchy of emotional aptitude, and to make associations between concepts of emotions.

Emotional Intelligence in the Workplace

The concept of emotion's influence on day-to-day life and even on business is accepted by prominent theorists (Gardner, 1983; Goleman, 1995). Emotion and its relevance in the workplace are gaining international recognition. For example, Asian employers increasingly view emotional intelligence as a vital job skill (Slater, 1999). Ashforth and Humphrey (1995) describe the pejorative view of emotion that is established in conventional thought, which positions it as the antithesis of rational thinking, as a simplistic stance on emotion. They recommend a change in the administrative paradigm to reflect the interdependence between emotion and rationality, the natural inclusion of emotion in any task-oriented activity, and the need for a holistic view of interactions in the workplace.

How Emotions Come to Work

Although efforts are often made to separate emotion from the workplace, the two are inseparable because people carry emotion with them wherever they go. Through suppression, emotions often come to work in more professional attire. Ashforth and Humphrey (1995) describe four kinds of suppression: neutralizing, using rational norms to keep emotion from emerging, is seen, for example, when we require completion of numerous forms before facing a contentious client; buffering, intentionally keeping emotion and rationality compartmentalized, may come across as "detached concern" and is often observed, for example, in physicians who want some degree of rapport with patients but who do not want to totally relinquish rationality. Other ways emotions can be suppressed include prescribing (applying "appropriate" emotional cues to the situation at hand—for example, a bill collector's voice conveys urgency and a flight attendant appears cheerful); and normalizing (creating a rational explanation for an emotional decision—for example, arguing that a proposal was rejected because of its high cost, not because of a dislike of the employee who suggested it).

Why Emotional Intelligence Is Important at Work

Methods of emotional suppression are often present in fields that espouse professionalism, including health care. Goleman (1995) describes a physician who buffered himself from the emotional trauma of one patient's tears by demanding that the patient leave his office. When emotions are suppressed at work, the destructive force of denying the emotions is compounded by the relinquishment of positive gains that can be achieved by accurately interpreting the emotional climate. "Knowing when to laugh at the boss's jokes, when to trust a coworker with a confidence, and when someone is on the verge of a nervous breakdown are, collectively, a form of smarts . . . vital to workplace survival," Farnham, Faircloth, and Carvell (1996) wrote in *Fortune*. However, emotional knowledge is not just about survival; it is about improving, raising not only the prospects of the individual but also those of the collective, and about promoting emotional and intellectual growth. Skills that lead to such improvement include being aware of others' feelings, being able to detect rising disagreements and prevent their escalation, and being able to achieve a "flow state" at work—that is, being able to accomplish work in a smooth, fluid manner (Csikszentmihalyi, 1997). In summary, emotions are always present at work; they can be dealt with or suppressed, used advantageously or detrimentally. How this is accomplished—and the result—depend on the emotional knowledge of the worker, team, or leader.

Authors and researchers explain further how important emotions are at work. Elfenbein and Ambady (2002) found that of the emotional abilities, emotion recognition was the most reliably validated and proposed that its implications are large for organizational effectiveness. Cherniss

(2003) presented nineteen examples of how emotional intelligence affected businesses and their bottom line. In the health care setting, Marvel, Bailey, Pfaffly, Gunn, and Beckham (2003) examined how relationship-centered care improved health outcomes. Gustafson (2003) and Freshman and Rubino (2002) point out how the competitive and businesslike atmosphere that used to dominate interactions between staff and the public must change to incorporate the relational needs of individuals.

The Impact of Emotional Intelligence on Nurses and the Organization

What scientist would not pay for the opportunity to increase his or her cognitive intellectual ability, if only to understand a theory in a new way? A scientist might wonder whether a slight increase in his or her IQ would lead to a significant advance in research or technical expertise. It is likely that if classes in increasing one's IQ were offered, we could expect eager participants from all occupations, from students attempting to do better on college entrance examinations to businesspeople seeking a competitive edge.

Some level of emphasis on IQ has been present through the years, but not without a bold disclaimer. Unlike college entrance scores or grades on arithmetic tests, IQ scores do not change regardless of the amount of preparation or study. Nevertheless, it has been intuitively known for some time that success is not directly attributable solely to the kind of intelligence measured by IQ tests.

Emotional intelligence is believed by many to be the determinant of who advances most quickly within an organization (Weisinger, 1998). The development of emotional intelligence theory coincides with changes in the workplace that intensify the usefulness of emotional skills. These changes include the globalization of the world economy, in which social and community interests may influence interactions (Kanter, 2003); the growth of information and its impact on work; the shift from individual effort to teamwork; and the rise of the transformational leader.

Emotional Abilities Can Be Learned

As I implied earlier in this chapter, attention to the emotional element is increasingly imperative for effective health care leadership. The propensity for rapid change that characterizes health care, as well as the critical, life-and-death nature of the business itself, is a likely contributor to emotional reactions in its leaders. Leaders must take the time to reflect on their own environment and assess emotional states (Goleman, 1998b; Chaffee and Arthur, 2002). It is possible that elements of the same emotional spectrum that, when managed appropriately, are thought to contribute to productive management methods, actually predispose leaders unaware of their emotions to less desirable managerial styles.

Fortunately, for executives, teams, and organizations, needed competencies for emotional intelligence can be delineated, acquired, and refined (Mayer and Salovey, 1997). To learn the desirable competencies, leaders must assess their own managerial style, determine their own level of emotional intelligence, and then seek to develop the skills that need improvement. Development of emotional intelligence skills that contribute to effective leadership attributes can conceivably result in a more productive managerial style.

Nurses and Nurse Leaders Can Benefit from Improved Emotional Intelligence

Nurses are the public face of the health care system, the people who are actually perceived as taking care of the sick. Despite the menagerie of staff members who interact with a confined patient on a given day, the patient's nurse is the coordinator of everything and is responsible for just about everything, at least in the eyes of the patient. Anecdotally, nearly everyone in a uniform is "the nurse" to many patients who are unfamiliar with various hospital roles. "The nurse" thereby takes on active and passive accountability for the patient's physical and emotional comfort. Collaboration, conflict resolution, coaching—all are leadership skills that can be used by any nurse, from the unit manager to the nurse caring for a group of patients postoperatively. Any nursing role can be enhanced by development of emotional intelligence skills.

The Emotionally Intelligent Organization of the Future

What can the emotionally intelligent nurse leader do, then, to enhance the work environment? How can he or she help to create the empathetic culture necessary to communicate and lead, a setting where workers' concerns are supported? Several major organizations, such as Federal Express and Southwest Airlines, have been able to attribute a better bottom line, at least in part, to more careful attention to workers' concerns. One symbolic example is that Southwest named the department that other companies call "Human Resources" its "People Department." Other emotionally intelligent organizations, including hospitals, have posted successes in the form of company loyalty, high safety marks, and low absenteeism. In a health care environment, the organization that encourages a more emotionally intelligent workplace is encouraging the same kinds of relationships between its workers that health care workers want to create with their patients. Such alignment of beliefs and behaviors, as I mentioned earlier in this chapter, is one way that organizations can move to the forefront in their industries.

The Institute of Medicine, chartered in 1970 as a nonprofit component of the National Academy of Sciences, recently issued a report on U.S. health care quality. This report calls urgently for a redesign of the system. Leadership is key to redeveloping health care (Institute of Medicine, 2001). Organizations of the future will represent a distinct transformation of the organization of the past, with hierarchical pecking orders giving way to effective working relationships. Future organizations will need to be oriented toward group and team action, and learners will have to learn in groups, continuing and extending current practices such as multidisciplinary teams that lead hospital practice and surgical teams that work and learn together. Leaders in these organizations will need multiple skills. For example, witness the growth of young physicians with PhDs and MBAs. These leaders, because they are multidimensional, will create a health care culture that is more relational than that of the past. The traditional hierarchy becomes less relevant when managers become more responsive and line employees more responsible, making the employee excuse "Hey, I only work here" passé and the distance of managers from customers minimal. As a result, the ability to accomplish goals and finish projects successfully with many partners is becoming a new measure of career capability that, for some, is replacing the concept of the career ladder.

Summary

Leadership styles can be related to emotional ability. Emotionally intelligent leaders create, share a vision, and set an example for constituents. In today's health care environment, the interface between leadership and followers is becoming increasingly collaborative, replacing the unilateral, top-down approaches seen in the past. Team interactions depend more and more on emotional skill for problem solving and conflict management. This chapter has given an overview of the concept of emotional intelligence and its significance in the workplace; next, we will explore the key role that emotional skill can play in specific aspects of health care leadership.

TEN THINGS YOU CAN EXPECT TO LEARN FROM THIS BOOK

1. The traditional dichotomy between emotionality and rationality needs to be reexamined and a new paradigm created, based on the increased need for emotional skill in the face of rapid technological advances in health care.

2. Emotional intelligence skills can be specifically linked to certain aspects of leadership style and developed and enhanced to increase leadership effectiveness.

3. Emotionally intelligent nursing leaders can foster an environment of creativity, an enjoyable work culture, and a sense of employee loyalty within an otherwise procedure-oriented work setting.

4. Nursing leaders who are emotionally literate have and share their vision of the ideal workplace, communicating this vision and inspiring others to believe that the vision or ideal can become a reality.

5. Emotionally intelligent nursing leaders do what they say they will do and operate consistently in all aspects of their role. They readily admit mistakes and also accept credit for a job well done. They provide a solid example and, through their actions, encourage others to follow their example.

6. Team membership or leadership benefits from emotional skill; in fact, without it, it is difficult for teams to operate harmoniously.

7. Emotional coaching fulfills a chief mentoring responsibility owned by nurse leaders.

8. Conflict, though often avoided and seldom enjoyed, is a very real aspect of health care as well as of leadership, and conflict resolution is enhanced by application of appropriate emotional skills.

9. Emotionally intelligent nurse leaders can foster emotionally intelligent work cultures, which have produced both tangible and intangible results at many major organizations.

10. The organization of the future promises to be oriented toward team action and relational skills rather than traditional hierarchy.

2

EMOTIONS IN A TECHNO-ILLOGICAL AGE

SOMETIMES OUR THOUGHTS turn to the unthinkable. What our fore-bears would never have thought possible a century ago has become, or is quickly becoming, a reality today. The far-reaching effects of progress can be both positive and negative: positive in the sense that we are able to do far more than we ever could, and negative in the sense that we are expected to. In addition, technology and the expansion of the reach of corporate and world powers have contributed to an increased need for awareness of what *could* happen.

The Necessity of Emotional Intelligence Today

The April 2003 issue of *Harvard Business Review* contains an article enti-tled "Preparing for Evil" (Mitroff and Alpaslan, 2003). This brief but sobering article reminds us of categories of events that can befall a busi-ness (or a nation or a financial system) in little more than the blink of an eye. Its emphasis is disaster preparedness, which many organizations are now examining more closely than ever before. The article presents "a timeline of major crises" spanning the past two and a half decades, includ-ing everything from terrorist attacks to transportation accidents to unpar-alleled natural disasters. It further classifies these disasters into three groups: natural accidents (such as floods and fires); normal accidents (recessions, stock market collapses, industrial accidents, strikes); and abnormal accidents (terrorist acts, cyberattacks, and the potential business losses resulting from intentional slander). While 80 percent of Americans surveyed in a 2001 Gallup Poll felt that nurses had high ethical standards (Malloch, 2002, p. 12), the article points out that this third type of crisis is occurring more and more frequently in recent years, especially in the financial sector, where corporate scandal and mismanagement have made headlines and "'ethical leadership' has begun to sound like an oxymoron" (Johnson, 2002, p. 1). Kramer (2002) underscores this idea of wavering trust in leadership, saying that our faith in the systems that used to provide us with a sense of security has been rocked by tragedies and scandals.

Given these types of unfortunate occurrences, it is little wonder that the editors of *Harvard Business Review* devoted an entire page in the same issue to explaining why "emotional intelligence is still smart" (*Harvard Business Review*, 2003, p. 95). The article indicates that some managers may dismiss emotional intelligence as unimportant, because in uncertain times, employees will "do anything to keep their jobs," so managers don't need to make efforts to create emotionally intelligent workplaces—as opposed to the situation in the 1990s, when many employers may have jumped on the emotional intelligence wagon in order to attract and retain good talent. In fact, explain the editors, "Emotional intelligence doesn't just spur growth and high spirits in boom times; it also protects you in harsh times. In fact, right now the smartest thing you can do with emotional intelligence is turn it on yourself" (*Harvard Business Review*, 2003, p. 95).

The authors point out that productivity can be bolstered by paying attention to employees' feelings. Sure, they may want to keep their jobs, but they will do better when their feelings are taken into consideration; as a result, the organization becomes much more resilient. Leaders, who in these trying times operate under close scrutiny, can use emotional skills to become aware of subtle innuendos that could imply danger for their own career and to avoid missteps by applying a bit of compassion or emotional management (*Harvard Business Review*, 2003).

Of course, it is a good thing that a leading business journal still upholds the concept that emotional intelligence is a key ingredient in leadership, and the article makes a valid point about the crucial nature of emotional intelligence in the maintenance of a leadership role. Because the concept of emotional intelligence is becoming more familiar, many are at least considering the emotional side of business and life. However, specific skills and abilities are critical for its correct application. This chapter will apply emotional intelligence specifically to improving leadership by improving staff performance and patient care in the midst of increased demands on staff, expanding technology, and the possibility of an unthinkable calamity. Leaders, after all, are the ones who ensure the very survival of organizations (Tyler, 2003).

Emotional Development in Children

"Crybaby" can be interpreted as downright derogatory. If a child is labeled as a crybaby, no doubt he or she is displaying or is known to display some kind of negative emotion inappropriately (by whining, bawling, or screaming), at least in the eyes of the adult or older child who creates the label.

One man—let's call him Jason—says he cannot display typical emotions of sadness or grief because he was ridiculed for this as a child. He claims that he has not shed a tear since he was about twelve years old, not even at the deaths of his parents, wife, brother, sister, and other close friends and family members. As a result, his children have never seen him cry. When they imagine what that might look like, it is disconcerting to them, almost scary. Here is a man who is seemingly exempt from that kind of emotional expression. This admittedly affected his children's emotional development and expectations as well as Jason's.

Jason can still point to a defining moment when his older brothers told him, rather emphatically, that crying was for girls and that boys should never cry. They laughed at him so much for crying that he made up his mind that it would not happen again. As a result, it did not: not during a six-year stint in the Marine Corps far from home, not at the births of his children, at his wedding, or at a plethora of funerals.

This example is purely anecdotal, but it is not fabricated; it is based on the real-life experience of someone that I know. Without consulting any research, most of us can likely recall how emotions were portrayed or viewed in our respective childhoods. Some families were free with emotional expression (positive, negative, or both), while others were more reserved and stoic. Consider family portraits. People nowadays are encouraged to smile when having their photo taken, while the subjects in older photographs may appear solemn. Culture may affect a family's emotional expression as well; some families express affection outwardly (lots of kissing and hugging), while others limit displays of fondness to brief touches or handshakes. Television and movies underscore these differences.

So what can we be sure of as far as emotional development is concerned? Do we just come into the world as empty emotional boxes, waiting to be acculturated by our parents, older siblings, and classmates?

Acquisition of Emotion

There are several phases of emotional development, according to Haviland-Jones, Gebelt, and Stapley (1997). Briefly, they are acquisition, refinement, and transformation. Emotion itself is described as "an organized mental response to an event that includes physiological, experiential, and cognitive aspects" (Mayer, Salovey, Caruso, and Sitarenios, 2001, p. 235). Acquisition of emotion occurs at or shortly after birth and essentially involves emotions and emotional expressions that are inherent in us as human beings. For example, a baby cries when he is uncomfortable and may display a form of anger when he is confined. Babies also display positive emotions—for example, by cooing and, later, smiling. These emotional expressions are not necessarily learned but rather are part of being human. Of course, we expect these behaviors and expressions to be tempered and regulated as a child grows up, but we understand and accept that they are a normal part of infancy. The point here is that we are born with an emotional basis of some kind. Acquisition encompasses the basic expression and perception of emotion.

Refinement of Emotion

The next phase, refinement, involves modification of emotional signals (such as crying) to produce more refined signals (such as more precise, verbal expressions of discomfort). Refinement is clearly influenced by cultural and family modeling as well as direct training. Consider the parent who counsels a wailing three-year-old, saying, "I can't help you if you don't tell me what is wrong" or who simply refuses to respond to nonspecific whining until the need is clarified. Refinement also involves learning to use emotions appropriately, in line with social expectations. Sometimes, emotions are minimized, exaggerated, or covered, depending on circumstances. Our earlier example was one of refinement: Jason learned to cover a particular emotion, in line with what he considered a social expectation. That learning has had considerable impact to this day. Refinement also involves the attaching of feelings to particular contexts and situations. During childhood, we learn to attach happiness, sadness, anger, or fear to certain events and contexts. These associations may differ from person to person. One person may associate holidays, for example, with joy and glad anticipation, while another remembers them as times of sadness or disappointment. These associations help form the basis of emotional context later in life (Haviland-Jones, Gebelt, and Stapley, 1997).

Transformation of Emotion

The third phase, transformation, relates to how emotion affects and transforms other processes, such as learning, acting, and thinking. It also involves the ability to change the emotional process based on experience, so that its context and meaning become more and more personal. This element of emotional learning is still the subject of much needed research, partly because it is so individualized (Haviland-Jones, Gebelt, and Stapley, 1997). The transformation phase of emotional learning seems to correspond to the higher abilities on the Mayer-Salovey-Caruso Emotional Intelligence Scale (Mayer, Salovey, and Caruso, 2000, 2002).

One can see where there are opportunities for learning and adjustment of emotions throughout the developmental stages. This partially explains why we are all so highly individualized in our levels of emotional learning.

Enter the profession we chose: health care.

Technological Advances in Health Care

We could have guessed that it was true; we have all probably joked, grumbled, or griped about it at least once in our career. We know that the amount of documentation and paperwork (or electronic charting) that accompanies a nursing procedure can be cumbersome. Excellent assessors that we are, our estimations were correct: a study by the American Hospital Association found that one half to one full hour of paperwork is associated with every hour of patient care. Health care providers are regulated by thirty federal agencies, while Medicaid and Medicare rules fill over 130,000 pages of text. Add to that the privacy laws imposed by the Health Insurance Portability and Accountability Act (HIPAA) and patients' increasing interest in their health care (and their right to see their health care information), and one can see how documentation and technical accuracy can very easily become the focus of what went on with a patient's care (Sokol and Molzen, 2002). Control, cost containment, and complexity, enveloped in uncertainty and chaos, are becoming the norm (Watson, 2000). Physicians also are affected. A study found that 31 percent of 4,500 physicians surveyed would choose a different career if given the opportunity (Neuwirth, 1999, p. 79). When the tired, disgruntled, and disenchanted physician is unable to maintain satisfactory relationships with patients, the quality of patient care suffers immensely (Neuwirth, 1999). We can infer similar impacts for nursing care.

Sokol and Molzen (2002) seek to explain the relationship between information technology and modern health care, particularly from the legal standpoint of medical errors and malpractice. They inform us that health care has been relatively slow to adopt technology, falling behind, for example, the automobile and steel industries. In one way, this may be advantageous, as "blindly following fads is a recipe for disaster" (Chesbrough and Teece, 2002, p. 127). As technology advances, health care systems adopt the new opportunities at varying paces; one facility may be years from converting to a "paperless" system, while others have surged ahead with computer-based medical records, handheld devices for charting, computerized physician order entry, and digitalization that allows routine tracking of patient whereabouts. A growing reality, telemedicine, is another technology trend that provides remote transmissions between multiple caregivers or between caregivers and patients. Some patients may even have clinical indicators such as blood pressure and blood glucose monitored via a telemedicine device (Sokol and Molzen, 2002).

It seems to be taken for granted that technological ability will increase in just about every industry, including health care, and that it must increase to contain costs, introduce efficiencies, and provide faster access to needed data. Few would deny that the health care industry, if it has not already, should make efforts to catch up with the rest of the industrialized world when it comes to technology. Perhaps the sheer individuality of each incident of nursing or medical practice has impeded achievement of this goal somewhat. The increased emphasis on quality, consistency, and avoidance of error, however, has no doubt accelerated it (Sokol and Molzen, 2002).

Turkle (2003) points out that in society at large, technology has moved from an acknowledged external presence to an intimate acquaintance. It is not unusual for computer game enthusiasts to "spend hours playing out parallel lives" (Turkle, 2003, p. 43), assuming fantasy identities in imaginary worlds created for them on the Internet; or for children to bond with artificial beings that appear lifelike, such as mechanical pets. In short, "technology is increasingly redefining what it is to be human" (Turkle, 2003, p. 44). Of course, technology is said to be what defines us as humans because it reflects who we are and what we are capable of producing. It is driven by our needs and desires. The idea that it defines us raises another question: who are we becoming, and what do we want? The ethical and emotional issues our technology can raise are just beginning to come to light (Flower, 2000). Technology, in defining us as humans, also demonstrates what we know and what we can do. On the obverse, the results effectively negate some of the human side. Earlier, I gave the example of how ATMs have replaced and supplemented many of the functions once exclusively reserved for bank personnel, but ATMs are only one example of how we interact with machines rather than people. Online credit reports, telephone prescription refill services, instant weather warnings delivered to our pagers, automated drive-through carwash bays, and pay-at-the-pump gasoline islands have provided us with options to replace the human touch in our everyday lives. There are countless additional examples of this trend. Additionally, sometimes we feel enslaved as instant response becomes more and more possible and expected. Pagers and cellular telephones are available to keep us close to work no matter where we are. This feeling of constantly being monitored, known as "techno stress," has been shown to contribute to anxiety and anger in the workplace (Helge, 2001).

Journals related to the health profession emphasize the need to prepare medical and nursing students for the technological age (including information technology) in health care (De Ville, 2001; McCannon and O'Neal, 2003; McNeil, Elfrink, Bickford, and Pierce, 2003). There is a concern that nurses are not properly prepared and that they do not have the foundation of skills and knowledge necessary to cope with the environments they will encounter after graduation. Notwithstanding these concerns, technological advances have been encroaching on the environment for some time. In many hospitals, electronic blood pressure cuffs—which record pressures and pulse, sound an alarm when limits are exceeded, and take and record multiple sequential readings—replaced manual blood pressure cuffs years ago; the manual cuff is reserved for instances when a patient's limbs are compromised or there is a need to verify a questionable reading by the machine. Even body temperature is monitored digitally (who can remember the last time they waited five minutes for a reading from a mercury thermometer?), and intravenous medications are delivered via preprogrammed pumps, sometimes three or four at a time. Mechanized alternating pressure stockings and passive joint motion devices have been around a long time, as have alternating pressure mattresses and beds, eliminating some of the need for repositioning and passive motion exercises that once took place much more frequently at the bedside by trained personnel.

Most would probably agree that these technological advances are good and that they promote efficiency, consistency, and quality in care. To nurses and other medical professionals or paraprofessionals scrambling to make rounds on a packed medical/surgical unit or seeing six to eight patients an hour in a clinic, the thought of manual vital signs and constant surveillance of each patient's position and motion would be overwhelming. We need technology to make our jobs possible, not just easier. On the other hand, one might ask the question, what will happen to the familiar infrastructure of our hospitals in light of these changes? The answer is that the familiar is rapidly becoming obsolete (Porter-O'Grady and Afable, 2002).

The Impact of Medical Advances

Along with the unquestionably technical aspect of nursing care comes the purely advanced aspect of medical care: that which is presenting patients and caregivers with entirely new ranges of options, hopes, and ethical problems. Because of medical, surgical, and pharmaceutical technology advances (for example, minimally invasive surgery, robotics, and nanotechnology), we are now able to offer to patients what we could not have imagined two to three decades ago (Porter-O'Grady and Afable, 2002). Transplants from living donors, in vitro fertilization, surgery in utero, reconstructive options, and costly medications that may retard but not cure a condition are only a few examples of the doors opened to us by medical research and technology. As technology and knowledge rapidly expand, we are presented with multitudes of additional possibilities that are new and that have varying success rates. Patients are faced daily with the question of whether to try something that may sap their resources, cause a degree of suffering, and in the end fail to work as intended or hoped.

This type of decision making can be both emotion-intensive and labor-intensive. One study (Byrne, 2002) examined feelings associated with a looming bioethical decision. Common themes for patients included guilt, anger, knowledge sufficiency, power, and frustration. Common themes for nurses included sadness, confidence, colleague support, ability to advocate, and satisfaction with the outcome. What are the consequences of a wrong decision? What if the rejected new treatment option would have made the patient better or at best, left her condition unchanged? What if the surgery is chosen and the patient loses function as a result, rather than gaining ground?

Life-or-death decisions can be especially cumbersome. We have the profound ability to sustain life through mechanical ventilation and cardiac support, but patients, families, and caregivers have individual views on the point at which life should or should not be sustained, views that may vary from moment to moment as a patient's condition or prognosis changes. There are cancer therapies that are potentially curative but not necessarily opted for in all cases; palliative treatment plans are sometimes chosen in lieu of these potentially disease-modifying regimens. Such decisions, which are not made lightly, can be fraught with uneasiness, resolve, peace, fear, guilt, anger, hope, disappointment, or overwhelming sadness and despair. In the middle is the nurse, who, knowing that the patient and family ultimately must decide, can only offer information, support, and respect. Through all of this, the patient's rights must be considered (Otto, 1999).

Cybersurgery, which may sound like something out of a twenty-fourth-century medical fantasy, is also expected to expand much like telemedicine has, following trends inherent in the technological aspect of health care. In cybersurgery, a physician would use computer-assisted robotic technology and telemedicine to perform surgery on remote patients (McLean, 2002). In addition, biotechnology is expanding rapidly, escalating the need for sharing of benefits with patient groups and the obligation to determine to whom the new technology—such as stem-cell technology and life-saving, expensive medications that most cannot afford—will be available. Recent advances in technology have also made it conceivable to manipulate genes, form vast databases of patient information, and even create "neo-organs" for later use (Gold and Caulfield, 2002; Flower, 2000). Such technological advances raise many ethical issues in health care.

Increased Focus on Health Care Ethics

In part because of the questions involved in new medical technology, there is perhaps more focus on nursing ethics than ever before. The American Nurses Association (2001) code of ethics provides a guide to ethical practice for nurses. The very first provision of this code calls for nurses to practice "with compassion and respect for the inherent dignity, worth, and uniqueness of every individual." Health, safety, and rights of the patient must be paramount (provision 3), but the nurse is also said to owe the same duties to self as to others, maintaining self-respect, wholeness of character, and integrity. In the medical field, these must be weighed against the boom in privacy and cost issues as well as potentials in new fields such as physical enhancement, cloning, genomics, and germ line therapy to ultimately eliminate "bad genes" (Flower, 2000).

The Most Important Ingredients of Nurse Training

The less time we spend at the patient's bedside, the more need the patient and family may have for our support, and in turn, the more need the staff may have for our support. In fact, say Zimmerman and Phillips (2000, p. 422), "with the emphasis in health care on implementing the latest technology and providing care in the shortest time interval, an important aspect of nursing, the aspect of 'caring,' may be lost." Compassion in leadership, says Kerfoot (2002), is incredibly important, as ethical decision making is made easy by simply putting people first. It is a conundrum that leaves the nursing profession once again wondering, "What are the absolutely imperative elements in nursing education today? Computer literacy? Fundamental legal knowledge? Ethics?"

CRITICAL THINKING AND MINDFULNESS. One skill that is becoming important in nursing is critical thinking. "Along with the evolution in the scope of nursing practice, there has been greater autonomy for nurses and a growing demand for expanded critical thinking abilities and the ability to solve problems and make decisions," says Cheryl Martin (2002) of the specific theory related to nursing practice. Martin cites the evolution of the profession into one that requires cognitive and relational skills and one in which nurses have moved from task orientation to skilled professionalism. She says that changes in teaching are imperative to develop nurses' critical thinking skills early in their careers. Mindfulness, says Epstein (2003), is that state of mind that allows us to reflect and have insight and presence; it applies to the cognitive, interpersonal, and technical aspects of health care. Exemplary practitioners will display this mindfulness, which involves paying attention to physical and mental processes while working (Epstein, 2003).

INFORMATION TECHNOLOGY SKILLS. Many health care professionals insist that information technology skills are necessary to succeed as a practicing nurse. McCannon and O'Neal (2003) assert, "One can conclude that integrating information technology content into undergraduate nursing curricula is imperative to help nursing students gain the necessary skills for successful employment." Nurses need this information technology advantage to review reports that are increasingly electronic, communicate with multiple departments and systems, and even to document their assessments and interventions with patients.

Critical thinking. Quick decisions. Efficient information handling. These sound somewhat like skills needed for the disaster preparedness discussed earlier in the chapter. In many ways they are. As nurses in today's environment, we must prepare for the unthinkable, which may come in the form of a deadly communicable disease, a victim of intentional abuse, a heart-wrenching opportunity, or a critical choice.

EMOTIONAL INTELLIGENCE. How do we prepare for the unthinkable, which these days can also be called the unknown? After all, we do not know what the next innovative medical breakthrough will be, any more than we know what the next act of terrorism will be.

We do not know many things. We do not know what external forces and pressures are driving each staff member we lead. We do not know what family and financial dynamics are present in the lives of each patient. We do not know which recovery will take a sharp turn for the worse, or which unfortunate mistake will send a new staff member's emotions into a tailspin.

In a particular situation comedy from the 1970s, there seems to be a round of laughter every thirty seconds. The actors and their situations create stirs of laughter within the audience that maintain the comedic flavor of the episode. It does not take a great deal of humor to start the laughter. Although the laughter must be intended to sound spontaneous, occasionally there is a shriek or loud chuckle within the laughter that is repeated as the laughter drones on. These distinct sounds are so similar that it is easy to believe that the laughter has been prerecorded and inserted at preconceived spots in the production.

As we also know, emotions are not always products of preconceived events. Think of the last time you laughed aloud, were extremely angry, or were terribly frightened. Each of these incidents was most likely a reaction to a stimulus or experience, not a planned display. We cannot can our emotions and save them for the appropriate spot in the comedy or drama of life, playing them and replaying them as the situation warrants. Life is an unscripted and essentially unpredictable production.

As we consider this, we should review what recent literature has said about emotional skill in an age of rapid change. While some journals stress the need for increased technical competence (De Ville, 2001; McCannon and O'Neal, 2003; McNeil, Elfrink, Bickford, and Pierce, 2003; Sokol and Molzen, 2002), others emphasize that emotional skill is needed now more than ever. "Human connection counterbalances stress and inspires the best in people," notes Segal (2002). She advises nurse leaders to "connect to your staff in a way that lets them know you understand and recognize what they actually do. Pick up the phone and make the time to listen. You can be interdependent with no loss of authority or respect and unburden yourself of stress at the same time" (Segal, 2002, p. 44). For all kinds of jobs, emotional intelligence outweighs the importance of technical skills and IQ combined at least twofold (Strickland, 2000). Simpson and Keegan (2002) ask whether we are forgetting about emotional connectivity as we connect to the Internet, networks, and voice mail. The more electronically oriented we become, the less need there is for face-to-face contact. E-mail, for example, makes it possible to hide behind technology instead of resolving issues face-to-face. Leaders should be especially attuned to this and be alert to opportunities to diffuse the negative emotions that might be brewing in such situations.

"As though we have time for that," some might think. Again, however, managing emotion is perhaps the most critical element of health care leadership today. Leadership style will affect the way nurses perform, the way they perceive their job, and the way they deal with their patients. Segal also asserts, "Good communication, especially that done with sick or frightened people, is almost entirely nonverbal." When we put ourselves in the patient's shoes, we may ask ourselves, "Which would I rather do: understand the technical aspects of the equipment I am hooked up to or have the feeling that my caregiver truly understands me?" Dry, lengthy explanations are no substitute for silent acknowledgments of one's grief or pain.

Not only do effective nurse leaders model this empathetic behavior for their staff, but they use it to interact with staff members and coach them to higher levels of emotional acuity. Affective learning is critical to the development of a caring perspective (Zimmerman and Phillips, 2000). The skills needed for success as a manager go beyond technical competence and tap into emotional competencies (Cox, 2002). "To be a self, to have an identity, is to be involved with others," Raingruber (2000, p. 44) points out. Emotional competency gives us a framework with which to better define emotional maturity. This framework can be useful for developing interpersonal skills and personal management effectiveness, as well as promoting a work environment that is productive and healthy (Cox, 2002). Current research shows that an employee's emotional intelligence is twice as important as technical skills and cognitive abilities (Connolly, 2002). As Cadman and Brewer (2001) put it, "The role of the nurse is evolving continually and 'portable' skills are the key qualities demanded by a health care system under pressure to compete" (p. 321). These skills include effectiveness in working as part of a team, the ability to appropriately recognize and respond to feelings, and the ability to motivate oneself and others (Cadman and Brewer, 2001).

Emotional abilities have been studied in a variety of ways. The Interpersonal Reactivity Index (Davis, 1980, cited in Schutte and others, 2001) assesses four ingredients of empathy, while Lennox and Wolfe's (1984) self-monitoring scale asks Likert-scale questions that allow respondents to assess their own responses to emotional situations. These are some examples of emotional indicators that have been used as early as the 1980s (Schutte and others, 2001).

Mayer, Salovey, and Caruso (2000, 2002) have presented a four-branch hierarchical model of emotional intelligence. Each branch of their model is said to build on the one before. As a review, the four branches that Mayer, Salovey, and Caruso (2000, 2002) test are as follows:

1. The ability to perceive emotion. This involves fundamental recognition of how one and those around him are feeling.

2. The ability to use emotional facilitation. This involves using emotion as needed to be able to communicate feelings or to use emotions in cognitive situations.

3. The ability to understand emotion. This includes understanding combinations of emotions and how they transition from one to another.

4. The ability to manage emotion. This involves modulation of emotions in oneself and others.

Why should we as nurse leaders focus on these emotional competencies? One reason is that these competencies are expected in good nurse leaders, whether explicitly or implicitly. In a study of attitudes toward particular characteristics in managers, "surveyed executives specifically preferred applicants who were team oriented, independent, organized and visionaries with strong interpersonal skills. They dislike and even terminated individuals who lacked these EI (emotional intelligence) qualities. Eighty percent of the nurse executives and 60 percent of the business executives admitted to removing someone from a management position because of lacking EI" (Connolly, 2002).

We will now take a further step and explain why each competency (we'll discuss the ones defined by Mayer, Salovey, and Caruso [2000, 2002]) is so important to our profession and to those commended to our care, especially now.

Using Emotional Intelligence to Cope with the Demands of Technology

"Our day to day leadership can better be described as managing chaos," says Hagenow (2001, p. 32), referring to the yet unparalleled transition in health care. Advances in communication capability, increased competition, nagging consumer demand for satisfaction, and the conflict engendered by competing priorities and budgets help to explain why (Hagenow, 2001). How can we, as nurse leaders, apply emotional skill under such complex circumstances?

Perceiving Emotion and the Need to Think Critically

The importance of critical thinking in nursing was mentioned earlier in this chapter. Zimmerman and Phillips (2000) cite that affective learning can actually encourage the ability to think critically. This is important in part because "as a client's status changes, the nurse must recognize, interpret, and integrate new information and make decisions about the course of action to follow" (Martin, 2002). The information we must recognize will contain emotional data. Times during which quick, precise decisions are necessary may also be the times when emotions are at their peak. When the most is at stake and critical decisions are most important, there will be a patient, a family member, or even a staff member whose emotions are aroused in one way or another. For the skilled professional, it should be impossible to ignore these cues. In one study, nurse leaders suggested that their ability to identify emotions in others was actually enhanced by working with the critically ill (Vitello-Cicciu, 2002). Perhaps this ability had to do with the intensity of emotions on the critical care unit.

Whenever a situation is critical or urgent, many nurses tend to focus on the immediate, taking care of the problem at hand and intentionally avoiding distractions. While this is necessary in some cases, every effort should be made to perceive the emotions of those in the room whenever possible. Not perceiving them is not going to make them go away. Is the patient angry or dismayed that his call bell was not answered right away? Suppose the patient has asked for a beverage and the nurse has deemed this request secondary in priority to the request of the patient in the next room for medication. The first patient may be upset regardless of the outside circumstances. An explanation of the outside circumstances may mitigate the patient's frustration, but only if that frustration is first perceived and acknowledged.

Is a family frightened that their loved one's prognosis may be more serious than is being outwardly acknowledged? Do they perhaps have another relative whose health took a similar course and died or underwent serious life changes as a result? In light of their previous experience, are they questioning their loved one's status, even though they have been told the prognosis is good? Perhaps they allude to others who "went bad" after having a similar procedure or "had this same problem a few years ago but didn't make it." This is the kind of chatter that may go on in waiting rooms or even in the patient's presence. Unless the caregiver perceives the fear inherent in these words, there will be no opportunity to allay it.

Recognition of emotion is especially important in situations where life-or-death questions are asked. It plays a large part in the ethical component of telling patients the truth. Take, for example, the patient who corners the nurse, demanding to know details of her condition that her physician had intended to keep quiet. This is an age-old example that is fraught with ethical as well as emotional implications. "How long do I have to live?" and "Is my daughter going to die?" are just a couple of examples of such emotional questions (Kinsella, 2001). Perceiving the emotions behind these questions can aid the nurse in handling them, especially when there are unknowns involved. The nurse may ask herself,

"Does the patient question whether he can trust me?" On the other hand, assess for anxiety (Dossey, 1996) or underlying concerns.

As nurse leaders, we must also be acutely present to the emotions that underlie the actions and attitudes of our staff members. When there is a problem or a change, we should always ask what emotion is involved. The answer may very well be that there is no emotion involved. For example, a problem may be solely the result of a learning deficit, physical illness, or poor communication. When we train ourselves as leaders to consider and perceive emotional components as much as we consider whether the staff member understood the instructions, we open up another avenue of opportunity to correct problems. In his book *Working with Emotional Intelligence,* Goleman (1998b) says, "The most effective people in organizations . . . naturally use their emotional radar to sense how others are reacting" (p. 167). The implication here is that emotional perception is not one of many litmus tests that we pull out in order to examine a situation. We perceive the situation through the lens of emotional perception in the first place. We should also mention that this lens allows us to see not only the emotions of others but our own as well. Sometimes people have difficulty because they do not even recognize the emotion driving their thoughts or feelings. Self-understanding, long a focal point of psychotherapy, can serve us here as we seek to improve our relationships with others (Raingruber, 2000).

Applying emotional skills to the critical thinking aspect of decision making, we can use the recognition of emotion to first perceive what is being felt by ourselves and others and then focus on what is causing the feeling, using that to assist in solving the problem.

Using Emotion and the Need to Effectively Communicate

The effective nurse leader must be able to recognize an emotion and then use it to communicate effectively. This use of emotions, called "facilitating" by Mayer, Salovey, and Caruso (2000, 2002), involves using emotions in mental processes or to communicate feelings. While emotions are ever present (even from birth, as mentioned earlier in this chapter), their use in the facilitation of thought can be enhanced.

As nurse leaders, we are constantly in situations in which we can use emotion to enhance our mental processes. One such situation is, of course, interacting with colleagues. We do this every day, on rote matters such as unit procedure and on more sensitive matters such as individual patient care issues. Each situation has the potential for emotions to be used to share our message more effectively. Let us look at one example of perceiving an emotion and then using it to enhance a communication.

At a nurse manager's meeting, suppose a colleague suggests that a nurse be transferred to your unit in order to avoid laying her off. You are aware that this proposal evokes anxiety in you, so you discuss your concerns about an unpleasant encounter you had with that particular nurse in the past (Vitello-Cicciu, 2002). As a result, you and your colleague are able to reach an understanding about not only what is best for the staff member but what is best for you as well. Further, if the nurse eventually transfers to your unit, this preliminary discussion with your management colleague may have served to calm any unresolved reservations you had about the employee, which will ultimately promote better relations between you and that staff member. It is easy to see how perception of emotion and the effective use of emotion to facilitate thought were key ingredients in this interaction. Suppose you had ignored the warning that your emotions were sending when you became anxious about the proposal of your colleague. If you had dismissed your intuitive misgivings as something more general, such as an overall reluctance to change, you probably would have missed that opportunity to create a more harmonious working situation. You might have inadvertently avoided the chance to clear up a previous misunderstanding about a fellow professional. You would have deprived yourself of the use of the most fundamental emotional capability we can implement and a powerful tool: perception of emotion.

The second misstep that you could have made in that situation would have been to recognize the emotion but fail to use it to communicate with your colleague. Suppose you were well aware that you felt anxious about the specific individual but did not take the time or the mental energy to ask, "Why am I feeling this way?" Asking such questions allows us to rehearse how different situations may work out and lays the groundwork for problem solving (Vitello-Cicciu, 2002). Or even suppose that you knew why you felt the way you did but chose to ignore it rather than discuss it with your colleague. Then, if the individual had transferred to your unit, your unresolved feelings might have hindered your working relationship with her, all because of a misunderstanding that had happened months earlier.

In patient care, using emotions becomes especially important. Returning to the scenarios of the frustrated patient or the worried family member, each of these situations could provide opportunities for the nurse to discuss and resolve emotional thoughts with the respective individuals. Indeed, perception of the emotion, while critical, has little effect if that perception is not used to think through the situation. If a nurse doesn't consciously monitor his or her own emotions, knowing that a person is angry or worried may lead the nurse to react internally to these emotions by either consciously or unconsciously avoiding the emotion in the future. For example, awareness that the patient became angry because his water pitcher was not filled quickly might lead the nurse to think of the patient as a difficult patient and to spend less time communicating with her. If the nervous family member perceives a nurse's unwillingness to acknowledge the worry, it may actually cause the family member to worry more. Nurses should be aware of their own perceptions and reactions and how to use them effectively, and their leaders can educate them on how to do so. In so doing, there are opportunities to master the skill of emotional understanding.

Understanding Emotion and the Need to Manage Crises

Earlier in this chapter, there was a brief discussion of crisis management and the events that might precipitate the need to put crisis or disaster management plans into operation. No matter how one prepares for a crisis, it is assumed that no one is completely ready for the details of a crisis as it unfolds.

In this context, we will think of crisis as anything from job burnout to an overwhelming explosion of events—that is, anything that may disrupt the normal flow of things and cause unexpected problems. While this is a very loose definition of the term *crisis,* the application to emotional skill is that preparation for anything of such a nature should include a fundamental knowledge of which events precipitate or contribute to which emotions and how transitions from one emotional state to another are likely to progress. There is an amount of reasoning present in understanding emotions—that is, in determining their meanings and implications (Mayer, Salovey, and Caruso, 2000).

Genetic risk testing is one technology that has raised a multitude of ethical questions. Such dilemmas as whether to disclose a parent's potentially harmful genetic diagnosis to a child of childbearing age present many emotional situations. Garrison (2003) relays an account of a mother who did not want her physician to disclose her diagnosis of Huntington's disease to her daughter. The daughter's ignorance of her own risk for the disease, let alone that of unborn children, obviously had implications for future generations, but disclosing the diagnosis was an option the patient did not want to consider. Because medical science has captured so much information about genetic risk, we now have the ability to cause or prevent emotional situations from occurring, based on the level of information we make available and to whom.

On the surface, the issue is whether the patient's wishes should be honored. In other words, would advising the patient's daughter of her risk, either directly or indirectly, breach the patient's right to privacy? Further, would withholding the information from the daughter increase her potential offspring's chances of genetic disease so greatly that the information should, according to duty, be disclosed?

There are ethical principles that govern such decisions, and volumes of literature and hours of study have been devoted to formulating a process that would help to resolve this conflict. However, this scenario contains a volatile emotional potential. The patient may be feeling some combination of fear, anger, guilt, grief, or other emotions, and these feelings may lead her to seek to hide her diagnosis, regardless of the risks to her immediate family. A practitioner who is skilled at emotional understanding could help the patient perceive her own emotions and understand how those emotions facilitated other emotions—or even a decision. After all, it is highly likely that this patient's wishes were driven not by scientific and medical facts but at least somewhat by emotion. Perhaps the patient does not even recognize the emotions she is feeling or how they are affecting the decisions she is making. She may, but this clarification would likely be helpful to both patient and practitioner. Decisions made while under emotional duress may be questioned afterward (Hughes, 2002), so it is worthwhile to help the patient become aware of all the factors in play at the time a decision is made.

The ability to understand emotions and the way they can transition from one to the next would help the practitioner to realize that breaching the patient's privacy, especially in the absence of talking about her emotions or even tacitly acknowledging them, might lead to an escalated emotion, such as rage, on the part of the patient. This understanding affects a practitioner's decision making, so the practitioner needs to make sure that his perception of the patient's emotion is accurate and also that the patient understands how the emotion is affecting her mental process.

Withholding information about a diagnosis from the patient may also have emotional ramifications. How the physician conveys the information will affect the care team. Open, honest care will not be possible if lies are building on lies, and credibility and trust may be lost (Hughes, 2002). This ethical dilemma has haunted practitioners and families for decades, partly because it is laden with emotional implications.

Staff members need to apply their understanding of emotions not only to high-stakes situations but also to the everyday perceptions and frustrations involved in patient-nurse relationships. The man who was angry about the water may very well become enraged if his frustrations go unnoticed and unvalidated. Tired, ill, and vulnerable, he may withdraw and become noncompliant. He may become angrier and more vocal about his frustrations. He may become more difficult because the nurse categorized him that way in the first place. The worried family may draw their own conclusions from the nurse's silence and launch themselves into panic mode, transferring their insecurity about the patient's condition to the patient himself.

Leaders should understand emotions, too, when relating to their staff. The nurse who is "having a problem" may have an emotional one. She may be having problems at home or a conflict with another staff member. There may simply be insecurity that has gone unrecognized or an issue with a patient's family member that is bothering the nurse. As leaders in health care, we watch those we lead providing medical knowledge to patients and sometimes forget that they are not immune from the same emotional turmoil as the patients and families whom they are supporting. We must understand how these emotions affect their thought processes and what consequences may result if the emotions are not addressed and resolved.

To review, the hierarchy of emotional aptitude thus far includes recognizing and perceiving what emotions are being experienced, being aware of how those emotions either have facilitated or can facilitate thought and communication, and understanding how those emotions can change and define relationships and events (Mayer, Salovey, and Caruso, 2000). The next step, managing emotion, can help pull it all together so that a common ground can be established despite the myriad challenges that consume our time, tax our cognitive resources, and make us vulnerable to crisis.

Managing Emotion and the Need to Establish Common Ground

Problem solving is inherent in nursing and health care. The very fact that a patient is in our care indicates there is some kind of problem or a potential problem to be avoided. Management of emotion involves not just recognizing and understanding emotion but using it to solve problems (Vitello-Cicciu, 2002). The regulation of emotion, indeed, can smooth many aspects of organizational and employee life (Grandey, 2000). Mayer, Salovey, and Caruso (2000, 2002) describe regulation of emotion as managing one's own emotions and assisting others in doing the same.

The use of complementary and alternative medicine has mushroomed in recent years. Patients may insist that they want to try an alternative therapy (for example, acupuncture, herbal remedies, or shamanic healing) in place of or in conjunction with a traditional therapy that their physician has prescribed. Some patients may forgo more proven therapies for this type of treatment, leaving physicians with ethical dilemmas related to the risks and benefits of supporting such choices (Adams, Cohen, Eisenberg, and Jonsen, 2002).

In addition, such ethical dilemmas may create conflicts between patients and practitioners (Adams, Cohen, Eisenberg, and Jonsen, 2002). If a physician is candid with her patient about the risks or nonproven efficacy of alternative therapies, emotional conflicts may ensue within the patient or between the patient and physician. At times, a patient's desire to use or avoid certain therapies relates to his or her spiritual beliefs or other very personal values, so such a situation may be laced with emotional implications (Adams, Cohen, Eisenberg, and Jonsen, 2002). This is another example of why an understanding of the use and management of emotions is so critical in this age, when medicine provides so many opportunities to patients. Emotions show up not only at the pinnacle of crisis but also in day-to-day management and prevention. The decision to have an elective oophorectomy or mastectomy to avert cancer is yet another example (Dimond, Calzone, Davis, and Jenkins, 1998).

Effective management of emotions enables us as medical professionals to control our own emotions when dealing with those of another. At times we may vehemently disagree with a patient's choice, either because of our personal beliefs or because of our medical knowledge. Mastering the management stage of emotional intelligence enables people to keep their emotions in perspective, as well as to help other individuals achieve emotional balance, even in the face of such conflicts.

Our man with the call bell could be handled appropriately with the right amount of emotion management skill. First, the nurse would recognize his own emotions about the situation and understand their potential, then manage them by not allowing them to disrupt professional patient care or his relationship with the patient. Second, a nurse skilled at the level of emotion management would be able to help the patient channel his building emotional state appropriately and prevent escalation to a state of withdrawal or noncompliance.

Our family who worried incessantly about their loved one could also benefit from the skill of someone who knows how to manage emotions. Again, the nurse should be able to put aside and manage his own anxieties associated with the family's worry, anxieties that may be preventing him from addressing their issues appropriately. He should then be able to help the family redirect their worry into more productive activities, such as positive, supportive interchanges with the patient and increased fact-finding communication with the physicians.

It should be apparent in both of these situations that the effectiveness of emotion management depends on successfully passing through the stages of perception, facilitation, and understanding of emotion. It would, after all, be very difficult for a nurse to help a family channel their worry if he did not recognize it or to place emphasis on calming the angry patient if he did not understand the thought processes to which his anger might be contributing.

Nurse leaders, as well, benefit greatly from the high-level skill of emotion management, for reasons that include those described for the other three skill sets. Difficult patient care situations provide natural ground for the use of emotional intelligence. In terms of leadership, often what the nursing staff needs is a venue in which to consider the ethical, medical, rational, and emotional contexts of a difficult situation and reach resolution. In such an ethical climate, there is opportunity for dialogue that promotes reflection on the problem at hand and eventual resolution. Nurses feel free to say what they need to say. A strong ethical climate promotes and requires trust, empowerment, inclusion, role flexibility, and inquiry (Olson, 2002).

Emotionally supportive climates are very similar to ethical climates. Chapter Six will expand on the inclusion of staff in decision making and the need to provide an open environment for discussion. Leaders should indeed be supportive of the emotional process that staff nurses must go through in order to recognize, understand, and cope with difficult ethical and emotional issues and should help them manage the process in order to provide effective care.

Summary

"Technology transforms work at a dizzying pace. People who have mastered their emotions are able to roll with the changes. When a new change program is announced, they do not panic; instead, they are able to suspend judgment, seek out information, and listen to executives explain the new program. As the initiative moves forward, they are able to move with it" (Goleman, 1998a, p. 9).

The "dizzying pace" underscored by Goleman affects the health care industry perhaps more than any other. Rapid changes are complicated by the intense emotional needs inherent in work with patients—not just the needs of patients, but those of caregivers and staff members too. Emotional needs in turn are complicated by technological advances with intense ethical and physical implications. "As time constraints, financial issues, and administrative burdens have shifted clinicians' focus from healing of patients to the mechanics of healthcare, many practitioners have been searching to reacquaint themselves with the qualities that form the heart of medical practice," says Epstein (2003, p. 2).

As nurse leaders, we must strive to increase our emotional intelligence so that we can support our staff in providing comprehensive, relationship-centered care to patients and families during this ongoing revolution in health care. Using Mayer, Salovey, and Caruso's four-step model of emotional intelligence (2000, 2002), the nurse leader can assess and monitor the progression of her own and her staff's emotional abilities.

TEN REASONS WHY LEADERS IN OUR AGE NEED EMOTIONAL INTELLIGENCE SKILLS

1. The current age requires us to grapple with the unknown and its ensuing emotional issues.
2. Work and our emotional response to it is perpetually being changed by technology.
3. Leadership becomes more influenced by emotion in the face of difficult decisions.
4. Staff interactions with patients become more influenced by emotion in the face of difficult decisions.
5. Advances in technology and medicine result in ethical problems that may have emotional implications.
6. Elements of emotional awareness are included in issues that used to be more purely scientific.
7. Assessment of a patient's situation is aided when one is aware of one's own emotions and those of others.
8. Situations call on us to use our emotions to support, not hinder, our critical thinking ability.
9. Proactive understanding of emotions and how they develop and interact can prevent crises and undesirable outcomes.
10. Times are replete with change and the need to make critical decisions, heightening the advantages of regulating and managing emotions.

3

EMOTIONAL INTELLIGENCE AND LEADERSHIP

MANY PEOPLE ATTEND leadership seminars and read leadership books for the same reason some buy exercise videos: they hope they will learn something new and different that will result in a quick, easy self-improvement. When people hear a fit celebrity touting how easy an exercise program is or a leader who turned a company around by following three simple leadership principles, they naturally want to hear more.

Unfortunately, such inspirational chatter soon proves to be little more than excellent marketing technique. Most of us know intuitively that effort is required to attain anything of value. Fortunately, for a demonstration of leadership effectiveness, we can look to two "spokespeople" who laid the groundwork for two health professions: nursing and psychology. They are Florence Nightingale and Sigmund Freud.

What Made Florence Nightingale a Leader

Florence Nightingale knew very early that she wanted to be a nurse. Today, we associate words such as *pioneer, visionary,* and *reformer* with her name and life. Few nurses graduate from their educational program without hearing about her, and many recite her namesake pledge at their commencement ceremony. Some, especially those outside the profession, vaguely accept that she invented nursing but know little else about her life. In reality, Florence Nightingale established the first nursing school, using donated funds, and it is widely accepted that she reformed nursing to initiate the profession as we know it today.

Hospitals and attendants to the ill, of course, preceded Nightingale, but they did not enjoy a very good reputation. She saw a need to reform the sanitary conditions of hospitals so that needless deaths could be prevented. Through the analysis involved in this reform, Nightingale applied the revolutionary idea that social phenomena and medical data could be objectively measured and subjected to mathematical and statistical analysis.

Florence Nightingale was a leader not because she created something out of nothing, but because she changed the status quo. Biographer Barbara Montgomery Dossey (2000) points out that Florence improved the conditions of soldiers and commoners against the societal expectations of the day, which treated women as delicate and unable to make decisions without help. In the mid-1800s, women of society did not involve themselves with hospitals. In addition, Florence was a child of society, having been reared in mansions and other properties inherited by her father and having been presented at court in London at the age of seventeen. Ladies of her stature were expected to marry well, but Florence sought something other than idleness (Dossey, 2000).

From the age of sixteen, she believed that she was called into God's service and pursued what that service would be. Nightingale's deep interest in her own work discouraged her from marriage, and she eventually disappointed a long-term suitor, choosing her calling over a society marriage. From that point forward, she dedicated her life to improving conditions for the sick and hospitalized.

There is no doubt that Florence Nightingale was a leader, but the reasons for this go beyond the obvious. Of course, she wanted to challenge the norm, which is a hallmark of anyone who ultimately allows change (Kouzes and Posner, 1995). However, what of the times when challenging the norm led to disappointment and failure? In Nightingale's case, those times led to acceptance of the disappointments as opportunities to learn and perhaps change more. After years of attempting to answer the call to service, she went into residence as superintendent of a formal establishment for the ill at thirty-three years of age. One year later, during the Crimean War, Florence was summoned by then Secretary of War Sidney Herbert, whom she had met years earlier, to nurse wounded British soldiers in the Barrack Hospital. What an opportunity, Florence thought, to prove the value that female nurses could add to the care of injured military troops. She enthusiastically assembled thirty-eight nurses, who descended on the facility, meeting with horrible conditions. The conditions faced by the military were unacceptable to Florence, and she focused on improving them even after her initial visit (Dossey, 2000).

"Two groups of people emerged from the Crimean War as heroes—soldiers and nurses" (Dossey, 2000, p. 183). Leadership goes beyond sticking with it when the going gets tough. Had Florence's determination stopped there, those wounded in the Crimean War would have been better cared for, but the reforms would not have lasted. For change to last, there must be a vision that translates to enduring action, and that action must begin with the leader.

Nightingale's vision was for betterment of hospitals and patient care. Her *Notes on Nursing,* published in 1860 and expanded and republished the following year, sold millions all over the world and is still in print. The Nightingale School of Nursing opened in 1860, when Florence was forty. Because Florence was chronically ill, she provided oversight for the school from her home, placing Mrs. Sarah Elizabeth Wardroper in charge of day-to-day school operations (Dossey, 2000). Her arrangement to carry on her work in this way demonstrated that even her own illness—the aftereffect of Crimean fever five years earlier—could not stop her vision.

For the first time, nursing had a professional, respectable image. "Ever since Florence Nightingale stepped onto the battlefields of Crimea," says Perra (2001, p. 69), "nurses have been leaders and innovators, using intuition, experience and practical knowledge to build the art and science of nursing."

Henri Dunant, founder of the Red Cross, credited Nightingale's work as having a great deal of influence on his ideas. In fact, Nightingale's work and vision had a great deal of influence on the ideas of many. She enlisted others in the vision she embraced and enabled them to act. Because of this shared vision, nurses have a profession that is held in high esteem. Because Nightingale herself was held in high esteem, there was an example to follow, even when she was too physically ill to carry out some of the work herself (Dossey, 2000).

In 1907, Florence Nightingale received the Order of Merit from King Edward VII, becoming the first woman to receive this honor (Dossey, 2000).

In 1910, writes Cecil Woodham Smith, "she no longer spoke" (Woodham Smith, 1951, p. 366).

The voice of a leader. It is as resounding as the heart it encourages, as far-reaching as the change it invokes. It is tuned by its keen sense of the voices around it and speaks back in a language they can understand. Its breath enters all that truly hear it, and when it no longer speaks, it can still be heard.

What Is a Leader?

Badaracco (2002) says that from the time we are children, we are taught to admire great leaders but that focusing on bold acts entrenched in our history is not the same as paying attention to the quiet capabilities of leadership. What is a leader, exactly, and how does one become an effective leader?

Authors, theorists, consultants, and managers have proposed multitudinous answers to that question, and just about all of them have been right. Most of us know that *leader* has more than one definition, at least in the practical sense. Goleman (1998a, 2000) further indicates that leadership can be defined in different ways by different people but that a leader's single most important task is to get results, although different situations call for different types of leadership. Birrer (2002) defines different types of leaders in categories such as specialists and achievers, investigators and developers. Four domains in one presented study (Robbins, Bradley, Spicer, and Mecklenburg, 2001) were industry knowledge, technical skill, conceptual and analytical reasoning, and emotional and interpersonal intelligence. The word *leader* is very often defined in terms of what a leader does or is skilled in rather than what a leader is.

To lead effectively, say Kouzes and Posner (1995), is to translate a vision into reality and then to sustain it through the empowerment of followers. Empowerment occurs when organizations allow the channeling of skills and talents into activities that support a defined vision. This is not purely a rational activity, not solely a function of knowing the business or understanding what the numbers mean. Some established leaders know the business very well and have agendas, visions, and goals, but are unable to communicate or inspire a sharing of that vision or to establish mutual trust. These leaders are unable to lead. They plan and envision, but they have not created the emotional bond necessary to inspire and help followers set and achieve goals around the vision.

Attributes of Effective Leaders

Many theorists have proposed attributes that characterize effective leaders. They imply that in order to translate a vision into sustained reality through actively involved followers, certain traits are helpful, if not mandatory. Gardner (1990) lists fourteen characteristics of leaders, including ability to motivate, confidence, assertiveness, flexibility, and physical stamina, but goes on to say that the required attributes depend on the leader's style, the demands of the situation, and the nature of the followers. Birrer (2002) says that leadership is qualified by such characteristics as equanimity, courage, focus, energy, and kindness.

Blake and McCanse (1997) define six key elements of leadership: conflict solving, initiative, inquiry, advocacy, decision making, and critique. All six, they say, must be present for effective leadership to occur.

These examples form part of a spectrum ranging from a broad list of characteristics that may be helpful depending on the situation to a narrow group of absolute musts for leadership. Pity the aspiring superleader who tries to master all of them! In reality, there are more so-called characteristics of good leaders than there will ever be time to perfect them.

WHAT DO LEADERS DO? Let us shift our attention once again from what a leader is to what a leader does. Shultz (2003) says that leaders assess social dynamics and take corrective action immediately where problems exist. Merely sweeping issues "under the rug" with the hope that they will disappear is an ineffective practice, but many managers would rather avoid problems than create discomfort by addressing them head on. Fortunately, managers can correct many problems through motivation and persuasion to adopt a compelling vision and follow a strong example. Staff members need to see opportunities for what could be, and how they can be an integral part of achieving that change. Kouzes and Posner (1995) outline five practices of leadership: leaders challenge the process, inspire a shared vision, enable others to act, model the way, and encourage the heart. These practices are neither characteristics nor skill sets; rather, they are manifestations of possibly infinite combinations of abilities and traits. However, examples of these practices are excellent examples of leadership in action.

THREE LEADERSHIP ACTIONS. Three common threads run through various interpretations of what makes an effective leader: leaders create, they share a vision, and they set an example. These threads align with the results that a leader should hope to achieve—that is, his or her vision carried out by followers because they embrace the vision themselves and are enabled to follow the example set by the leader. The three denominators also encompass some characteristics of leaders but not so much so that the characteristics can be distinctly categorized. This makes sense, because leaders who do what they need to do to be good leaders may possess a variety of character traits.

The Leadership of Sigmund Freud

In the late 1800s, when Florence Nightingale was pioneering today's nursing, a talented medical researcher was developing many of the concepts of modern psychoanalysis. His name was Sigmund Freud, and today we know him as the father of psychoanalysis.

Freud devoted his energies to the study of human nature and concluded that humans are self-centered beings. Freud's constructs of human nature hold a significant irony; considered separately, they leave the leader bewildered and directionless. However, Freud himself was a masterful leader who had a devoted following and an impact on Western thought that has far outlived him.

HE CREATED. Freud was a leader who created. He challenged the process of the day, was willing to experiment, and was willing to make mistakes. Freud recognized the intellectual paucity of neurological research directed at tracing psychic disturbances to physical causes, which was accepted in scientific circles at the time. He proposed a less scientific approach to research because he felt that the convergence of clues about the inner workings of the psyche was sufficient confirmation of fact to justify theorizing. He had seen in his own practice that physical treatments, such as hydrotherapy and electrotherapy, were futile in treating supposedly physical diseases. Not only did Freud challenge established modes of investigation, but he also challenged established therapeutic modes.

In challenging the status quo in psychiatry and neurology, Freud experimented freely, trying hypnosis and, later, free association and dream interpretation, despite the fact that neurologists of the time generally viewed hypnosis as a fraudulent technique that endangered the patient (Miller, 1993). He did not let opposition or failure stop his progress. In an age when psychoanalysis was officially held to be of ill repute, Freud participated in establishing leadership within the International Psycho-Analytical Association to advance the cause (Freud, 1935). In addition, although he believed strongly in hypnosis, his own failures in inducing hypnosis in patients led him to turn eventually to dream interpretation and free association as therapeutic alternatives.

When a leader creates, he or she must also create the climate for followers to want to participate. It is not sufficient to challenge the status quo or attempt to change it if constituents have no interest. This is perhaps more challenging than going against the norm, because it involves changing the perspective of people other than oneself. Freud believed that his patients expected great things of him, and that belief in him fostered self-confidence and his ability to accomplish his goals. Similarly, Freud sought to engender self-confidence in others by expecting great things of them and giving them the resources to accomplish their goals, even if they did not coincide with his own (Freud, [1914] 1972). He desired most of all to be a leader among leaders, not to monopolize power. In this spirit, he sponsored the informal discussion group that met in his home, the establishment of professional societies, and the foundation of a new journal in which fellow psychoanalysts could publish their findings and expound their theories.

HE SHARED A VISION. Through his work, Freud spoke volumes to the dynamics of human motivation and communal interactions. Freud's vision began as a narrowly defined one, in which he strove to alleviate the mental ailments of patients who consulted him as a neurologist in private practice, yet it became all-encompassing. Freud described psychology as his consuming passion (Miller, 1993). His ultimate goal became to enable individuals to understand their own history so that they could make choices.

Today we refer to Freud as the father of psychoanalysis, not because he was the originator of key ideas about sexuality and the development of the psyche or the therapeutic benefit of talk; he was not. He freely admitted that he had derived some of his ideas from others, including Charcot and Breuer, and he made a point of giving them full credit for their work (Freud, [1914] 1972). What marked Freud as the father of psychoanalysis was that others found his own conviction so compelling that they came to him asking for training. Freud never actively recruited adherents to his theories, but nonetheless, his fervent belief, his intellectual prowess, and his lucid writing style drew others to him from around the world.

Freud once pronounced, "We have the truth, I am sure of it" (Freud, [1914] 1972). It is quite significant that Freud referred here to a collective "we," not a self-aggrandizing "I."

Freud's daughter Anna shared Freud's vision and worked toward a common purpose. She ultimately became a pioneer in the psychoanalysis of children. Other psychoanalysts, including Heinz Hartman and Erik Erikson, advanced her ideas in their own work, making major contributions to current thought in developmental psychology. Once Freud's ideas gained a foothold of legitimacy in hospitable environments in the United States and Switzerland, the trickle of adherents to his theories became a torrent. Soon, Freud's work was applied to education, art, history, religion, anthropology, and sociology (Appel, 1995).

Freud was a visionary and a creative leader by virtue of his message and his means. Many a leader with great potential has stopped with a message, albeit a grandiose or a carefully crafted one. An organization whose leader is merely a visionary without the means or motivating factors to carry out the vision will produce, simply, an organization with vision. A leader who carries the vision to reality by creating an environment for change can only do so in tandem with the motivation of his constituents. In other words, it is insufficient to have a vision or to create the means to carry out the vision, if one does not lead.

HE SET AN EXAMPLE. Followers are only followers because they are following something or someone. The leader must set an example for others to follow, without expecting followers, albeit dedicated to the vision and eager to get started, to set the example for them. Even self-directed work teams become such because they have a strong example to begin with: a leader or strong guiding principles. Example is a crucial point of leadership, the make-or-break element, no matter how strong the vision or how ripe the environment for change.

There is a distinct transition of power that must occur when a leader sets an example. The followers have to feel the ability to follow the example. Freud was a masterful leader in the sense that he set a beautiful example, enabling his followers and constituents to act because he gave them a framework for taking action.

We may think of setting an example in terms of the old adage many of us heard in childhood, often in jest. "Do as I say, not as I do." This statement left many of us squirming in our conscience, because people naturally want to do as others do. Today's leadership theory boldly denounces the practice of walking any walk other than that expected of followers. Simply put, this involves honesty and credibility.

Freud was a scrupulously honest leader. Although in his day, psychoanalysis was still subject to trials and the truing up of conflicting avenues of thought, the very process of psychoanalysis required an unrestrained approach to what was often the bitter truth. In addition, conflicting theories and the ripples created by challenging the norms of the day often resulted in dissension between Freud and his followers. Constant intellectual battles ensued, some of which created breaks in professional relationships. Freud discussed even these with honesty, giving due credit to the merits and strong detail of the theories of others while supporting his own through truthful comparisons.

Freud proved himself an honest leader, then enabled others to act through collaboration and the sharing of information and power. He said, in effect, "Do as I do." Although Freud did much of his work in isolation, he studied with others in order to advance his own theories throughout his career. In turn, he provided an environment of collaboration for others through weekly discussion sessions at his home and later through offers of collaboration with medical institutions and professional societies. He tirelessly supported and worked to help other theorists who had been met with rejection in the psychoanalytic movement. In fact, for ten years, he had no followers largely because of a similar rejection (Freud, 1935). However, over time, he shared the personal power of his expertise with others, which enabled them to act and ultimately to advance his theories, creating what we know as modern psychotherapy. One man, no matter how brilliant, no matter how visionary, no matter how creative, no matter how powerful, could not have done this alone.

Why Nightingale and Freud Are Leaders Today

Sigmund Freud and Florence Nightingale were both stellar leaders in their day and remain so in our day because, as beneficiaries of their respective examples, we are inspired and empowered. Their leadership styles may have been sharply distinct. Their immediate followers may have varied in education and social status. Their characteristics may have reflected distinct differences in their early lives and environments. However, we recognize them for three unmistakable commonalities: They each had a vision, which they shared with others; they each created the environment and means to carry out that vision; and they each set an example, which empowered their followers. Despite differences in details, these are the things that leaders do which make them great leaders.

Emotional Skill Supports Effective Leadership

Today, says Watson (2000),

> Nursing's dormant, value-based vision of caring and healing and wholeness is emerging from the dark side of history to help to reestablish light and balance in systems and society that are out of balance. As nursing leaders rethink nursing's place and purpose, it is about to emerge from the dark and reenter the health care arena at this turning point in history. As it does, we see that new life, new germination, and new light are being brought into those spaces where there has been institutional darkness. Nursing's value-guided vision of care—caring for the human condition, for the embodied spirit seeking wholeness and healing—must gain voice as part of the nursing leader's true vision [p. 2].

What better time is there than now to focus on emotional intelligence for the "light and balance" we are seeking?

"We are living in a period of profound transition," observes Hagenow (2001, p. 30). "The changes are perhaps more radical than those ushered in by the second industrial revolution . . . or the structural changes triggered by the great depression in the 1930s. Health care leadership has been equally affected by these cultural shifts in our society." Why? For just a few reasons: business competition, interpersonal and ethical conflict, consumer demand for perfection in products and services, overwhelmingly large volumes and speeds of communication, and technological complexity (Hagenow, 2001; Perra, 2001). "The new world we live in" is a common phrase (Freshman and Rubino, 2002, p. 7). Nurse leaders everywhere must not only absorb and understand change as individuals, they must also lead through it while maintaining morale, employee satisfaction, and quality.

Leadership development is described as a make-or-break issue in companies all over the globe (Dearborn, 2002). Some might say that the most important element for good leadership is trust. *Trust* is quite a subjective term. Our loss of it is underscored in government regulations and reimbursement models that monitor and manage the practices of health professionals (Malloch, 2002). "There is a huge interest in leading with values and ethics," Jay Conger was quoted as saying at a recent leadership seminar, referring to the management world's reaction to the Enron scandal (Giganti, 2003b, p. 9). As the world becomes increasingly interdependent, relationships rather than individual results will create leadership (Ulrich, 1996). Relationships, which are traditionally formed to get needs met, can be breeding grounds for mistrust (Malloch, 2002). Correlations have been found between the quality of interpersonal relationships and emotional intelligence (Schutte and others, 2001). Relationship skills require some mastery of emotional skills and are needed for the three leadership actions of creating, sharing a vision, and setting an example described earlier. The good news is that creating, sharing a vision, and setting an example are not limited to people with a prescribed personality or leadership style. Even better news is that many of the abilities required to create, share a vision, and set an example are learned abilities, not merely natural talents. They are emotional abilities.

Leadership Effectiveness and Style Are Tied to Emotional Skill

EI (emotional intelligence) is widely accepted as foundational to getting along with others in the workplace, as well as a primary managerial and leadership competency (Freshman and Rubino, 2002). A study performed with 280 college students (Moss, Rau, Craig, and Strack, 2000) revealed the abilities or characteristics that they felt typified someone they classified as an outstanding leader. As part of the survey instrument, students were given twenty statements about characteristics of leaders and asked to rank them on a Likert scale of usually, sometimes, rarely, or never. Several of the abilities on the survey were emotional in nature—for example, awareness of feelings and their effect on others and the ability to build trusting relationships. Over 90 percent of respondents selected such abilities as usually describing their selected outstanding leader.

The students were then asked to rank in order of importance a series of leadership characteristics. Nearly half (48.2 percent) felt that treating others with dignity and respect was the predominant attribute of an outstanding leader. This overshadowed other attributes such as a strong desire to achieve results, seeking to understand issues from different viewpoints, implementing innovative projects, and acting with confidence.

This study demonstrates the intuitive knowledge of a group of college students, most of whom had been employed for fewer than five years. We do not know whether the respondents' outstanding leaders were professors, parents, employers, or leaders recognized by the world at large. What we do know is that these students placed a high emphasis on the importance of emotional abilities in leadership. There is an assumption that the selected outstanding leaders were admired individuals who generated some level of loyalty on the part of the students. Regardless of whether we can study the effectiveness of these leaders, we know that a great deal of their perceived effectiveness can be tied to emotional abilities.

Further correlation has been shown between emotional intelligence and leadership style, specifically among health care leaders. In a study of health care executives who self-assessed their leadership style through a series of descriptors, those choosing a team management style garnered higher mean scores on the Mayer-Salovey-Caruso Emotional Intelligence Test than did those choosing other categories (Moss, 2001). Goleman (2000) points out that leaders can increase their flexibility within a leadership style by learning about and developing emotional intelligence. Hagenow (2001) says that the climate of today's health care leadership requires emotional intelligence because of the potential for conflict and the need to foster cooperation in health care organizations. Now more than ever, the function of leadership is more about human empowerment (Hagenow, 2001) than about red tape and function. Additionally, emotional ability, according to U.S. News and World Report ("The Secret Skill of Leaders," 2002), is often called on by leaders in times of crisis as they sort through emotional reactions and help constituents cope.

Background and Definition of Emotional Intelligence

What did Mayer, Salovey, and Caruso have in mind when they developed their four-branch model of emotional intelligence? By their own account, they proposed to dispel the multitude of definitions of emotional intelligence that were being discussed in educational, business, and behavioral science circles. In the 1970s, emotions began to be studied as having influence on thought, and during the ensuing twenty years, the term *emotional intelligence* was used sporadically. However, by the last decade of the twentieth century, the field was quickly emerging as its own scientific arena. When Goleman published his *Emotional Intelligence* in 1995, a work based loosely on the prior research of Salovey and Mayer (1990) and others, he popularized the field so much that the term gained a popular meaning, as Goleman applied the scientific concepts of emotional intelligence to elements of social behavior. The result of this and other attempts to popularize the concept was a plethora of definitions of the term, most of which referred to personality traits such as warmth, motivation, persistence, and social skills (Mayer, Salovey, and Caruso, 2000, 2002). In popular writings, "emotional intelligence" has come to include assessment of "motivation, non-ability dispositions and traits, and global personal and social functioning," (Mayer, Caruso, and Salovey, 1999) rather than actual indicators of emotional ability.

In 1997, Mayer, Salovey, and Caruso recast their 1990 model of emotional intelligence in a way that would more succinctly clarify the abilities involved—and not involved. They focused on measuring emotional ability as one would measure a cognitive intelligence, using as a basis for their decision the fact that self-reports of ability are rarely correlated with actual performance.

The researchers over the next three years constructed and perfected their four-branch model to include the following: emotional identification, emotional facilitation, emotional understanding, and emotion management. These four are postulated to be hierarchical in nature; that is, the categories of ability can be arranged from lower to higher, with perception or identification of emotions as the lowest level skill and management of emotions the highest (Mayer, Caruso, and Salovey, 1999). The researchers then broke the branches into specific tasks, or abilities, which could be measured in a test setting. Tasks include associating the degree of association of a picture with a certain emotion; indicating which emotion is likely to follow a series of events; and choosing actions, given a situation, that would result in a desired outcome. Respondents must choose the right answer to each problem. Their scores at each branch level tell much about their emotional ability, and the task-level scores provide insight into specific areas for development (Mayer, Salovey, and Caruso, 2000, 2002). Table 3.1 illustrates the levels of feedback from Version 2 of the Mayer-Salovey-Caruso Emotional Intelligence Test.

THE ABILITY TO IDENTIFY EMOTIONS. Emotional identification, or emotional perception, is the most fundamental of the branches of emotional ability. It involves attending to and decoding emotional signals

Table 3.1. Levels of Feedback from the Mayer-Salovey-Caruso Emotional Intelligence Test (MSCEIT), Version 2.

Emotional Intelligence Quotients			Further Diagnostic Information
Overall Scale	Two Areas of the MSCEIT	Four Branches of the MSCEIT	Task Level
Emotional Intelligence (EIQ)	Experiential Emotional Intelligence (EEIQ)	Perceiving Emotions (PEIQ)	Section A: Faces
			Section E: Pictures
		Facilitating Thought (FEIQ)	Section B: Facilitation
			Section F: Sensations
	Strategic Emotional Intelligence (SEIQ)	Understanding Emotions (UEIQ)	Section C: Changes
			Section G: Blends
		Managing Emotions (MEIQ)	Section D: Emotional Management
			Section H: Emotional Relations

Source: Mayer, Salovey, and Caruso, 2002, p. 8. Reprinted with permission from Multi Health Systems.

accurately, in faces, tones of voice, and artistic expressions and scenes. Individuals who demonstrate this ability are able not only to recognize and express their own feelings but also to recognize and appraise those of others around them. In fact, Mayer, Salovey, and Caruso (2002) cite research that indicates a direct relationship between the ability to assess emotion in oneself and the ability to assess it in others.

These researchers are also quick to point out that fundamental to appraising emotions is attending to them. That is, one cannot draw conclusions about emotional expressions and what they mean without being able to accept them for what they are. Many people have difficulty paying attention to the expression of negative emotions, for example, because they are uncomfortable being confronted with such emotions. The tendency to avoid paying attention hinders accurate perception (Mayer, Salovey, and Caruso, 2000, 2002). This will be especially relevant later, when we focus on the critical nature of this skill in leadership.

THE ABILITY TO USE EMOTIONS. Using emotions, or emotional facilitation, is the second branch of the Mayer-Salovey-Caruso model (2000, 2002). They define this skill as the ability to use feelings to assist in reasoning and decision making. This is especially important in creative problem solving. Although some emotions, such as fear and anger, have been associated with short-term detriment to cognitive abilities, Mayer and his colleagues propose, based on their research, that such emotions actually supplement the cognitive system's ability to prioritize based on urgency and importance (Mayer, Salovey, and Caruso, 2000).

Furthermore, emotions, when used synergistically with cognitive thought, may be applied to enhance reason and productivity. For example, skill in facilitating or using emotions provides insight into which activities one performs best when one is feeling a certain way emotionally. This supports a purely reasoned approach to using moods to enhance cognitive abilities, as opposed to the concept that mood governs abilities. Although mood and emotion can and do change the way an individual thinks, being, in essence his "window on the world," the ability to know how emotions affect thought and to use them to facilitate appropriate thought is crucial. From their research, Mayer, Salovey, and Caruso point out that shifting viewpoints brought on by fluctuations in emotion may foster creative thinking and that mood swings can foster greater creativity (Mayer, Salovey, and Caruso, 2000).

THE ABILITY TO UNDERSTAND EMOTIONS. Emotional understanding is the third level of emotional ability constructed by Mayer, Salovey, and Caruso (2000, 2002). They differentiate emotional understanding from emotional facilitation this way: "the emotional facilitation of thought branch involves using emotion to improve cognitive processes, whereas the emotional understanding branch involves cognitive processing of emotion" (2000, p. 107). The ability to understand emotions involves knowledge of what leads to a given emotion. For example, disappointment may lead to grief if the disappointment involves a loss. On the other hand, irritation may lead to anger if the source of irritation is not removed. While many people can say they have experienced any of a set of given emotions and can describe the emotion in terms of reactions and feelings, understanding the relationship of one emotion to another may prove more difficult. This skill is important for the sheer reason that self-understanding and our understanding of others can only be improved by knowing how emotions combine and change with time and circumstances (Mayer, Salovey, and Caruso, 2002).

THE ABILITY TO MANAGE EMOTIONS. Emotion management is the fourth branch of the Mayer-Salovey-Caruso model (2000, 2002), and, like emotional understanding, it is classified as a higher-level ability. Managing emotions involves managing them in oneself and ultimately being able to help other people manage their own emotions. Mayer and his team draw a defining line in the area of emotion management to squelch a popular concept of the skill. Many people think that managing emotions means repressing or rationalizing emotion. Although sometimes it is appropriate to contain emotion, the goal of emotion management is not to continually sweep emotions under the rug. Rather, emotion management involves knowing when to feel the feeling and how to use feelings judiciously rather than act on impulse of emotion. Because of this, the skill of emotion management enhances problem solving by invoking abilities such as awareness and use of emotions (Mayer, Salovey, and Caruso, 2002), and it aids in decision making by helping us cope with negative consequences of a decision (Mayer, Salovey, and Caruso, 1999). Although their model describes emotional intelligence as spanning both the cognitive and emotional spectrum (Mayer, Salovey, and Caruso, 2000), the levels at which cognition affects emotion appear to advance with each stage. For example, one might infer that managing emotions requires a higher level of cognitive effort than perceiving a particular emotion in oneself.

Three Leadership Actions, Four Emotional Skills

Leaders who create, those who share a vision, and those who set an example set themselves apart from other leaders. Why? Such leaders combine the key ingredients of knowing where they want to go and enlisting the buy-in of others to get there. These ingredients involve emotional intelligence skills, in addition to other skills such as business knowledge and analytical ability. Sometimes, this involves changing the mind-set of those in a position of higher authority. This "leading upward" and "marshaling the people above" are abilities that health care leaders need to instill in their own organization (Useem, 2001a, p. 58). It is no longer enough to assume that top-led organization will automatically prosper; the challenges have become too myriad.

Leaders Who Create

"Many executives try to change organizations," says Hirschhorn (2002), adding, "Few succeed" (p. 98).

Bureaucratic methods are no longer effective in leadership, because they squelch creativity and hinder the process of making decisions (Eisenstat and Dixon, 2000). Leaders who create need emotional ability to create. This means that they should be able to identify, facilitate, understand, and manage emotion in order to create opportunities and the environment for change.

EMOTIONAL IDENTIFICATION. "Leaders should be led by the group's needs," says Michael Useem (2001a, p. 53). Identification of one's own emotions, as well as the emotions and needs of others, is pivotal to other emotional abilities (Mayer, Salovey, and Caruso, 2000, 2002). Creating a new environment or a new status quo involves change, and change involves emotions that must be dealt with early. One such emotion is complacency, which often hinders and hampers truly beneficial, substantial organizational reform. Just ask anyone who has tried to get a new project off the ground with insufficient funding, only to be told, "We just don't have the budget to work that in next year." Behind that statement, someone is saying, "Show me why this is more important than all the usual, normal things we keep paying for year after year." Once a sense of urgency is established, budget constraints seem more malleable. Without a sense of urgency, even the most glaring needs for improvement may go unnoticed because things have gone unimproved for so long that no one notices that things could be different.

Being able to identify emotions lets us in on the fact that people are complacent in the first place. It lets us see that they are more comfortable in their comfort zones and identify the degree to which they are going to resist change. They may express fear, disdain, or even disgust at yet another initiative. Attention! What they express is what we must manage if we are to lead.

Identification of emotions in oneself is very closely related to one's ability to identify it in others (Mayer, Salovey, and Caruso, 2000, 2002). Knowing how we feel about change or about a particular change is foundational to going forward with the change, because if we repress those emotions, we will encounter them in an uglier form later. Some leaders are fundamentally resistant to change—that is, they are conservatives who tend to come around to change more slowly than others do. Yet that does not mean that they can refuse to move, hoping the world will someday revolve to meet them once again where they are today. These leaders most of all need to identify their own emotions in relation to change, because every time an opportunity to change occurs, they are naturally going to want to resist it, and there is an underlying reason why. It may be fear of failure, anxiety about the reactions of others, or even a sense of grief over leaving the old ways behind. Whatever it is, they need to identify it.

EMOTIONAL FACILITATION. Once emotions are identified, they must be used to facilitate thought (Mayer, Salovey, and Caruso, 2000, 2002). This is especially important in creative leadership. Challenging the process is challenging. There are times when we are more able to engage in grueling, uphill-battle initiatives than others are. Very few of us can go full steam ahead at all hours of the day and night, with no regard for how we are feeling emotionally. Some people, including some of your team members, will give you 100 percent as long as they are feeling confident, secure, and happy. The minute they are feeling sad, insecure, or distrustful, their work becomes more laborious, painstaking, and slow. These shifts apply to us, too, and it is important to understand what they (and we) do best under these circumstances and to create an environment that supports these natural fluctuations. Recall that mood swings promote creativity. I propose that it takes skill—emotional skill—to make that happen.

EMOTIONAL UNDERSTANDING. Emotional understanding, the first of Mayer, Salovey, and Caruso's emotional skills requiring conscious processing (2000), is a crucial skill for the leader who creates. Understanding emotion allows us to anticipate roadblocks that are likely to be caused by emotion and, in turn, to visualize likely solutions. For example, consider political battles that may ensue over a significant change within an organization. These battles can be emotion-driven and fueled by the slightest provocation. Say someone on our team who is pushing for the change is on the radar screen of someone not on the team who is resistant to change. The opposing force zeroes in on a known weakness of the most vulnerable team member, exposing a small oversight in the planning of the new idea and maybe even making a big deal out of it in front of the right people. The team member, perhaps insecure, albeit beginning to become more comfortable with change under strong leadership, suddenly spirals into the death grip of self-doubt on the heels of what is probably a minor mistake. If you know the path down which self-doubt takes a person, and what emotion leads to it (for example, embarrassment), as well as where it goes next, then you have likely taken a huge step toward salvaging the contributions of a key person on your team, as well as the creative energy behind it. This is emotional understanding.

EMOTION MANAGEMENT. The ability to manage emotions is the ultimate goal. Without identifying them, facilitating them, and understanding them, we lack the key components of managing them (Mayer, Salovey, and Caruso, 2000). Part of creating an environment that allows team members to change the status quo involves helping them manage their own emotions. A pattern becomes noticeable in the three previous stages of emotional intelligence: they each seem to involve *knowing*—for example, knowing what an emotion looks like, knowing how it helps us, and knowing how it progresses. The ability to manage emotion requires some *doing* on our part as well. Once we as team members know what we are feeling, how it is useful, and what it can lead to, we need to be able to regulate those feelings in ourselves and others to achieve the desired result.

Leaders Who Share a Vision

Earlier in this book, the proposal was made that effective leaders engage in three actions: they create, they develop and share a vision, and they set an example, thereby enabling others to act. That order has been used consistently, and the order may seem unusual, as we typically think of vision setting as the first step in achieving any mission or objective. However, it should be reemphasized that simply having a vision does not equate to leadership and that many visionaries have failed miserably in their attempts to lead, despite stellar plans and goals. The reason for this is a link that many visionaries miss or expect to happen effortlessly: the vision must be *shared*. Eisenstat and Dixon (2000) identify one of the "silent killers" of good leadership as an ineffective senior management team—ineffective, that is, in that their strategic direction and priorities are unclear in the face of inconsistent demands imposed by the system in which they are operating, be it finance, health care, or anything else. The senior management team must share a vision with the rest of the organization. Further, they must involve the organization in the change process.

Having a shared vision is not a natural result of having a vision. In fact, it is just the opposite. The vision of those above naturally causes speculation among those below, the degree of which varies according to factors such as trust, stability, and corporate culture. People ask, "What does this mean for me? How will this affect my colleagues? What are the alternatives? What am I going to have to give up?" These questions are all driven at least partially by emotion (Kotter, 1996). Whenever a company or a department changes its vision or resets its priorities, look out below (and above)! A change in paradigm is uncomfortable.

If you have come to think that leadership is all about change, you are half-right. Half is about current and future change, but half is about managing the past. The past includes any ruts that staff was in and can no longer be in, old philosophies, old cultures, old attitudes. The old stuff eventually stays behind, but attachments remain as long as the people who hold them. That is what visionaries fail to realize when they assume that a team of workers will simply embrace their vision. Planning for change means planning for the fallout of having to manage people's old ideas and emotions.

How is this different from creating an environment that fosters change? The answer lies in the result. Leaders who create cause two things to happen: the environment becomes ripe for growth, and the people become ripe for growth. Leaders who share a vision actually change the mind-set of the people and the environment; not only do they foster the ability and willingness to change, but they also give direction as to what change should happen. In addition, they engage the minds of their followers, persuading them to share and move toward the vision. This magnificent feat also, as one might imagine, involves emotional skill.

EMOTIONAL IDENTIFICATION. Let us apply Mayer, Salovey, and Caruso's hierarchy (2000, 2002) to leaders who share a vision. First, it is crucial in this visionary aspect of leadership, perhaps more than in any other, that a leader be able to identify his or her own emotions, express them, and perceive them accurately in others. Recall that Florence Nightingale identified early that she felt called to nurse the sick. By that account, we are not given much to go on in regard to her emotions on the topic. However, imagine how important it would have been for Florence to give the emotional aspects of her calling due consideration. Why was nursing the sick and improving sanitation so important to her? What specifically continued to drive her, despite the political and social obstacles she faced?

Why, indeed, did many of us choose health care as a career or management as a pursuit? Were there emotions involved? Can we tie our rational decision to go to nursing school or advance within the organization to factors that are other than rational? In many cases, probably. Many of us can probably identify a sense of anticipation, compassion, happiness at the prospect of a salary increase, or pride in our competence as contributors to our career path. The same applies when we attempt to put a fresh coat of vision on an old, established avenue of thought. There is a reason we want to make a change, and we may have to dig to find the emotional elements, but they are there. As leaders, we must answer the questions "What emotions of mine are driving my vision for my department, team, or organization?" and "Can I identify the emotions in my team that will either support or hinder the vision?"

EMOTIONAL FACILITATION. I stated earlier that sharing a vision among a team is perhaps the most challenging of the three essential leadership actions, because it often involves a complete change of paradigm for team members and not just a change in action. When we share our vision, we often give team members very little autonomy to come up with a vision on their own. Perhaps that is why, even though a vision may have been well communicated, there are often renegades who are determined to do their own thing regardless. It is not that they have their own vision; it is just that they do not see the need to subscribe to ours, necessarily.

Persuading people to make a paradigm shift requires extraordinary emotional intelligence. Once we have identified the emotions that our colleagues are or might be experiencing, it is necessary to apply a definitive approach of knowledge and action. We must know how these emotions will facilitate their thought and then address the issues that arise from those thoughts.

After a big meeting in which the CEO has outlined his goals for the hospital for the coming year, one unit manager remarks to another, "It's the same old thing, year after year. And then we go back to doing the same old thing, year after year." What a testimonial to the CEO's failure to share a vision! Why? Because, for one, the CEO did not know about or chose not to acknowledge feelings of apathy, mistrust, and doubt, feelings that led to a somewhat conscious decision to make no change, year after year.

While this example may be extreme, there are other smaller instances of failure to subscribe to a beautiful vision, which also involve emotional processing, whether conscious or unconscious. People let their emotions tell them what to do all the time, even if they do not realize they are doing it. If their emotions tell them it is impossible to go where the company expects to go, or if they resent being told they need to change, many will figure out ways to make do in the old paradigms while giving lip service to the vision. In that case, there is no shared vision.

A shared vision means just what it says. It indicates that the team actually has the same vision as the leader. Once that is accomplished, it is reasonable to assume that everyone will be working toward the same thing without prodding or coercion. Many managers do not think it matters whether their employees feel they need to do something, as long as they are doing it and doing it well. It goes without saying this is a hugely mistaken line of thought, which is evidenced in sagging production, high absenteeism, and issues of accountability and responsibility. An age-old quandary of managers is how to get employees to feel as passionate about their individual job as the manager feels about leading a successful team. The answer: understanding and managing emotions.

EMOTIONAL UNDERSTANDING. The first two levels of emotional skill, identification and facilitation, allow us to know something about what is going on, almost without conscious thought. We now enter the realm of having to consciously do something about it. When we understand emotions, we are processing what already exists against a backdrop of scenarios. Understanding involves realizing that the team members who feel that sense of skepticism will combine that skepticism with whatever is thrown their way next. If it is an unkept promise, the skepticism may migrate toward overall distrust. If it is a display of personal interest by the leader, the skepticism could conceivably soften. Can we do something about the emotions of our team members? We certainly can!

EMOTION MANAGEMENT. This does not refer to manipulation but rather to good management. Few people want to be known as manipulative, but manipulation and emotion management may seem to go hand in hand. Here is the key: we will manage our emotions; they will manage theirs. If anxiety about any type of change is prominent, we learn to recognize and manage our own anxiety in therapeutic ways (Dossey, 1996), and we pass this skill along to others. And we give them the tools to do it. As leaders, our work is cut out for us. Let us develop the emotional skill that allows us to help our team manage the emotions that stand in the way of the shared vision and get on with the work at hand.

Leaders Who Set an Example

Eisenstat and Dixon (2000) say that leaders are often selected for their clinical expertise but have not had the leadership experience or example to manage continual and rapid change.

Earlier in this chapter, I pointed out that leadership is half about managing the current change and half about managing the past. Create the ripe environment and successfully share the vision, and the past is taken care of. Now comes the onward and upward: taking team members where we very much want them to go, for their own sake as well as the team's. This involves setting an example and allowing empowerment.

EMOTIONAL IDENTIFICATION. At this point, the eyes of all are on us, the leaders. It is hard work to help people want to change, then to give them something they want to change *to*. Now, if we think that getting to this point required skill and finesse, we are in for quite a surprise. Leading by example is the moving forward of all we have set the stage for by creating an environment ripe for change and sharing a vision. Can we expect followers to go forward without our example to follow?

We can expect it, but it will not happen. They are going to follow as we lead, however that may be. It takes a lot of work to get buy-in and trust in order to create followers who are willing to help realize our vision. While we do not plan for our troops to abandon us just when we have gotten them prepared for battle (that would be unthinkable!), in order to keep them with us, we must be certain that we are ready to do exactly what we have told them they should do. Therefore, it is important that we identify at the outset those forces that assist us in and hinder us from doing just that.

Recognizing the forces for and against our vision requires emotional identification. Further, it requires us to identify the emotions that might keep people from actually following us and carrying the shared vision through to fruition. Take the distrustful manager who has just heard the CEO deliver the same powerful message of vision for the umpteenth time. Let us imagine that the CEO or someone leading under his capable direction pulls the manager aside a few days later and practices uncanny emotional skill. She observes that the individual has doubts and is complacent, she knows that that complacency is keeping the manager from performing well, and she talks the manager through the reasons why. What has occurred in the last year or two that has dampened the manager's own vision? Why is he no longer emotionally tied to the mission of the company? The executive then helps the manager to think of the ways this type of complacency might be affecting his staff's productivity and enthusiasm, and coaches him to manage his own attitude and emotional bias so that he can be a better leader. In fact, by the time he is finished with this individual (perhaps weeks later), the manager is a full-fledged disciple of the vision. Perhaps he is a key employee whose dedication is perceived to be crucial to the success of the company. Perhaps his coming to terms with the new vision is thought to be a magnificent turning point that will result in getting things done.

Let us now imagine that that same manager is now left to his own devices and assumed to be the proverbial team player. However, the heroic individual who lifted him out of his preliminary doldrums and into a new perspective may have stopped too soon. The emotions that kept the employee from believing in the vision and wanting to change must continue to be identified, used, understood, and managed if the change is to continue. Managing the past is simply not enough.

EMOTIONAL FACILITATION. Leaders who set an example see what emotions stand in the way of going forward and know what to do about them. Someone may have a consistent problem with anger, for example, that manifests itself in different ways, hindering the person from wanting to do anything the leader suggests. Perhaps an earlier mishap or circumstance led to the ongoing anger. Now, it may be that any stumble along the way results in intense anger toward another person or situation. This emotion as well as others must be recognized and appraised for what they are and, even more important, not swept under the rug. This is hard for many leaders. They assume that a happy employee is a productive employee without stopping to realize that if this were true, production would fail miserably, because employees are not always happy. Happiness is not the only emotion employees feel. Facilitating emotion is not about making people happy but rather about knowing how people and their work are affected when they are, to take one example, not happy.

EMOTIONAL UNDERSTANDING. Now let us return to the topic of setting an example. Setting an example means demonstrating that an emotion such as anger (or fear or anxiety or elation) is not an excuse for consistently ineffective performance or for abandoning the task or mission at hand. Setting an example means demonstrating that you as the leader know exactly what will happen when you are angry or when someone else is sad or distrustful. This is vastly different from denying that such emotions exist. You can pretend the anger or the anxiety is not there, hoping and assuming that equilibrium will soon reoccur, or you can accept the emotion for what it is, figure out what it does, use it to one's best advantage, and willingly admit that it will return.

Some managers have difficulty leading by example because they do not understand emotion. The truth is that a leader's example is such because it prevails through all types of occurrences, not just the happy, productive moments. In addition, leaders who understand emotion know how emotions are naturally going to progress. Imagine a manager who storms through staff meetings with a "do it or else" approach. One staff member glances at another with chagrin. Another scowls in the corner. What likelihood does the manager have of rallying her team behind her? Although the answer may seem abundantly obvious in the context of the question, the answer may not be so clear to the manager, who, like many in authority, equates the use of power with effectiveness. Therefore, instead of understanding that the scowling employee in the back may eventually become enraged, given the right mixture of circumstances, the manager may interpret his facial expression as a natural by-product of having to do what the boss says, ignoring an opportunity to address the scowling employee's concerns in an effective way.

EMOTION MANAGEMENT. Leaders who lead by example, in contrast to the ineffective manager in the previous section, benefit from understanding emotions and where they may lead, in order to interpret the responses to what they do. Further, they learn to manage their own emotions and, by doing so, teach others to do the same. Recall that emotional identification, facilitation, and understanding are simply building blocks for emotion management. They are all key elements in example setting; the primary goal is for followers to be able to manage the emotions that confront them daily. Emotionally intelligent leaders who lead by example should produce emotionally intelligent followers. After all, "If your words don't stick, you haven't spoken" (Useem, 2001a, p. 56).

Leader Self-Care

As leaders, we deal with constant demands. Being a leader increases our responsibilities, as well as our accountability both to those we are leading and those who are leading us. Increased responsibility and increased accountability also increase the skills we need to handle the emotional aspects of our jobs and the emotional aspects of making our teams successful. Perhaps the most obvious need of leaders is for development of emotional skill within themselves, especially the skill of managing their own emotions (Goleman, 2000; Dearborn, 2002).

Lachman (1998) provides additional suggestions to help nurse leaders take care of themselves while watching over those under their leadership. The suggestions include identifying your core beliefs and values, making sure that you are taken care of in addition to everyone else, and taking care to understand how you perceive an issue before responding. Using these self-care tips requires emotional skill, too, which is a primary reason that the nurse leader should have it.

In addition to self-awareness, leaders should also understand how others perceive them and their leadership style and make sure that it is congruent with how they perceive themselves (Dearborn, 2002). This focus on one's own leadership style and effectiveness involves self-directed learning, experimentation, and feedback from others.

Summary

Florence Nightingale and Sigmund Freud are still regarded as leaders and pioneers today, despite the fact that they did not practice in today's rapidly changing health care environment. Today, leadership literature has exploded, with authors, researchers, and professionals expanding on and theorizing about the qualities and actions that leaders must possess. One characteristic that is becoming more prominent in the literature is emotional intelligence.

The three chapters that follow will expand on the principles of emotionally intelligent leadership in the health care setting. As a nurse leader, it is important to understand what it means to create, to share a vision, and to set an example—activities that are largely facilitated by emotional skill.

TEN CRITERIA FOR EMOTIONALLY INTELLIGENT LEADERS

1. They recognize the inherent need of those doing the work to have input into the task at hand.

2. They encourage and demonstrate creative problem solving and thinking.

3. They recognize that employees need valuable insights and information in order to do their job well and feel they are making a significant contribution.

4. They set an example, being careful to downplay the distinction between management and nonmanagement.

5. They exemplify and foster commitment to the organization as a whole, and they expect the same from their followers.

6. They give credit freely for successes; they accept responsibility for mistakes.

7. They include followers in designing expected outcomes and goals.

8. They realize that people need to succeed, and therefore they facilitate learning.

9. They envision a better future and share this vision with followers.

10. They focus on continual improvement and change for the better.

PART TWO

INTELLIGENTLY CREATING, SHARING A VISION, AND SETTING AN EXAMPLE

4

LEADERS WHO CREATE

WE EXPECT HIGH PERFORMANCE, but failure will do when necessary. The leader who can reconcile himself or herself with that credo, paradoxical as it may seem, has accomplished an exceptional feat. To create an environment in which mistakes are openly admitted and corrected, where risk is necessary, where failure is an expected and even welcomed by-product of risk, and achievement is the ultimate result should be every leader's ultimate prize. In fact, failure is not tolerated in many high-performance work environments. We have been conditioned, through quality controls and other consistency standards, to treat less-than-best products as seconds, scrap, or, in the service industry, "learning opportunities."

"Creativity involves a great paradox," notes Stonecipher (1998, p. 371). "On the one hand, it depends upon thinking differently—and that often begins with selecting the right principle—the right idea or the right connection—and then applying it in a new setting." Many people have heard how Thomas Edison struggled to create a working light bulb and about his multitude of prototypes, but perhaps fewer know that Edison's finally successful invention had its roots in the work of Sir Humphrey Davy decades earlier. Edison improved on what Davy had started by heating the element in a vacuum, in which it was less likely to burn up (Stonecipher, 1998). Edison's ultimate success was a combination of innovation, elaboration, and failure.

Those who learned chaos theory in the early 1990s or earlier can probably relate that in at least some aspect of their job there was some element of chaos that needed to be organized or systematized (Vinten, 1992). Truly, the realization that chaos, disorder, or a faulty process exists is often impetus for creative change, the result of which may not be readily apparent. In fact, the idea that chaos is present in business as well as science should attune us to the need to be more creative and to the understanding that failure can be expected. In reality, however, few people tend to identify failure as part of their long-term career map. It would be hard to find the medical professional who wants to spend eight months going back to the drawing board to create a new patient education process or the manager who wants staff turnover to reach higher and higher levels each year. As much as we talk about risk and what to do if (heaven forbid!) at first we do not succeed, most of us would be perfectly happy to succeed the first time, enjoy the applause, and then get on with the next exciting project, especially if a monumental solution is reached in the process.

Joe Torre, who has managed the New York Yankees baseball team since 1996, realizes that life, and work, is not like that. In an arena where competition is keen and performance statistics are dialed up on scoreboards for spectators to scrutinize like Wall Street ticker symbols, one would expect failure to be a no-no. Nevertheless, "Joe doesn't put added pressure on you or act differently toward you because you're not hitting well or playing well," former American League batting champion Paul O'Neill told *Fortune* magazine (Useem, 2001b, p. 69). In baseball, when a team performs poorly for one game, they look at the pitcher or maybe the second baseman who dropped an easy fly ball. When a team performs poorly for a season, they look at the manager. Joe Torre has to reconcile that kind of pressure with his heartfelt belief that the guy who could not catch the fly ball today is still a valuable part of the team who has to get right back out there tomorrow (Useem, 2001b). He lives in a world where change is encountered as often as a player's off night and where emotion management could be the difference between pressing on to victory and declining to defeat.

In a commencement address to University of California graduates in Berkeley, Peter Chernin, chairman and CEO of FOX Entertainment, promoted creative leadership as the key to his personal success. "Creative leadership," he said, "rests on (an) ability to reach people by getting outside yourself—before you're imprisoned within yourself, which is a remarkably boring place to be" (2002, p. 247).

Kouzes and Posner (1995) studied personal-best leadership cases of executives in many fields and noted an overwhelming trend: most of the personal-best leadership cases were about managing a change, even though the executives who submitted recollections of their most stellar leadership moments were not prompted as to the nature of the experience they should expand upon. Because change often takes us out of our comfort zone, it is no wonder that many executives considered leading a change to be the accomplishment that they were most proud of.

Although much has been written about creativity and about leadership, studies and theories combining the two were scarce until very recently (Goertz, 2000; Sutton, 2001). Now, *innovation* is a buzzword in many organizations, and *creativity* has a plethora of individual definitions (Poste, 1997). At the same time, unfortunately, changing nursing practice can be difficult because many nurses lack the confidence or leadership skills to promote change (Chapman and Howkins, 2003). Additionally, many norms and values, the basics of nursing, have become ingrained because health care as an industry fails to attract change agents (Bradford and Sutton, 2003). Some of these basics—patient-centered care, do no harm, nurse the patient, not the machine—are valuable, but some of the older expectations of health care—that it moved at the patient's own pace, that it had deep pockets, that it was primarily for the cure of illness instead of the promotion of wellness—must change if the system is to survive (Bradford and Sutton, 2003). Fortunately, people who have ideas lay a foundation for innovation that leaders can build on. Nurse leaders can build their effectiveness by creating an environment ripe for change, creating followers who participate, and building constituent ability to manage change. These are the leadership skills required to manage in this changing world, and they can be strengthened by actions that involve identifying, using (facilitation), understanding, and managing emotions (Mayer, Salovey, and Caruso, 2000, 2002).

Creating an Environment Ripe for Change

The culture or environment of an effective organization must nourish innovative ways of problem solving. *Culture* in this sense refers to beliefs and values that are not only shared but also manifested by leaders and members of the organization (Andriopoulos, 2001). In various writings, strong leadership is cited as a precursor to innovation, creativity, and motivation (Evashwick and Ory, 2003; Rugh, 1999), as is effective teamwork (Arthur, Wall, and Halligan, 2003) and a creative organization as a whole (Eskildsen, Dahlgaard, and Norgaard, 1999). The need for such active mechanisms to create or manage change is due, in part, to the fact that avoidance of change is common, as evidenced by such statements as "We've always done it this way" and "I don't know if I'm comfortable with that." One of the biggest drawbacks to planning a major change is the staff member who continually asks, "How will we reconcile this with what we are already doing?" While this issue must be addressed at some point, the time for doing so is *not* before the change is defined. Change will not occur when people expect that the status quo will not be disrupted.

Sutton (2001) offers what he calls "weird ideas for managing creativity" (p. 97). For example, rather than rewarding success and punishing failure, he recommends rewarding success and failure and punishing inaction. When it comes to the need to innovate, he encourages debate rather than conflict avoidance, defiance of bosses and peers rather than obedience, and looking away from past methods of solving the same problem. Says Sutton, these unconventional ideas tend to work because they, like innovation itself, are not in line with the primary activities of most organizations. Explained another way, most organizations rely on tried-and-true methods to make money and solve problems. One has to become radical to innovate.

The tried and true can be very influential. A multidisciplinary team of managers at a small hospital was meeting to discuss written patient communications. Six months before, standardized communications, including letters describing the hospital's services and providing visitor information; general health and safety information; materials designed to provide information for families and caregivers; and discharge preparation sheets, had been developed over a period of three months and circulated through various approval committee members before becoming part of patient admission kits. Now, half a year later, the team was meeting to determine whether any changes needed to be implemented in light of cost, effectiveness, and patients' response to the information.

One team member, a marketing manager, spoke immediately after the meeting facilitator had stated the objective of the meeting, which was simply to discuss possible revisions to the communication package. The marketing manager wanted to know how the changes were going to affect existing materials and the work flows involving distribution of the materials to patients. Because she had heard that someone had suggested doing away with the discharge instruction sheet due to its sparse utilization, she noted that a certain physician group that admitted large numbers of patients to the hospital used it almost exclusively and would be sorry to see it go. Perhaps the hospital could retain that form for that group of doctors.

The manager's response indicated a resistance to change. She was attempting to reconcile the change with the present-day procedures and realities. However, she had forgotten one small detail: no one had decided on a change yet. The meeting facilitator very tactfully guided the manager to discuss the changes needed as though the past or the present were not an issue and assured her that impacts on the current communications package would be discussed in light of the team's recommendations and that appropriate actions would be taken at that time.

We intuitively know that like the marketing manager, people are generally resistant to change. As leaders, we need to be prepared to create around this natural resistance.

Look for the Perfect Opportunity to Change, Then Change People's Mind-Sets

The irony here is that although we tend to resist it, change is a major element of the universe. People cannot control the fact that change exists, but they can have influence over its circumstances (Porter-O'Grady, 2003), keeping in mind, of course, that the perfect opportunity implies that something is going to be different when all is said and done and that people's mind-sets are delicate objects that need to be handled with care. This means knowing what the emotional attachments are, acknowledging the ones that mean trouble, and knowing how these emotions will hinder or promote the project. Further, it involves anticipating whether a certain action or decision on the manager's part will stall progress or cause people to come out from their shells. It includes, ultimately, being able to manage one's own emotions and those of others—specifically, through synergistic contribution of supportive emotions and healthy control of destructive feelings—so that the project is successful.

Continually Ask Whether the Present Situation Is Good Enough

When you question the present situation, be prepared for the fallout. Someone, maybe even yourself, is attached to the present. Realize that the same conscience that puts one in touch with oneself also helps us align our strategies with principles that urge us toward something better (Covey, Merrill, and Merrill, 1994). When instructed to change the present in some way (for example, develop a new medication record or a new staffing model), the manager must first *identify* his or her own feelings toward the present practice so that biases toward change can be dealt with up front. Badaracco (1997) recommends that we ask ourselves how our intuition and feelings define the situation. If we like something very much, we are less likely to want to make radical changes to it. If the changes need to be made, we need to understand how our feelings toward the status quo will either help us *facilitate* or actually hinder a mind-set toward change. If the change needs to occur and our feelings will hinder the change, we need to *understand* and *manage* the feelings so that the change can occur.

We are often afraid to challenge an existing process, especially if we are comfortable there. That is the first sign of a leader who creates—being the first to develop a need for a change. The creative leader risks comfort by asking, "What could we be doing better around here?" This type of leader also challenges complacency by stepping up the sense of urgency felt by those around him or her (Kotter, 1996), which may result in another project, another subcommittee, or another reorientation to process.

When a leader challenges the existing process, the manager who is handed an assignment involving change will have emotional attachments to the present process, just as the leader did, and those emotions will need to be managed. No matter what the change, the leader must always be attuned to the emotional spectrum of followers, act to understand and manage those emotions, and help the followers to do the same (Goleman, 1998b; Mayer and Salovey, 1997).

In the case of the new communications package, let us say that the project leader is relying heavily on the marketing manager to redraft some of the materials, but the manager seems to be stalling. In fact, one week has passed, and the agreed-on outlines have not been started. The project leader is having a discussion with the marketing manager today (Monday) and must give a status report to her boss on Thursday. It turns out that the manager has not had time to draft or outline any new communications. The manager again refers to discomfort with some of the suggested revisions but indicates that this has nothing to do with the lack of attention to the project. It is mainly a lack of time and other pressing priorities.

The project leader recalls the same concerns about change from the meeting a week ago and realizes that she overlooked something earlier. During the earlier meeting, she did not give appropriate attention to the feelings at hand. Now the project is delayed, and those feelings seem to be playing a major role in the delay, although the manager does not admit it. The project leader had been so eager to get the project off the ground and to be successful that she had failed to acknowledge, *or identify,* the mind-set of the involved individuals. She realizes that she should have addressed the concern immediately, in a separate meeting if appropriate, because the emotion is now involved in the *facilitation* of a negative reaction to the project and causing a delay. Next time, she will be more attentive to emotional signals and understand how the underlying emotions can derail the sense of urgency she wants to convey.

The project leader can still salvage the critical steps involved to accomplish the goal. To do so, the leader must *understand* that her next actions will make or break the situation. Inside, she is furious that the manager has taken this lackadaisical approach to getting the project done. Nevertheless, she realizes that the manager is entrenched in apathy and may become very divorced from the project at the slightest affront. The project leader must *manage* the delicate situation and the emotions involved—both her own and the manager's. She is able to regulate her own emotions and address the manager's concerns about change, calmly refocus her on the necessity of getting the work done, and obtain agreement for a specific deliverable by Thursday. She has successfully changed the mind-set of the manager.

Expect Resistance, and Function Better Because of It

Many young managers believe that a key measure of their success is acceptance by their followers and the smooth implementation of their projects. As a result, some are deeply discouraged at the slightest hint of challenge from those they are leading or of resource-driven challenges to the project. The desire to be accepted can be so strong that some inexperienced (and experienced) managers rely on force or power to carry out their edicts. Not knowing how to handle resistance any other way, they assume that sometimes people just need to be told that this is the way it is going to be, even if they do not understand or like it. Not understanding that leadership always entails adversity, they will often quit a project too soon if the current infrastructure seems not to support it. Effective leaders expect resistance; by acknowledging it and managing the underlying emotions, they improve their processes and their team's ability to implement change.

The health care field is certainly a good testing ground for this theory. In fact, almost everyone who encounters the health care system is asked to change something, be it their smoking habits, the amount of sleep they get, or what they swallow every morning. Doctors and nurses continually hear the reasons why these changes are impossible. Health care has silently subscribed to the principle that patients should just change because it is the right thing to do. We all want our patients (and staff) to smile and say, "Oh, thanks for telling me; I will definitely begin doing that, now that I know it should be done." It just does not work that way. Nor does the apparatus to facilitate the change just instantly appear because it should. Financial issues, time constraints, and social influences continue just as they did before change was recommended. These factors often make it difficult for patients, and staff members, to try something different, change a behavior, or start a new lifestyle.

Managers who do not find resistance along the way can be sure of one of two things: either they are not really trying to change anything or they are not paying attention. As uncomfortable as resistance may seem, it is a barometer of the opportunity inherent in the change itself.

Many revered leaders of the past are best known for their ability to effect a change in spite of resistance. Often that resistance came from culture itself (as in the case of Florence Nightingale); other times, it came from followers (as in the case of Freud, who parted ways with some constituents over disagreements on theory). Winston Churchill is another such example. His desire to convert the navy's principal fuel supply from coal to oil encountered challenges. Oil was not a commodity to be had easily, and during wartime, there was even less of a guarantee of securing the precious fuel. Churchill used this opportunity, and purchased an interest in an oil company that secured not only the needed resources to better the navy but a profit for the country in years to come (Hayward, 1997).

In all three examples, we note that these respected leaders pressed on, in spite of adversity. As leaders, we may encounter adversity in the form of a budget crunch, a lack of staff, or an unwillingness to change on the part of the staff. How will we handle the external factors that affect our team?

Emotional know-how can get us through situations that are seemingly insurmountable. We must, of course, first *identify* what the challenges are and how we view them. We must recognize that when we challenge the current process, the process is not going to lie down and invite us to change it. Resource issues are going to surface. People are not going to have time to do one more thing, and money is going to hide behind the necessity of carrying on the current procedure. How will we react to this resistance? Will we *use* it to *facilitate* a firmer resolution to change the status quo, or will we cower and remain in the current situation, convinced that change was never really a good idea because it did not take into consideration the problems it would create? Our response will dictate whether we innovate or not.

Get Out and Vote

Around election time, we often hear people say, "If you don't vote, then you can't complain about who gets elected." That is true of leadership as well. If you did not lead, then you cannot complain when things are still done the same old way. Challenging the process and standing up to adversity, admittedly, are not easy feats; *understand* your own comfort level and those of your followers, then seek to *manage* those emotions. Change will come.

Creating Followers Who Participate

We said earlier that many companies do not tolerate mistakes or at least do not flaunt them. Along these same lines, many managers are not proud of the mistakes they or their staff make. Some environments are so intolerant of mistake making that people are tempted to cover up their errors rather than own up to them and do what is necessary to achieve an ultimate quality result. They would rather conceal their flaw and have it show up later than admit that there may be something wrong with their process, even if it is likely to happen again. The result is ultimately the same; if something is wrong, it will reveal itself eventually.

The result of an environment or leader who does not tolerate mistakes is a group of fearful team members who are afraid to make a move, especially if that move requires some degree of risk. In addition, while creating an environment ripe for change is something the leader absolutely must do, the followers must cultivate and sustain the environment. They are the ones who will get the job done. How, then, do we create followers who are willing to take risks, while banishing old fears, wherever they came from, that mistakes are absolutely not OK?

Treat the Whole Thing as an Experiment

Patience, or lack of it, is frequently touted as a virtue or blamed for bad decisions. "I'm just an impatient person," one might say, explaining why something was done hastily or prematurely. On the other hand, patience and flexibility are lauded as qualities in leaders who allow experimentation (Rugh, 1999; Hanna, 1999; Goertz, 2000). There is a fine art to being able to take one's job just seriously enough to accomplish a quality result yet not seriously enough to be devastated by a failure. Often, the two seem in direct opposition to each other: quality, after all, is often the deciding factor in purchase decisions where all other factors are essentially equal, and one flaw or setback could mean loss of a competitive edge. Moreover, in health care, flaws are discouraged, zeroed in on by meticulous attorneys, and protected against in quality management procedures.

For these reasons, it may be difficult for leaders to grasp the concept that everything is an experiment, but once they do, and once they successfully relay that message to their teams, they will most likely be endowed with a team that produces its best work and isn't afraid to move forward.

The word *experiment* may conjure up images ranging from structured, respectable research to young chemistry students mixing noxious chemicals and joking about blowing up the science lab. Some may feel that it downplays the seriousness of the need for change. Actually, experimentation allows room for improvement before things get too serious, before it is too late to change course. A change will be harder to accept if the concept or its implementation has a major flaw. A spirit of experimentation allows us try a change on for size before committing the whole organization to it.

ENCOURAGE RISK TAKING. "I work in a business where failures are not only frequent but necessary," said Peter Chernin, referring to the television industry, in which professional critics and critical audiences alike are empowered not just to influence programming but to determine its destiny (Chernin, 2002, p. 247). Even in health care, failure is painfully necessary: we learn as novice nurses what method of IV access is the quickest, but not without perhaps several frustrating tries. We develop our "system" for distributing medications and charting patient progress only to have it disrupted by the unexpected chiming of an all-too-familiar monitor alarm. The individualized nature of each patient and her problems creates a learning ground for us each time we walk up to the bedside. As leaders, we must be careful to encourage appropriate degrees of risk taking. This is a concept that has been around for years, but it still is difficult to implement. Scott and Bruce (1994) state that in studies on work groups in the 1950s, fear of personal censure proved a strong discouraging factor against innovation. This fear has not gone away, despite advances in leadership theory. To realize that this is true, all a manager need do is recall one or two sheepish, embarrassed employees obliged to admit that they had made a terrible mistake or a bad judgment call. It is almost as though something in our core being punishes us for not getting it perfect the first time. Added to that, the culture and environment of health care is not one that applauds failure. If it were, then fewer people would be shaken by their own human error. Naturally no one wants to compromise a human life or the quality thereof, and most medical mistakes are at least minor steps in that direction. Some errors require filling out forms or reports that are kept somewhere as a permanent record of the mistake. In short, the stakes are simply too high for many nurses to want to experiment.

One manager tells new managers under her mentorship, "I come to work expecting to make at least one mistake a day. When I make my first mistake that day, I know that it is a normal day. Sometimes I make more than one mistake per day. The important thing is to make sure they are not the same mistakes each day." Hearing this little speech seems to bring a sense of relief to new managers, who often say on their first or second day, "I just hope I don't make too many mistakes before I learn what the job is all about." What they do not realize is the note of paradox in their statement. If they accept that managers learn through making mistakes, do they think that at some point they will have learned what they need to know and thus will stop making mistakes? Do they think they will stop needing to learn? Too often, we believe that the adage "We learn from our mistakes" applies only when we are not talking about ourselves.

Another concept is that "people who win big, fail big" (Olesen, 1993, p. 141). However, would Babe Ruth, who struck out 1,330 times in his career, have believed that at first? Would Walt Disney, reeling from a job termination because of his lack of good ideas, have pictured himself as the entertainment mogul he eventually became? An entire nation may have been shocked to learn that Abraham Lincoln would eventually become president after he was demoted from captain to private during the Blackhawk War (Olesen, 1993, p. 141). The connection between perceived failure and eventual success is not easy to perceive immediately. As leaders, we must remind learners of this connection and of its practical application within the ever-changing health care environment.

"Creativity does not exist in hostile environments where all of one's time is spent thinking about survival," asserts Kerfoot. "Highly synergized workgroups that have developed safe environments in which to practice can be the most creative" (1998, p. 181). Safe environments encourage employees to take risks. No one wants to risk patient safety, but that is not the kind of risk supported. Rather, a spirit of experimentation encourages planning for a change in hopes that it will result in improvement but with no guarantee that it will.

In planning for change, it is most important that we *identify* how we feel about conducting our particular experiment without a guarantee of success. Then we must be certain we know how our team feels about it. If someone is not willing to invest a single hour in anything but a sure thing, we have a problem, because there are few sure things in life. Therefore, we need to work with that individual to help him understand the experimental nature of the plan and that under no circumstances would we consider the outcome or even the method of getting there a sure thing. There are too many variables. What we need to do is *facilitate* an emotional state that will aid in getting the work done in spite of the possibility that the desired result may not occur. If that state is the absence of fear about having blame laid for making a huge error in resource allocation, so be it. If that state is excitement about the prospect of the change, then we must work on motivating the staff member. Ultimately, our goal is to have the new ideas for change come from the followers themselves.

Many people think that emotions are based solely on events. If something bad happens, it seems that bad emotion will ensue. In addition, happiness seems to come from positive circumstances. This makes it even easier to understand why failure is so commonly feared. No one wants to experience the negative emotions that are sure to follow, not to mention the fiscal or relational damages that might occur.

The fact is that events do not lead directly to emotion; there is an intermediate step: thought. That is, events generate thoughts, which generate emotions (Olesen, 1993). The intermediary role of thought in this instance is so powerful that it can be the deciding factor in how we perceive the opportunity created by not succeeding the first time. It is crucial for the leader to understand how thought generates emotion and, even more important, how emotion facilitates thought and action. In effect, the leader must observe which thought patterns are developing among followers in the face of a bad decision and take steps to help followers modify subversive thought patterns.

Thomas Edison configured about five thousand light bulbs before he found one that worked for a reasonable length of time (Olesen, 1993). Imagine where we might be if after the hundredth light bulb Edison had thought, "I must have been a complete idiot to think this would work. To avoid being laughed at and to avoid wasting any more of my time, I am going to start working on another project or maybe just go into another line of work." We would be about 4,900 light bulbs shy of a stunning metropolitan night sky, a vibrant concert stage, or a warm reading lamp late in the evening. Fortunately for us, Edison identified his roughly five thousand missteps as opportunities to learn five thousand things that didn't work rather than as failures (Olesen, 1993, p. 149). As leaders, we must develop the same mentality and pass it on to our followers. When they fail (and they will), what they are thinking will lead to what they are feeling, and what they are feeling will facilitate the attitudes and actions they pour (or don't pour) into accomplishing the goal.

HONOR NEW IDEAS.   The command-and-control style of leadership has typified nursing culture for decades, but that is quickly becoming an ineffective leadership mechanism (Kerfoot, 1998). As leaders, we must be attuned to new ideas presented by our followers, for two reasons. First, people tend to be attached to their ideas as a part of themselves. Ideas that are presented as rational solutions to a problem often have a personal meaning for the originator. People like to feel that they are making a contribution, and presenting an idea gives them a sense of personal accomplishment.

Second, listening to our followers' ideas has the very desirable effect of making them active participants in the change. We must be careful not to brush off new thoughts presented by our constituents, even if they seem to be just thinking aloud. It is important to understand the factors underlying the presentation of ideas. For example, a team member may mention a solution to a harrying problem under his breath, so that only the leader and one or two other people hear it. What happens if the idea is squelched? Two things. First, the idea may not be a bad one, and thus an opportunity is lost. Second, the team member may not understand the value of his or her contributions and may be struggling with feelings of doubt, insecurity, or unpopularity. Considering his idea, especially if it surfaces as a solution, will go a long way toward turning that team member into an active participant. The skill required to encourage new ideas in this way involves *understanding* of emotions and how they interface with one another.

Along those same lines, in order to honor new ideas, we must be very careful not to consider ourselves the ultimate expert on any subject. While we cannot leave behind the basics of nursing while innovating, we must be aware that even better ideas exist. "Major inventions are very rare," Stonecipher (1998, p. 370) reminds us, "and even then, they are not a complete departure from the past."

Resistance to innovation, or the fear of being wrong, is frequently reflected in hyperprotectiveness of a current system. One health services vendor was so sure that its reporting methodology was correct that it consistently failed to listen to the suggestions of a difficult but very profitable customer. The customer was known as a constant complainer, and usually any advice proffered by that customer was thought of as nagging. No one wanted to admit that perhaps the customer might actually be right. The customer continued to be a constant source of worry for the vendor, because it did not want to employ the customer's ideas and feared losing the customer, which never seemed satisfied.

The vendor's leadership should have stepped in and seized a golden opportunity that was masquerading as an annoyance. Because top management was sensitive regarding its methodology and deeply loyal to its executive advisers, no one wanted to delve into the notion that perhaps the experts could be only half right. Even more regrettably, the vendor lost the opportunity to create common ground with the customer based on valuing its ideas. Instead of giving the customer's ideas and suggestions due consideration, the vendor repeatedly explained that they had tried all that before and that they had found their methodology to be the most valid. As a result, the relationship with the customer continued to be one that was deemed hypercritical, because any suggestion made by the customer was automatically framed as an uneducated opinion.

As leaders, whether dealing with customers or with staff, we must constantly guard against being the "experts" in our field. The quiet person in the back of the room or the customer who always keeps us on our toes may just have something. We must not approach his or her idea from the mind-set that we already know the answer. We do not. Our team does.

Encourage What Cannot Be Done

"I can't" is essentially taboo in the achievement-oriented society that is business. Moreover, it is disconcerting for family members of sick patients to hear that we cannot help them. Therefore, most of us do everything we can, trying hard not to say, "I can't."

Yet we hear it time and time again, if we just listen.

No one ever said that setting a new standard or changing an existing way of thinking was easy, but motivating employees to do what they consider impossible seems to take a whole new kind of managerial muscle. If team members do not see the need for change or the possibility or opportunity inherent in change, chances are that they will be thinking "I can't"; our job as leaders is to convince them that they can.

We can begin by expecting just about every change we advocate to lay the groundwork for some impossibility thinking. However, because most of us are professionals and most of us expect our team members to step up to the plate and be team players, we will miss quite a bit if we expect whining and complaining as cues that team members aren't completely ready to change. Listen for the "I can'ts" out there, and you will be ready to establish a framework of possibility for the doubters in your ranks.

People say "I can't" by doing any or all of the following:

o Continually bringing up the benefits of the old process or system long after those concerns have been addressed

o Stalling

o Referring to competing priorities

o Making suggestions after a course of action has already been firmly agreed on

o Hosting off-line discussions with others about the negative aspects of the change

o Ignoring the change itself; acting as though nothing is different

If team members are saying, "I can't" in any of the preceding ways, it is time to take immediate action! If we do not, progress will be seriously stalled. Still, encouraging what cannot be done is one of the most challenging aspects of leadership.

We encourage our team members to do what they do not believe can be done in several ways. One is by setting an example, which we will discuss in Chapter Six. Other methods include coaching, follow-through, and the use of well-placed motivation. Another way is by creating a change-ready environment. We must create the possibility of change for our team members. As leaders, we must do this in spite of the doubters. Whether no one or everyone doubts that what we are suggesting can be done, it remains our responsibility to create the possibility. We do this in two ways: by helping our team members to see what the change means to them and by helping them see that it is simply one manifestation of the phenomenon of continual improvement, not an earth-shattering event.

Kouzes and Posner (1995) point out that "What's in it for me?" is a question that cannot be ignored. Imagine, for example, that the second shift of ancillary staff is pilot-testing a new call schedule and that you are in charge of the pilot for your unit and two others. The goal is to develop staffing patterns that allow efficient scheduling while taking peaks in late evening admissions into account. Some staff members are, of course, resistant to this idea, preferring to never be "on call" and viewing it as either a potential unwanted schedule disruption or an opportunity for the hospital to reduce their working hours based on fiscal need. In planning this exercise, you as the leader must take into account how the team is feeling about this change. In addition to the concerns just listed, the team may have questions about how the new schedule is going to work. First, listen to the concerns and questions, then use them to design the new schedule. True, it may not work in the end, but this would be difficult to determine at the outset: perhaps it will work, and perhaps it will not. In order for the change to have its best chance for success, you must convince the staff that it can work, even though you may be proven wrong later. Remember that change is not always a sure thing, not always dead on target.

Once we *identify* how the team is reacting to the change, we must understand and help them understand how they may be *using* those emotions to set up their overall response. If they feel betrayed by the organization, expect impossibility thinking to skyrocket. For example, if members of your second shift feel threatened by the possibility of losing hours, you can expect them to come up with all kinds of reasons why their presence at work should not be interrupted regardless of ebbs in workload.

If you can use your knowledge of the team's emotions and concerns to identify the magic solution to their questions at this point, you have mastered the dilemma that has plagued leaders for decades: how do we position negative necessity so that people embrace it as positive progress? The answer: sometimes we do not. When answering your team's question "What's in it for me?" answer it honestly. The answer may make anyone with a background in sales and marketing cringe, but your goal is not to sugarcoat the truth. People are much more likely to respect the leader who says why something has to occur and how it will affect them than the leader who paints a pretty picture that fails to materialize. Team members do not want to be told that everything will be OK, only to find out later that they were lied to in order to obtain buy-in. However, when answering "What's in it for me?" be alert to the emotional courses that will naturally follow. *Understand* that your demeanor and attention to the needs of your team members can actually make the difference in whether they escalate negative emotions or proceed to productive management of these emotions.

All of these interactions need to occur within a framework of the constant nature of change (Kouzes and Posner, 1995). Often, teams and individuals forget that change is not just something we conjure up because we are bored. The necessity of change is ever present, waiting only to be acknowledged. When the need for change slaps us in the face, we may be more inclined to understand its necessity, its urgency, even its possibility. That is not always what we are dealing with as leaders; often, needed change is subtler, requiring us to seek buy-in when no one understands what is wrong with the way things are. For whatever reason, people often develop the mind-set that once something changes one time, it is a permanent arrangement, no matter how permanent they thought the last arrangement was. However, imagine a squirrel thinking, "Wow, what a winter that was. But it sure has been warm lately. I guess it will be summertime forever. I guess I'll never have to store up nuts again." Like the more astute squirrel, who realizes that fall lurks around the corner in accordance with natural law, our teams must acknowledge the reality that change will come around again. When they do, we will have a much easier time saying, "Team, this is it, another advance in the scheme of things," and we will spend less time trying to convince them that change must happen—again—when it never really stopped in the first place. Then it is easier work on the possibility, because we are not so focused on the necessity.

Expect Much of Your Followers

Some leaders, including many inexperienced ones but perhaps just as many veterans, are afraid to expect great things from their followers. They may feel that expecting too much will cause followers to feel pressured, put upon, or bossed around. In reality, the opposite is true. When we fail to expect things of our followers, we send a message of incapability that may pervade their attitudes toward their own job. Granted, there are people with a work ethic so strong that what we say, do, or expect really does not make a difference. Every leader covets these individuals. Nevertheless, we do not have to micromanage in order to achieve these same outcomes from those who are not as self-motivated. We simply have to understand what it takes to keep them going in this change-friendly atmosphere we have created. We need to expect them to do something, something big.

As leaders, we must provide what people need to do their work, asking several questions: "Do people need resources, or information, or access to new people? If they had these, could they get on with the work? And would we let them?" (Wheatley and Kellner-Rodgers, 1996, p. 38). This produces an implied trust. In other words, "I trust that you can, therefore I expect that you will." If I ask you to make photocopies, I trust that you are able to do that without inordinate waste of toner, paper, or time. If I did not believe this to be so, I would ask someone else. Likewise, if I ask you to give Mrs. Hill her Demerol injection, it is because I trust that your knowledge of nursing is such that you will practice good technique and not place the injection improperly. If I ask you to create a task force to make sure the unit is the cleanest in the hospital, I trust that you can achieve this result for the unit.

For many leaders whose reputations are riding on what they delegate to others, letting go can be one of the hardest exercises imaginable. Essentially, it involves entering a cake that we did not actually bake in the big bake-off. We must be constantly on guard that we are not sending task force–capable people to the photocopier because that way they won't fail. We must put our team in a position to do a good job, then expect that they will. They can tell if we expect that they will not. Expectation does not imply an alternative or an opt-out clause. Often, what we expect is exactly what we get.

Allowing Followers to Manage the Change

Managing change involves much more than it implies. Change is present when it is getting ready to happen, when it is occurring, and when it has just occurred. This concept is really about *transition* rather than sudden change, which we are more familiar with in day-to-day life. Leaders must realize that people they allow to promote and implement change will need to deal with the transition that follows.

Allow Teams to Prosper

Perhaps one of the most difficult tasks a leader faces is developing the team, a task that goes far beyond selecting people with complementary strengths to manage a certain initiative or situation. Team members do not always automatically blend to form the model team. For teams to reach their full potential and become great, they require coaching and principle-based leadership (Fisher, 1993). When teams are given appropriate coaching, their members are developed individually and as team players. They are coached to work together effectively (Fisher, 1993).

One thing that is important to remember is that creating an idea or a concept for change, through creativity or excellent judgment, is only the first step; infiltrating that change through the organization is often even more challenging (Berwick, 2003). The result has to do, in part, with sharing a vision (discussed in Chapter Five), but it also has much to do with allowing the team to manage the change.

Fisher (1993) describes self-directed work teams and points out ways to help them develop. One of the more obvious ways is through continual coaching—developing individuals and the teamwork among individuals. In lieu of absolute veto power on the part of the leader or the handing down of commands, coaching implies creativity in leadership. Team members are asked what problem they want to solve and how they would best go about solving it. The team leader's job is to guard the external boundary that surrounds the team—interfacing with other areas of the organization, protecting against opposing fronts, and bridging communication gaps with crucial external players (Fisher, 1993). Teams come into maturity through an evolutionary process that involves investigation and preparation stages before implementation, then continual improvement. The challenge for leaders is in adapting to these stages of team transition (Fisher, 1993). This requires a keen awareness of what the team needs from its leader, as well as the realization that what the team needs may be different at different times.

Open the Floor and Promote Constituency

Perhaps nothing impedes followership (what followers do) more than faulty downward communication from leaders. Many books have been written about good leadership, but few have been written about good followership. Articles about executives like former General Electric CEO Jack Welch and Microsoft mogul Bill Gates abound, but people are assumed to have less interest in understanding how followers contributed to a success. We often conclude that the leader is responsible for making it happen, so we want to read all about his or her technique. When it comes to the lowly followers, we gather that they were mere by-products of the leader's ability. The purpose here is not to criticize business journals that seek out the pinnacles of the corporate ladder but to open readers' eyes to the sheer value of those people we call followers, henceforth referred to as constituents.

When we are leading effectively, we are not expecting people to literally follow us—that is, to do exactly what we are doing. In line with the great expectations mentioned earlier, we cannot expect great things if we are simply demanding mimicry. We begin to transform followers into constituents by communicating well.

It is an accepted principle that a leader must communicate with those assigned to his or her leadership. Many people see it this way: "What I don't tell you, you won't know, and in order to do a good job, you must know, therefore I must tell you." Obviously, as a leader, you must tell your team when there is a new policy so that they will know that there is a new policy. Having good followership depends on the fact that you can be counted on to do that.

What is sometimes not so obvious is that the floor must be open in order to provide an atmosphere of constituency and empowerment. That means the same thing in this context as it does in a conference presentation: when the lecturer finishes droning, the real communication begins. Realize three things: constituents have questions, constituents have ideas, and constituents need feedback. After your "lecture," or direction, is given, communication has barely begun. The floor must perpetually remain open.

CONSTITUENTS HAVE QUESTIONS. Constituents will continue to have questions long after you wish the question-and-answer period were over. At a press conference, when the president of the United States smiles, nods, waves, steps from the podium, and says "Thank you," he means, "I refuse to answer one more question, and this time I mean it." Leaders do not have that luxury when they open the floor to their constituents. They must anticipate and address the questions that are being asked, even when they are not being vocalized. Knowing what the questions are requires the ability to identify emotional cues.

For example, a common mistake of managers is to assume that getting a project off the ground is where the effort should be concentrated. In reality, facilitating the management of the project takes much more effort, although it usually can be spread over a longer period of time. Once our constituents are aligned with the change we are creating, things do not go into autopilot mode. We must continually identify and manage the emotions that are present, which may change over time.

Be especially attuned to the emotions that arise from heightened expectations. When we empower work teams to get a job done, we create all sorts of uncertainties. We wish that this were not the case and that people would simply bask in our trust. However, many people, we must admit, are more comfortable with followership and less comfortable with constituency. Leaders should be aware of their constituents' negative responses (self-doubt, feeling overwhelmed, fear) as well as their positive responses (increased job satisfaction, increased sense of job ownership, heightened interest) to becoming active participants in managing a change and should be available to entertain the questions that arise out of these responses.

CONSTITUENTS HAVE IDEAS. Earlier in this chapter, I discussed giving merit to the ideas of others as a catalyst for positive change. The same principle applies here, as the change is put in place or in the stage of ongoing development. Constituents must constantly feel that their ideas are valued, and this must indeed be so.

CONSTITUENTS NEED FEEDBACK. As leaders, we often take for granted that our constituents understand how we feel about the job they are doing, because if we were not pleased, we would let them know. We must take every opportunity to provide constructive and supportive feedback to those we are leading. This is usually far more important than rote recitation of the "fact of the day." What constituents do not know, they can somehow find out from someone else who does, but what they could have done better with adequate feedback is lost forever if we do not provide that feedback. Kouzes and Posner (1995) describe feedback as a bridge between our expectations and our constituents' belief that they can do what we expect them to do. If we recognize the emotions that can arise from people's varied reactions to expectation and possibility, as well as the emotions that arise from our own propensity toward trust and delegation, we are better equipped to visualize the gap that we are trying to bridge and to bridge it well.

Share Ownership with Constituents

In fostering constituency, we might think of renting a car (or an apartment, a house, or a tuxedo) versus owning one. Although this is an elementary example, it may serve to enlighten us about ownership as it relates to the work of our constituents.

A nervous groom visits the formal wear shop, often with an excited bride in tow, to select his tuxedo for the big ceremony. If he doesn't plan to ever squeeze into a cummerbund again, chances are that he will choose to lay down a deposit for his garb as well as that of his groomsmen and promise to return the paraphernalia by a specified day and time. He signs an agreement saying he will return the tuxedoes in good condition (in other words, not destroyed) and leaves the garments at the shop for alterations.

On the business day after the wedding, the groom may return the tuxedo to the shop with white icing smeared on the vest, a small rip in the hem, or a gaping hole in the seam of the right front pocket from a desperate last-minute search for the bride's ring. Does it matter? It depends on whom you ask.

The truth is, we all know the answer to that question. It matters to the person who owns the tuxedo. That person is the one who must clean, repair, or mend the damage done by the groom. It is true that in many rental situations, the renter is somewhat responsible for repairs, but these provisions notwithstanding, the owner is still the loser if something happens that is not addressed or repaired. Security deposits are held to protect owners from damage done by renters, as unintentional as the damage may be.

The message for leaders should be clear. Ownership defines where the responsibility for the job lies. On your health care team, there are no deposits that will protect you against loss due to carelessness or lack of motivation. That is, you cannot have your staff sign an agreement that they will foot the damage for you if they fail to come through on a project for which you are responsible. If you are responsible for the outcome and you want the person doing the job to be responsible for the outcome right along with you, give that person ownership, not a lease.

To do otherwise serves both you and your constituents unjustly. If you are holding team members to a higher level of responsibility, it is only fair to allow them to own that which they are responsible for. In other words, you should say, "This is your effort; you deserve credit for it." Whether you receive credit for it as a leader is unimportant. That your leadership led to the success should be implicit throughout the success without your saying a word. Furthermore, if you do not allow ownership, you set yourself up for damages to your property against which you are unprotected as well as less motivation toward optimal performance on the part of your team.

You must *identify* any reservations you have toward allowing your team members to own their responsibilities, along with the credit that goes with them. You must also allow your constituents to be responsible for any negative results of their work. Because some constituents may fear responsibility for failure (although they are extremely willing to bask in credit for their successes), it is important that you identify and understand the emotions confronting these team members, as well as your own emotions in regard to the situation, so that you can manage them and give ownership where ownership belongs.

Know What Is Going On, and Discuss It Often

Sometimes when team members do not like how they are being led, they refer to being micromanaged. They feel that if their manager is not pleased with what they are doing, he or she is paying too much attention to what is going on and possibly getting too picky about the details. People who think of themselves as professionals (as most nurses do) usually prefer to be given some professional latitude rather than examined under a microscope to make sure they are not doing something wrong. For this reason, leading professionals presents a set of challenges for managers that managing nonprofessional staff may not. Although our intention may be never to micromanage, our constituents' perceptions of our efforts often walks a fine line between too much supervision and not enough support.

At the same time, as leaders we need to be aware of what is going on. Responsibility and job ownership notwithstanding, if it is our unit, our shift, or our meeting, we are responsible for it 100 percent of the time: we have to be able to appraise the situation almost immediately or know where to get the answers in order to make effective decisions.

Knowing what is going on requires that we understand where our constituents are without giving the impression that we are investigators. For many managers, this can be a difficult venture. First, we have to correctly place expectations and ownership of team efforts, as I discussed earlier in this chapter. If my expectations have never been high, and I have not given ownership to my constituents, I am fully responsible when the unit secretary does not put the admissions records in the proper format or when the medications are only given as scheduled 50 percent of the time. By having expectations and giving ownership, I do not relinquish my ultimate accountability for the actions of my staff, but I increase the likelihood that when I seek an update on a project, it will present itself readily without my having to excavate it from a mire of confusion about roles and responsibility.

Leaders should be apprised of progress even when there is not a problem. As with feedback, progress appraisal that is reserved only for situations in which correction is needed can lead to distrust and reluctance on the part of constituents. Consider the following case:

The house supervisor approached a nurse manager one night just after the beginning of third shift. The supervisor asked, "Where do you usually keep the crash cart on this unit?" The nurse manager's first response was to wonder why the supervisor was asking such a question. Everyone knew that the crash carts were located immediately outside each supply closet. As far as she knew, this was universal throughout the hospital. Instead of repeating this very fact, the nurse manager immediately glanced down the hall. She started to say, "Why? Is something wrong? Is ours missing?" Catching herself and not wanting to display any sign of paranoia, she confirmed that her crash cart was placed correctly and then answered, "Outside the supply closet, down at that end of the hallway." The supervisor then explained that just recently, she had discovered that another unit was unwittingly out of compliance with this placement procedure, and she was merely confirming the understanding of unit leadership throughout the facility.

The nurse manager's reaction typifies that of a staff member who feels he or she is approached only when there is a problem. As leaders, we must avoid any semblance of solely investigatory interest. That is, we must make sure that we are not giving our team reason to believe that if we ask a question, we are investigating a problem that involves them. One way to ensure that this does not happen is to make routine assessments of how things are going, even when nothing seems to be going wrong. It would seem ill intentioned to feign interest in what our colleagues are doing on a regular basis, just so that we can more easily wheedle the truth out of them at those times we are looking into a problem. However, getting to know our constituents and what they are doing provides us with the benefits of being able to identify difficulties they are encountering, both within themselves and with the task at hand; help them to facilitate their actions with regard to how they are feeling; and manage situations and emotions coming in to play. In short, it makes us better leaders, brings us closer to our team members, assists in accomplishing the purpose at hand, and helps us mentor and coach our constituents.

Summary

Change, creativity, and innovation are accepted concepts in business society, so much so that their relevance is underrated. Especially in the past two decades, they have come to be known as key ingredients for a good leader. However, many people are resistant to change, including many leaders. This, combined with the fact that health care does not encourage risk taking at the practice level, makes some nurses and administrators even more reluctant to innovate, even when a problem is apparent. Again, we turn to the emotionally intelligent leader to infuse innovation into areas where it may not seem natural.

Leaders who create embrace innovation by creating an environment ripe for change, followers who willingly participate in the change, and constituents who readily manage the change. To manage change, leaders must be ready to admit and even embrace the probability that change will come less easily to some than to others—even to the extent that some will have significant resistance to change. There are few situations in which emotional skills (identifying emotion, using emotion, understanding emotion, and managing emotion) are more valuable.

The next chapter discusses the crux of the change—the vision itself—and how the effective health care leader can share it with an empowered team.

TEN CRITERIA FOR LEADERS WHO CREATE

1. They seek out opportunities to change, asking what could be better about the present situation. They do not wait for change to come looking for them.

2. They change the mind-set of their followers. They understand that people have ties to the old ways of doing things, and they work with these feelings to create new ways of thinking.

3. They expect resistance, because they realize that resistance is part of change. They work with the emotions that cause resistance in order to facilitate change.

4. They treat opportunities to change as experiments. They encourage followers to try to produce new ideas, even though some of the ideas will be unsuccessful.

5. They identify and manage impossibility thinking, recognizing it in many actions other than saying "I can't." They deal honestly with the change they are proposing and remind followers of the constancy of change.

6. They expect much from their followers. They realize that one of the highest forms of trust is expectation.

7. They make constituents out of their followers, expecting them to take an active role in managing change.

8. They open the floor for questions, ideas, and feedback. They realize that this form of communication facilitates effective management of the emotions surrounding change.

9. They allow constituents ownership of their part in the process at hand. They realize that ownership fosters accountability and responsibility for outcomes.

10. They are aware of what is happening because they discover it every day. They create an environment of concern for individuals and are in tune with the dynamic processes they are managing, so they have less difficulty approaching team members when something goes wrong.

5

LEADERS WHO
SHARE A VISION

THE EFFECTIVE LEADER is not only creative but is also able to share a vision with constituents. Often vision is seen as a luxury: something that we use when we are not trying to put out fires and have time to make things better. We will see, in the pages that follow, that there is no time like the present to lead with vision and pass it on.

The Necessity of Change

Change happens. Sometimes change seems to occur naturally and imperceptibly. Winter turns to summer so gradually that once we are sweltering in the August heat, we may have a difficult time remembering that we ever needed coats and gloves. Industry has provided several survival mechanisms, such as air conditioning and the thermostat, which allow us to ease into such transitions with minimal discomfort. We have learned about the predictability of seasonal change and have developed systematic ways to respond to it.

Change in business does not always happen that way. Change happens either because someone decides it needs to or because someone is forced to make changes in order for the business to prosper or survive in the current environment. At times, the change is unpredictable, and very often, it is perceptible and sudden. People must create their own mechanisms to adapt to the change, and these responses vary with the person and the situation. There is no universal antidote for the stark difference between today and yesterday or even for the gradual transformation between the two.

Why Do Leaders Need to Influence Change?

The National Center for Healthcare Leadership identified six traits of effective health care CEOs, including leadership, collaboration and communication, and learning and performance improvement (Beckham, 2003). More and more, we find that these traits are expected not just of CEOs but of department heads and team leaders. No doubt, one of the reasons that these traits are so necessary is the constant change faced by the health care industry and its organizations.

One item that was absent from the list of desirable CEO traits was vision. Perhaps having a vision is assumed to be an ever-present expectation for senior executives. But it is still a necessary one. The same is true for nurse leaders at all levels. Today's nursing science is especially affected by the need to integrate change and to have a visionary reason for doing so. One influential factor is the need to deliver evidence-based care, based on national standards and aimed at improving and documenting quality of care. This alone requires understanding and clear direction to implement (Rycroft-Malone, Harvey, Kitson, McCormack, Seers, and Titchen, 2002). In addition, medical science, including that of nursing, is multifaceted and complicated (Taylor, 2003). Good nursing practice does not simply fall into place without vision. After all, someone needs to understand what needs to happen for the patient—healing, relief of suffering, improved wellness, restoration of function—and then establish a plan, often with others, to make sure that vision becomes reality. On a much grander scale, nurse leaders must see the needs for their unit and organization and not only make plans for the changes needed, but also carry them out. Change will happen whether the leader plans for them or not: the leader is in a unique position to influence change to support a compelling vision.

How Do Leaders Influence Change?

Often, change means simply doing what needs to be done (Place, 2002). People who influence change do so either deliberately or unintentionally. Effective leaders do it deliberately. They know what they want to achieve and are skilled at achieving it through people. Their desires equate to their vision.

We rarely make changes because it is the thing to do. In other words, few people sit around making sure they change at least ten things a day. Change in and of itself is futile unless it leads to the fulfillment of a defined purpose, or vision. Most change is the result of either a conscious or an unconscious vision of a desirable result.

The term *vision* still has a certain mystique, although its use has exploded in recent years. Leadership books everywhere extol the virtues of vision. It is not unusual to find great leaders referred to as visionaries. Florence Nightingale herself was called a visionary (Dossey, 2000), and examples of her vision abound. After all, practically everything she did was groundbreaking.

Today, great visions are touted in a multitude of entrepreneurs, overnight successes, and quests for number one. Simply having a vision no longer guarantees anyone a place in industry history. Deciding that an organization could stand to change, deciding that one wants to go somewhere in health care, or deciding that things should be better are more the expectation than the exception.

So what sets great leaders apart from ordinary ones? They share their vision. They transmit their vision to the people working around them. Their vision catches on in a way that is nothing short of phenomenal.

There is plenty of competition for the attention of those who are doing the work. Opportunities are as diverse as the people who pursue them. Loyalty to the company has been replaced, at least in part, by the draw of personal achievement. People are not standing around waiting for a great vision to follow; they have visions of their own.

In fact, vision is not a basic managerial skill, according to Jim Collins' description of leadership levels (Collins, 2001b). He describes five levels of leadership: the first is the "highly capable individual," the second, the "contributing team member," the third, the "competent manager," the fourth, the "effective leader," and the fifth, the "executive," a level that requires an almost paradoxical combination of humility and resolve (Collins, 2001b, p. 70). It is only to those at the fourth level of his hierarchy, the effective leader level, that Collins assigns the defining characteristic of a compelling vision that inspires followers to higher performance. Those at the first through third levels can perform well without this distinguishing feature, but vision helps define the effective leader.

Sharing a vision takes talent—specifically, emotional talent. Sharing a vision involves getting the attention of people who may be focused on their own plans and goals and perhaps are not in tune with the needs of the organization. Further, it entails motivating people based on one's vision.

Vision does not automatically flow from the top down. Some leaders who have great plans and goals for a company, department, or unit may not understand this. In many cases, those individuals will be left wondering why their plans and goals never came to fruition. Rather than being effectively shared, a vision may be hidden or articulated but not acted on.

A vision hidden from everyone is as effective as a secret recipe that has been lost in a roaring blaze.

Six Actions of Leaders Who Share a Vision

What sets someone apart from his colleagues in this unique way, establishing him as the type of leader that influences change by sharing a vision? Let us explore six actions that can undergird the nurse leader attempting to proactively influence change in her organization.

They Act as the Visionaries of Their Organization

"Having a vision of what is possible is the currency of leadership; it's what sets the leader apart from the manager, whose emphasis is on the implementation of someone else's ideas," says Taylor (2003, p. 44). If someone identifies another person as a visionary, it is highly likely that that person's vision has made an impression. We remember Florence Nightingale as a visionary primarily because she has had such profound impact on many of our careers, even in the present day. We do not remember her simply because she had many different ideas. While the impact may well be more important than the new idea, the idea must constantly be present.

Often, a visionary must fight uphill. Although the chief executive officer should undoubtedly be strategy-oriented, he or she should never be considered the sole visionary of the organization. People with very little explicit authority can attain and nurture a very influential standing. If a person lacks the positional power to assist in driving the vision, he or she must often convince the masses one by one of the substance behind the vision.

WHO ARE THE ORGANIZATION'S VISIONARIES? How do we identify a visionary, especially one whose vision is rising through the ranks rather than coursing downward? Fisher (1993) describes what he calls "change-influencers" as people who take three basic actions. They envision what the future can be; they discuss what the future can be at every opportunity; and they work and support selected processes to ensure that the vision materializes. Unlike the CEO, who can stand before the organization and describe his or her vision with defined authority, the team leader, unit manager, staff nurse, or support staff member often, through a series of small steps, creates their own scenario in which to reside, in which to act the part, so to speak, of having the vision come to be. This takes work and dedication, and true visionaries will pay the price to see their goals become reality.

Managers and others who understand this principle can use it to full advantage, often with considerable success. There is no time like the present to lobby for an improvement. Informal meetings, decision-making sessions, and conversations in the corridor all provide many opportunities to promote one's vision. The astute leader will be political while being passionate about his or her vision. Emotional acuity is key when a person is attempting to influence change.

CONTINUAL VISIONARY BEHAVIOR. One nurse manager believed very strongly that a specific change should occur on her unit, so she went after it fiercely and held on tenaciously. She spoke of the proposed improvement to several of her colleagues, even when her issue was not the topic of the hour. This meant catching them on the way to other meetings, during rounds, and during report. Whatever the situation, she never missed an opportunity to promote her vision. She did it in politically correct ways, of course, not by badgering fellow employees with her agenda. Her technique was seamlessly executed. No one felt she was trying to hammer anything into his or her head or that she was nagging them with data. Yet in every person she spoke with, she engrained a form of brand recognition surrounding her vision.

She also lived her vision every day. She thought of herself as representing the principle behind her vision, almost as though she had voting rights in some virtual parliament involving the unit's future. As a result, she drafted policies that supported her vision, she discouraged actions that did not support her vision, and she worked behind the scenes to change impediments to the realization of her vision. The behind-the-scenes effort took the majority of her energy but also garnered the biggest payoff. Her vision was ultimately achieved, because she had laid the groundwork from within.

Having a vision (for oneself, for an organization) consists of multiple tenets, one of which is knowing where one stands and knowing what one's personal convictions actually are (Yukl, 1998). Visionaries should have a keen sense of who they are, what the organization or department is, and, most important, who their team is. This is indeed the first and most basic skill of emotional intelligence: knowing what is perceived or felt and what to call it.

For one individual or leader, what is perceived may be that there is more capability within a group or team than is being utilized. For another, it may be a nagging sense of unrest that progress is not being made toward a desired result. In both cases, there is a foundational sensing of the future, an emotionally educated guess as to what the future will or should look like.

Rational or predictive thought often fails to lead us to such conclusions; this is why emotional intelligence is so critical for leadership. For example, we can base a scientific prediction only on events that have already occurred, even if the predicted event is unprecedented. If someone were to predict that the sun would burn out in a certain number of millions of years, he or she would need to determine the rate at which other heavenly bodies are assumed to or are known to burn out or at least base calculations on certain proven facts about energy and solar structure. When it comes to forming a vision of the future, the confines of rational prediction can be extremely limiting—as much as they would be if we were asked to cause an object to materialize out of thin air. A vision is rarely based on previous events; rather, it is based on future ideals. Therefore, although a vision must be based somewhat in reality to be accepted, it may also contain elements that are not proven but only intuited.

HOW EMOTIONAL KNOWLEDGE INFLUENCES VISIONARY BEHAVIOR. Reflecting on the importance of emotional intelligence in forming visions returns us to a basic point that that has been stressed throughout this book: understanding of the interactions of emotions, of people and their emotions, and of oneself and one's own emotions can be a key element in sound decisions that involve the future. In other words, understanding what the future will be or should be in any particular case involves making very reasoned guesses about the human and emotional forces that will react en route to the future. The catch is that we do not have a chart or predictable model to follow. One of the distinguishing features of emotional intelligence is the multitude of variables that can be present in almost any situation yet still lend themselves to intelligent processing of the scenario. There are human responses, interpretations of human responses, hidden responses, interpretations of hidden responses, what is said and what is not said. . . . The list goes on and on. Would that we could add two numbers and multiply by a factor to find out where to go next! However, if we learn as much as we can about emotions, we can apply that knowledge to a plethora of unpredictable situations as they arise. In addition, most conflicts and conundrums fall into anything but mathematical categories. We need emotional intelligence to venture far into the future with any degree of confidence.

They Hold a Vision of the Ideal

Being satisfied with the status quo forces us into conserve mode. If we are happy with the way things are, why change them?

This was discussed earlier along with creating an environment that fosters change. Now, we will focus on the actual change impetus itself: the vision.

ENTREPRENEURIAL THOUGHT IS KEY TO CREATING A VISION OF THE IDEAL. The Institute for Johns Hopkins Nursing, which reunited education and service, was created because leaders thought like entrepreneurs. The leaders of this initiative had a vision to reconcile some of the gap between education and practice that had been widened by the movement of education out of hospitals and into universities and technical schools. Their ideal was the institute, a joint venture of two entities—Johns Hopkins School of Nursing and Johns Hopkins Hospital Department of Nursing—so that education and practice could work hand in hand to jointly advance nursing as a profession. This endeavor integrated the knowledge that nurses are natural creative problem solvers, although they are not always in a position to solve problems beyond their individual clinical practice (Sabatier, 2002). They did what many who start a new business do: they established a mission statement, formed a business plan, created a budget, and defined their resources. They went through an approval process with both the hospital and the school of nursing, both of which had to approve the idea and share the vision that the nurse leaders were attempting to promote. As a result, The Johns Hopkins Institute for Nursing was born in 1995 (Sabatier, 2002).

Nurses can capitalize on their own entrepreneurial skills just as those at the Johns Hopkins Institute did. To do this, it is helpful to think of the end result of a vision, the ideal, as a new organization just like the Johns Hopkins Institute. This new organization may represent the combination of two current practices to form a new initiative, the formation of a committee to specifically address an opportunity, or the development of a new approach to efficiency. Often nurses forget that they have entrepreneurial skills, especially when their days and nights are filled with clinical duties. However, the same ability for innovation that characterizes meeting patients' needs can also meet a departmental need; the same ability to plan and organize can also create a successful initiative.

Emotionally skilled nurses have insight into how their emotions influence their thoughts and affect particular behaviors (Mayer, Salovey, and Caruso, 2000, 2002). As they envision the ideal, their emotions may either be motivating or discouraging. At this stage of forming and promoting a vision, it is important that both team and leader realize how emotions are affecting the will and ability to innovate and support the vision wholeheartedly. Nurses should highlight their own problem solving and visionary skills and carry them forward into their department and their organization.

THE QUALITY OF THE VISION MATTERS. Those who have no vision at all cannot be expected to facilitate change, but for those who do advance a vision, the quality of the vision itself cannot be overlooked. Visionaries are idealists to the ultimate degree (Kouzes and Posner, 1995). They do not settle for what looks feasible, reasonable, rational, or possible. They are not merely predicting the natural course of events, in which transformation is likely to evolve without effort. They see something that they want for the organization, no matter how far-fetched it may seem, and they pin themselves to it. If they want better employee satisfaction, the employees they envision are not just happy; they are ecstatic. If they want more efficient, timely patient care, they are pushing for much more than a just-in-time result. Idealism by its very nature lends itself to optimism: the belief that something can or will be better to a certain degree. The mere presence of idealism indicates that a goal is present. We often temper the goal with realism because there are facts and realities that, no matter how lofty our ideals, will influence the end result. Collins (2001a, p. 69) reminds us that "facts are better than dreams" as he cautions us that facing brutal reality is critical to making good business decisions.

A quality vision, then, includes both fact and idealism. Nurses and nurse leaders should learn to incorporate both in their vision for their organization. One way to construct a quality vision is to establish a picture of what can be (the ideal) that incorporates what must be (the facts).

A quality vision achieves a delicate balance between fact and ideal. The two elements temper and complement each other. This can be applied to broad visions as well as minor, more specific ones. Suppose a nurse leader wants her staff to become experts on particular clinical topics and publish articles on these subjects. The nurse leader should imagine the end result of this vision—published articles—and then consider the facts that affect the vision—staff knowledge, time available, and organizational policies related to publication by employees. Emotionally, the leader may strongly believe that the vision is possible: the facts help her manage the emotional aspect and create a realistic, quality vision. At the same time, the emotionally astute leader can realize that because writing may be new to some nurses, there may be resistance, and she can prepare for how to meet this resistance with guidance and encouragement.

DRAFTING AND REFINING VISION AND MISSION STATEMENTS. The visionary leader must know exactly what his or her vision contains and what it means to the organization. This is the first step in bringing about organized action around a vision. Some recommend that a formal vision statement be drafted, including a mission and guiding principles (Wall, Solum, and Sobol, 1992; Kouzes and Posner, 1995; Kotter, 1996; Mintzer, 2003). There may be no more concrete way to establish a formal vision, especially since departure from core principles is identified as the cause of a lapse of attention to what is important in carrying out the vision (Beckham, 2003). This statement should not merely be drafted, framed, and hung on the wall. It should be refined as often as needed and kept dynamic (Silversin and Kornacki, 2003). In fact, people should be constantly asked what they are doing to bring the organization closer to the vision and what problems they are encountering along the way. This establishes a mentality focused on the vision (Mintzer, 2003).

A vision statement may contain a mission statement, a glossary for clarification of terms, and a set of guiding principles (Wall, Solum, and Sobol, 1992). The mission statement is simply a statement of the department or organization's purpose or goal. The mission statement encourages involvement with and relationship to the goal. If it is seen as "our mission," then some form of ownership has been established.

Even if there is not already team or corporate buy-in to the vision, Covey (1991) recommends a personal mission statement. This keeps a visionary leader who must inject the vision into an organization focused on the vision and mission at hand, and it gives concrete evidence of a purpose and plan.

In the mission statement, the team or individual considers who they are (or want to be), what they do (or want to do), whom they (want to) do it for, and why they (want to) do it. A mission statement can be bland, but it should not be. Ideally, it is charged with energy and enthusiasm. It could be defined as inspiring (Wall, Solum, and Sobol, 1992; Yukl, 1998; Pfeffer and Sutton, 2000).

Guiding principles are value statements that define how the work is carried out and secure a common understanding of direction (Fisher, 1993). Wall, Solum, and Sobol (1992) outline six cultural elements that the guiding principles of world-class organizations have in common: customer focus, obsession with quality, continual improvement, high participation levels, teamwork, and ethical integrity. Guiding principles are road maps for carrying out the mission and vision. They are invaluable in making values-based decisions that arise during the course of change. As such, they should not be lightly created any more than should the mission statement. Mission statements and guiding principles require buy-in from those involved. Whether that includes one individual or five hundred, the statements require consistency, thoughtful consideration of every detail, and attention to their implications on and in the work culture.

"IDEAL" DOES NOT MEAN "PROFOUND." "*Family, work, neighborhood, freedom, peace*" (Strock, 1998, p. 35). In the early years of Ronald Reagan's administration, it would have been difficult to avoid those words when describing the values of the president we now recognize as the Great Communicator. Common though they were, these ideals were the threads of what came to be known as Reagan's vision (Strock, 1998). Common though they may have been, they were nearly profound.

An ideal need be neither complicated nor mystical. It simply must be ideal. If the ideal is simple, we should not complicate it. In the early 1980s, family, neighborhood, work, freedom, and peace were not new concepts, but they were certainly not stale. In a time when government was growing ever larger and political unrest had laid a heavy hand on the face of democracy throughout the world, Reagan emphasized his guiding principles as those that would promote stability, personal individuality, and opportunity for unoppressed growth. Yet in an era during which each decade seemed to represent an entirely new set of circumstances, Reagan was not given to an entirely new concept of the world. He relied on traditional values as though they were profound innovations.

We have now seen that a vision can range from simple to lofty. What determines where the vision falls on that spectrum? The answer is the same emotional aptitude that determines the ideal. There is a vast difference between knowing what is and knowing what can be. Knowing the present is essentially a function of keeping informed. Knowing what can or will be is a factor not of psychic powers but of incredible foresight that can be bolstered by emotional intelligence. Reagan saw the past in a special way, and because of this, he could see the future. That is, he looked at what people were going through, what they had gone through, and how they had reacted and adapted, and he applied learnings from those experiences to determine what he believed was a better experience for Americans and the world (Strock, 1998). One could tell that he actually envisioned America and the rest of the world enjoying democracy and the benefits of family, community, and self-sufficiency. Many Americans liked what Reagan saw.

Reagan used emotional skills when he envisioned the quality of life inherent in freedom and democracy. Emotional skills are critical in forming and holding a vision because of the need to see and appreciate the intangible outcomes. Nurses can use emotional skills to ask, "how does the current situation make me and my colleagues feel?" "How do these feelings affect patient satisfaction?" "What will be the emotional result if this pattern continues?" "What will be the emotional benefits if it changes?" Framing a vision in terms of its effect on the quality of individuals' lives can help everyone identify with the relevance of the vision more closely.

They Communicate the Ideal to Others

People change their actions not so much because they receive an analysis that shifts their thinking but because a truth resonates within them and influences their feelings (Kotter and Cohen, 2002). When the ideal is communicated, it can influence the emotions that drive others to action. This aspect of sharing a vision also supports Mayer, Salovey, and Caruso's (2000, 2002) skill of using emotion to facilitate thought.

In part because he mastered the skill of influencing people's emotion, Reagan was able to effectively communicate his ideal to others. People liked the ideals that he fostered for them. As does any leader, Reagan faced opposition from all corners, but he is remembered by many as an effective leader who accumulated remarkable achievements in his eight years in office.

What else contributed to Reagan's success in relaying his message? After all, people with acute imaginations and high hopes can be viewed as anything from entertaining to living in a fantasy world. Creativity is praised in childhood, often equated with mischief in adolescence, and considered very cautiously as we become adults. While children can pretend and imagine, adults, after all, are thought to be better grounded in reality. Next, let us explore the idea of promoting the ideal when it does not seem real or attainable.

THE IDEAL IS NOT ALWAYS REAL. Kouzes and Posner (1995) refer to formulating a vision as "imagining the ideal" (p. 94). That means just what it appears to mean: imagining something that is not yet real but that the visionary believes can come to be. Kouzes and Posner go on to define a vision as "an ideal and unique image of the future" (p. 95). Nothing in that definition even hints of reality. The future is not here, nor is the image tangible.

Many people have a vision but are afraid that it is not real enough to transfer to those around them. One relevant analogy is that of Noah and the ark (Genesis 6–9). The story says that because no one in Noah's time had experienced deluges of rain, Noah had a difficult time convincing anyone that there would be a flood that would destroy all living things. When the flood came, his foresight resulted in his safety. But multitudes of others based their reactions on the only reality they knew; they did not grasp the vision that Noah had been given and were not prepared when the waters came.

Sometimes our visions representing an ideal are so far removed from reality that we may have the same difficulty that Noah had in convincing others. If no one understands where we are coming from, it could be because they have nothing to base it on. Alternatively, it could be that we are not skilled in communicating the vision. Because visions are not always based in reality, it is best to develop our communication skills.

WAYS TO MOVE A TEAM FROM THE OLD TO THE NEW. How can leaders persuade their team to trade their old viewpoint for a new vision? Perhaps more than any other area, this is where visionary leaders fail. A vision that looks impossible can be compared to a drastic, tangible organizational change. The difference is that the vision is not yet tangible. Wall, Solum, and Sobol (1992) and Kotter (1996) outline methods for helping a team from the old to the new, which also can be applied to vision sharing. These methods include keeping everyone informed of the vision and what changes will take place in roles, procedures, and goals; displaying decisiveness; communicating the ideal with excitement; involving others in the vision and decisions related to it (empowering employees); and being on the lookout for conflict.

Keep the Team Informed. Keeping the team informed may almost feel like overcommunicating for a time. In reality, there is little danger of overcommunicating when a team is crossing new ground. People want to know what to expect, especially when a radical change is imminent or there is no baseline for comparison. They may need persuasion that the vision is real and that results are possible. Anything that seems concrete or familiar can help to fill the knowledge gap. Processes, time lines, outlines, and milestones help employees digest the proverbial elephant without oversimplifying the tasks needed to reach the goal. Reinforcement of the goal itself and progress toward the goal help to underscore the vision and promote its validity.

Display Decisiveness. Decisiveness is key when communicating a vision, and emotional literacy plays a major role in the intuition inherent in solid decisiveness (Cooper and Sawaf, 1997). It is difficult to trust a leader who appears to shift between resolves. Whether the vision is dead wrong or entirely on target, it is better to make a decision about when to start and when to change course than to never fully commit to the vision. The leader reacts to his own indecisiveness in much the same way as constituents will. When there is an air of indecisiveness, advancement toward the vision is slow, suspicions are high, and constituent buy-in is tentative. The leader need not promulgate this by her own indecisiveness. It leads to a cycle of uncertainty.

Decisiveness was one of Reagan's communicative traits. Of his decision to issue an ultimatum to thousands of striking air traffic controllers, he said, "I think it convinced people who might have thought otherwise that I meant what I said" (Strock, 1998, p. 42). This was a powerful episode in a series of tough presidential decisions. Reagan's communication and decisions were also tied to his vision. His vision included change he knew was coming at the end of the century, and he continually communicated his vision of a more democratic world in terms of values that Americans understood. The actions of executive leaders should be tied to their vision and implemented decisively.

Whether or not one agrees with Reagan's actions, one has to admit that Reagan was a man of resolve. Resolve is a key factor in getting ideas recognized and adopted. People are wise to the indecisive, and they will often trust someone who is firm about something they do not necessarily agree with more than someone who wavers on a much more palatable action. Your constituents, those you lead or have the opportunity to lead, are also appreciative of decisiveness. As well, they respect and are strengthened by three other traits of a communicator: identification with them, listening to them, and respecting them (Kouzes and Posner, 1995).

Communicate the Ideal with Excitement. Perhaps as critical as decisiveness is an element of excitement in the communication of a vision. A leader's excitement in sharing a vision gives constituents an added impetus to adopt the vision. A vision that is articulated well and coherently and enthusiastically presented generates further excitement among constituents (Taylor, 2003).

A bold voice goes a long way in communicating a vision and integrates decisiveness with excitement. Boldness in sharing a vision characterizes belief in the vision because there is an unwavering internal commitment. If a patient were dying or suffering, a nurse would be expected to use a voice strong enough to be heard and to obtain appropriate care for the patient. Unfortunately, this expectation of nurses is not always carried into the venue of the dying or suffering department or organization. Nurse leaders should be, in fact, just as urgent about these issues as they would be about patient issues (Barden, 2003).

Involve Others in the Vision. Think about communicating with those you are leading in much the same way that you would about dressing for a job interview, a formal event, or a reverent occasion. Just as we would not slap on our gardening attire for these venues, neither should we slap together shoddy, unpolished communication that is inappropriate for our audience. No doubt a teacher or adviser in high school or college let us all in on the secret about first impressions and professionalism. We must respect our constituents enough to address them professionally, even if they are not acting professionally. This does not mean speaking in lofty language or talking down to them. It means acknowledging their value as human beings.

In the retail environment, this respect for others might be known as good customer service or just common decency, but it is one element of establishing support for a vision that cannot be taken for granted. It means that we do not reward certain behaviors by displaying different levels of respect. Meting out respect based on someone's actions or attitudes may have implications for an associate's discipline and self-confidence, but it is an ineffective way to establish one's credibility as a leader. In the meantime, speak as you would be spoken to. Act as though others want to hear what you have to say. Accept opposition with resolve. Cling to principles despite opposition. Offer several chances to buy into the vision. Treat constituents as though they will.

Expect Conflict. Speaking of opposition, there will be some. Accept it. Learn from it. Acknowledge it. Do not cower to it, but do change because of it if that is appropriate. In addition, know the people you are leading. Know them and their capabilities. Know their emotional constitution. Know what will make them come along. Study them in terms of who they are, as well as who you want them to be. Keep communicating the vision, and keep expecting buy-in. Expect that they will contribute, and then show them how. When they come around to your vision, show your appreciation.

They Convince Others That They Can Contribute to Success

Truly, invention is difficult, but getting the word out and disseminating the invention is even more challenging (Berwick, 2003). "If there's a clear and distinguishing feature about the process of leading," note Kouzes and Posner (1995), "it's in the distinction between mobilizing others to do and mobilizing others to *want* to do" (p. 31). This statement specifically refers to mobilization toward a vision. It takes on additional meaning because it is talking not just about the vision itself but also about the people who are carrying it out. In other words, people may be more likely to participate when they are convinced of their own abilities. Believing something to be possible does not make it doable. The nurse leader skilled in emotional understanding will likely understand that lack of motivation leads to more lack of motivation, and that a person's emotions must be managed if she is to benefit fully from helping the vision become reality.

USING THE PAST TO MOTIVATE FOR THE FUTURE. The leader must have an understanding of what motivates people intrinsically as well as extrinsically. It is easy enough to see how adequate rewards can help bring about results; just ask any commission sales team. Less clear are the devices needed to cause people to want to succeed, especially when it involves a higher level of performance than they are accustomed to.

One way to motivate people is to help them believe that they are capable of carrying out the vision. Perhaps one of the most familiar is providing examples of previous successes, either their own or those of others. Many people are inspired and enlightened by stories of everyday heroes, and by the same means, many people are convinced that success is not reserved for the strongest and ablest of society.

Leaders who are motivating teams should use examples of past successes, paying particular attention to the difficulties the team overcame to reach the goal. No one is blind to the fact that obstacles arise when pursuing something better. Effective leaders face this head-on instead of attempting to sidestep these realities.

ACKNOWLEDGING CHALLENGES. As the initial drafts of this text were being written, the United States had just experienced perhaps the most significant challenge in its history. Within the space of two hours on September 11, 2001, terrorists had used commercial airliners to effect the slaying of thousands in New York's World Trade Center, in Washington's Pentagon, and in Pennsylvania. American and world leaders have quickly rallied those who believe in democracy to the vision of eradicating terrorism from the free world. At the same time, words and phrases such as *sacrifice, long, hard-fought battle,* and *not always an easy course* have been standard inclusions in almost any speech or discussion about how the vision will be carried out. Leaders know that difficulty lies ahead.

This is an extreme example but nonetheless a relevant one. When people consider the challenges they may face, the vision becomes more real and more personalized and, in effect, more shared. Very few people believe that they can do practically anything without problems, but hearing the leader admit that they will have challenges along the way provides a sense that the leader has thought through these obstacles and still believes the team can do the job. Some leaders fear that acknowledging obstacles will cause the troops to retreat in discouragement. Actually, the troops are too smart for that. A lofty goal with no obstacles along the way hardly seems real, much less achievable, and they probably will not buy into it.

BUILDING CONFIDENCE. While leaders need to acknowledge obstacles, they also need to build the confidence of their constituents. People do not all come equipped with autonomic, pulsed doses of "I can do it." Motivational speakers would starve if this were so. Based on the work of University of Texas professor Roderick Hart (1984), Kouzes and Posner (1995) say that the key to motivation is in the language the leader uses. They mention four types of words used by leaders: realistic words, optimistic words, activity words, and certainty words. As I discussed earlier in this chapter, motivating people to work toward a vision involves making an intangible vision concrete, conveying optimism that the goal can be realized, expecting action, and displaying assurance that the goal will be reached (while acknowledging possible difficulties).

DEFINING WHAT SHOULD BE DONE. One of Britain's early experiments in public welfare was the establishment of workhouses, established in the early 1800s to provide those seeking public aid with shelter and sustenance in exchange for menial duties. The problem was that so many flocked to the workhouses that they were overrun with people who were sick, disabled, elderly, blind, or chronically ill. By 1861, approximately one-third of the workhouse population consisted of medical patients (Dossey, 2000). These individuals were not sent away for treatment but were cared for in the workhouse community by physicians and nurses who were underpaid and inadequately trained.

Agnes Jones had studied nursing at the Nightingale Training School for Nurses, having been inspired by Nightingale's work in Crimea. Jones eventually became known as the pioneer of British workhouse nursing, an initiative that Nightingale carried further after Jones's death in 1868 (Dossey, 2000). Nightingale had a vision for the care of the sick in workhouses that she believed to be achievable. Using her gift for systems analysis, Florence stated her vision succinctly and boldly: "So long as a sick man, woman, or child is considered administratively to be a pauper to be repressed, and not a fellow-creature to be nursed into health, so long will these most shameful disclosures have to be made. The care and government of the sick poor is a thing very different from the government of paupers. Why do we have Hospitals in order to cure and Workhouse Infirmaries in order not to cure?" (Dossey, 2000, p. 296).

It was more than just a rhetorical question: Florence's summary of the current situation was a call to action; in fact, she quickly proposed legislation to realize her vision. Her steps were clear and visible: to separate the sick and otherwise physically or mentally infirm from the regular population during their infirmity, to manage all workhouses centrally to ensure more consistent training and administration, and to support the care of these individuals through public finance.

As leaders, we must not neglect to communicate what our constituents really want to know: what they can or should do. This should be intrinsic in the fabric of the vision. Note the realistic, action-oriented tone of Nightingale's call to aid the workhouse infirm: if we do not want shameful disclosures to continue on the grounds of deplorable conditions in workhouse infirmaries, we must change things. She described reality, which was the antithesis of the ideal, but the direct opposition of real and ideal was made abundantly clear in Nightingale's strong statement. She provided contrasting scenarios, different ways of doing things, consequences for inaction, and a follow-up with specific initiatives that could be taken. We should lead our constituents as concretely and comprehensively as Nightingale did. In addition, in doing so, we should make them part of what we are doing.

They Inspire Others to Partner with Them

It is one thing when someone believes you have a great idea. It is entirely another when someone believes in your great idea.

THE DRAW OF CHARISMA. Charismatic leaders have a knack for taking their vision and making it the vision of their followers. How they do this has intrigued students of leadership for generations. Theories and explanations abound for why and how leaders possess or attain personal charisma (Yukl, 1998; Kouzes and Posner, 1995). Certainly, it is a trait that most leaders desire, because charisma is often the "something" that propels a leader from brilliant to beloved, from innovative to infectious. If there is a catalyst that facilitates a reaction in the face of adversity or challenge, charisma may very well be it.

One theory, that of Meindl, attributes charisma to the phenomenon of social contagion. That is, in the face of crisis, people will normally seek out a leader who speaks and acts heroically. This leadership trait is attractive, perhaps because of the need to identify with someone who exemplifies mighty, even self-sacrificial aspirations that the followers themselves may be inhibited from displaying. The reaction of followers is said to spread like a wave, capturing the majority in a rush of emotion or identification with the leader (Yukl, 1998).

Other theories attribute charisma to social identification or self-identification. That is, the need to attribute desired characteristics of others to oneself or to feel a sense of belonging may drive followers to closely identify with and support the leader. Still another theory proposes that the desire for charismatic leadership arises from a need for structure and guidance and, more specifically, from a deficit of personal or group direction (Yukl, 1998).

Many of the theories have in common certain leader behaviors. Charismatic leadership is said to usually arise out of a condition of crisis or disenchantment of some sort, but it can also be seen in situations of a less dramatic need for change. When five major theories of charismatic leadership were compared, these leader characteristics were common to at least three of the five (Yukl, 1998):

○ Innovative vision

○ Unconventional behavior

○ Impression management

○ Model behavior to imitate

○ Confidence in followers

These are certainly not unusual or novel traits; most of us have seen them before. What, then, in the combination of these characteristics causes a desire on the part of followers to adopt a shared vision?

Winston Churchill, the British prime minister during World War II, may shed some light on this question. He was known as a great innovator, someone whose vision reached far beyond what seemed practical, and a communicator who was anything but conventional. Yet he surged forward during a very adverse time, being patient with himself, understanding his own capabilities as well as those of others around him, spurring others to believe what he knew to be true, that there could be success even in the midst of adversity. It was a time when one could only imagine the military capacity we have today, yet Churchill made a foundation for his effectiveness in his willingness to look beyond current reality to what could only be imagined. Believing that the British military could greatly improve, Churchill diagrammed the organizational chart and put the Naval War Staff into place just before World War I, converted the Navy's principal fuel to oil—which allowed them to go faster than coal did—and he founded the Royal Naval Air Service. Perhaps Churchill is best noted for his development and improvement of the tank, now an indispensable part of our military, which he developed and used despite the initial skepticism of those participating in the project (Hayward, 1997).

"The act of innovation is both cognitive and emotional," says Goleman in *Working with Emotional Intelligence* (1998b, p. 100). "Coming up with a creative insight is a cognitive act; but realizing its value, nurturing it, and following through calls on emotional competencies such as self-confidence, initiative, persistence, and the ability to persuade." Goleman goes on to say, "Throughout, creativity demands a variety of self-regulation competencies, so as to overcome the internal constraints posed by emotions themselves" (1998b, p. 100).

"Overcoming internal constraints" beautifully describes the art of emotion management. Truly, the skill of regulating one's own emotions and helping others to do the same (Mayer, Salovey, and Caruso, 2000, 2002) involves overcoming many internal hindrances. Perhaps no general idea can be better applied to the concept of garnering partnership surrounding one's vision. In fact, when are we more often called upon and actually expected to attain the highest level of emotional management than when we are gathering and persuading constituents and supporters? Goleman further states that people who get things done usually possess a "high emotional intelligence level [and] . . . see that a variety of elements—most of them human—have to come together to make something new happen. You've got to communicate with people and persuade them, solve problems with them, collaborate" (p. 101).

Let us now compare the abilities described by Goleman with the characteristics of charismatic leaders listed earlier in this section. As I noted there, theorists who have written about charismatic leaders have tended to find that charismatic leaders have certain traits in common: innovative vision, unconventional behavior, impression management, model behavior to imitate, and confidence in followers. The first two traits seem to make up the nuts and bolts of having a vision in the first place: innovation and unconventional behavior were described earlier as having a great deal to do with insight; foresight; and the ability to see how forces, some of them human, will interact and thus to predict what the future might be, could be, or should be. The last three traits are largely about managing people, and they round out the qualifications of the capable leader who understands not only what needs to happen but also the people who will make it happen.

This description of leadership is not by any means a new concept. Emotional intelligence, being a relatively new field of study, brings science to some truths that great leaders knew far before modern civilization. In the fifth century A.D., Attila, king of the Huns, described leadership as "influencing people, processes and outcomes" (Roberts, 1987, p. 18). He went on to point out the incredible influence a leader must have over the people he or she is leading: "Chieftains and leaders in every subordinate office are responsible for establishing the atmosphere in which they lead. This atmosphere may have periods of change even as the seasons change. Nonetheless, unlike our lack of influence over the weather, our leaders can and must influence and control the spirit of our tribes" (Roberts, 1987, p. 61).

Our constituents are not like the weather, which tends to change according to natural patterns and is difficult to influence on a broad scale. They are more like air conditioning systems, which can be influenced as long as we perceive that this is needed. An outdoor thermometer can do little more than tell us that it is miserably hot or cold. An indoor thermometer can actually work in tandem with a thermostat to regulate the tolerability of the air. As leaders, we must be like both the thermometer and the thermostat. We must be able not only to perceive but to regulate in response.

THE VALUE OF LEARNING.   Learning also facilitates partnering. The more people understand about a change, the less they will resist it. Therefore, the leader needs to assess whether the organization is a learning organization.

In learning organizations, employees are allowed to grow, and they also feel that their work has value. There is a pervasive spirit of open, clear communication within collegial relationships at all levels, and this mindset fosters mutual resolution of issues. Employees feel they can take risks, ask questions, and share openly with others in the organization in order to understand and to accomplish goals (Reinick, 2002).

If the organization is indeed a learning organization or has the potential to be one, the nurse leader should encourage constituents to pursue the vision with even more freedom and capability. Just as we would feel comfortable asking questions in a classroom setting, team members can feel comfortable asking questions in a learning organization.

If opportunities for learning and sharing in the organization are less than ideal, the leader should encourage constituents to infuse opportunities for learning into the organization's culture bit by bit. A team might do this by creating an interdepartmental forum where views are expressed and acknowledged, or asking for feedback from the entire staff on different aspects of unit policy. One by one, learning opportunities will begin to create a learning organization. Team members who are working on these types of initiatives should be acutely aware of the reactions of other staff members to the increased openness and make sure the staff does not fear they will be penalized for sharing their views.

THE NECESSITY OF MULTIDISCIPLINARY COLLABORATION. Another aspect of partnering involves multidisciplinary interaction. Health care workers have always been expected to exercise some degree of collaboration, but how the organization executes this collaboration strongly influences its ability to share and implement a vision. In order to carry out a vision, nurses need to collaborate with social workers, physicians, occupational therapists, and those in other disciplines. Thus nurses should hone the ability to reach a consensus (Bronstein, 2003). Due to the nature of multidisciplinary practice, there will usually be conflicting priorities and goals. The key in vision sharing is that these priorities do not conflict fundamentally; in other words, each discipline should contribute toward the same desired outcome. While conflict will certainly occur, there is little room in a shared vision for lack of consensus. Bronstein (2003) emphasizes the importance of moving toward a common goal and collaborating. Multidisciplinary perspectives—of social workers and physical therapists, for example—may foster different views on an issue or an aspect of patient care. Priorities and focus may be different. In the clinical setting, a physical therapist may be just as concerned about the complications of immobility as the social worker is about social isolation caused by confinement. When working with a team of clinicians or even nonclinicians, the nurse leader should remember that the priorities of each discipline can engender emotional responses, so the leader should prepare to help resolve any conflicts that arise. In administrative settings, for example, nurses and physicians may disagree on unit practices simply based on each discipline's perspective. Something that makes life much easier for the nurses on the unit may cause added work for the physicians making rounds or vice versa. Managed care itself creates such emotional battles. Physicians feel their duty is to treat the patients; HMOs feel that their duty is to manage care efficiently from the standpoint of cost and quality of care. Both want more stable, quality health delivery systems, but there are two very fast-held views. The nurse leader must consider the views of everyone who will potentially be impacted by a vision or plan and be alert for, and help to resolve, conflicts.

They Demonstrate How Activities of the Present Translate into Reaching the New Goal

Leaders who align activities with established core values are able to harness authority and facilitate the flow of information (Feifer, Nocella, DeArtola, Rowden, and Morrison, 2003). Leaders at all levels can assume the role of facilitator. Facilitators are individuals who champion and perform specific actions through a variety of methods. They may take on a specific role or perhaps more than one role in an initiative, requiring them to have multiple attributes and skills. They have a knack for weaving together the evidence of need to change with the actual implementation of change (Rycroft-Malone, Harvey, Kitson, McCormack, Seers, and Titchen, 2002). Facilitators demonstrate how activities of the present can translate into the desired outcome for the future because they are intent on making this happen, and they apply their energy to effecting the progressive realization of the ideal. Think of the ways you have seen the word *facilitate* used in the past. "What can I do to facilitate a rapid transition?" "Joe facilitated the meeting this evening." Facilitate actually means to make something easier. That is what facilitators do: they make things easier for everyone else by pointing the way. They are like the global positioning systems present in many cars today. While these systems will not do the driving for us, they are quite useful in giving turn-by-turn directions. Their directional help begins at point A and ends at point B, and they provide the help we need at the point we need it. If we are in Manhattan and wish to drive to Albany, the positioning system calculates how to get to Albany, but it will tell us first how to get out of Manhattan. How lost we would be if the system began by instructing us, "as you approach Albany, take the third exit from the main highway"!

Good facilitators realize that the team needs to be able to make it easier to get from point A to point B and that they *must start at point A*. There is incredible value in the present: it is all we have to work with.

By understanding that people need to relate to the present, a facilitator has already applied some emotional knowledge: understanding the need for security and familiarity that most of us have. By helping constituents manage the emotions related to change, the facilitator can help them tackle the changing health care environment and manage their own initiatives so that they make the changes most important to them and their practice.

MADELEINE ALBRIGHT TACKLES THE CHANGING WORLD. When Madeleine Albright became secretary of state during the Clinton administration, it quickly became apparent that the world had changed and was still changing in terms of the type of work she would need to do.

The struggle today "is a confrontation not so much of armies as of values and emotions; of reason versus hate; of faith versus fear," said Albright of world relations (Lippman, 2000, p. 212). Albright was describing the new priorities that had emerged since those pursued by her predecessors, including threats of terrorism, environmental decline, and international criminal activity, which were weighty but nebulous concerns that almost seemed to dwarf the pinpointable nuclear and military hazards of recent days. One thing that was and still is unique about the new priorities was that response mechanisms were yet scant, unlike the country's ability to react to military challenges of the past.

Albright found herself at the end of a cold war and at the beginning of a new vision. It was indeed one of necessity, as many visions are, but it was also one of subtle immediacy, and at the core of it, in Albright's own words, was "a confrontation . . . of values and emotions" rather than of traditional threats. Albright understood how the present world situation precipitated a need for a new vision and formed her new vision based on the current situation. Certain values and emotions needed to change, and Albright saw the need to start with point A.

THE NURSE LEADER TACKLES THE CHANGING HEALTH CARE ENVIRONMENT. Madeleine Albright's recognition that a new vision was necessary required a skill that all leaders should possess: understanding the environment so well that it is clear when a different course is needed. It is fundamental to the process of understanding why nurse leaders are often asked, "Where do we go from here?" The nurse leader is then charged with helping constituents to understand clearly what is going on, gracefully move from the past to the future, and use their current abilities and comfortable processes to guide them into the ideal situation.

Leave the Past Gracefully. Although constituents may know about the leader's or organization's expectations of them for the future, their main concern is often instead what to do right now. In many contexts, including health care, it may be that not only is the way of doing things changing, but so is the reason. Keep in mind that many followers have no idea what to do because they are not accustomed to the new paradigm. First, they need to understand what the new paradigm is, whether it be budget, regulatory changes, a new health crisis, or something else.

Explain Clearly. Next, the leader needs to be able to explain the new paradigm to constituents. She does not need all the answers or even the ultimate solution, but understanding of the challenge is imperative. In referring to the new paradigm described by Madeleine Albright, Sandy Berger, who was Bill Clinton's national security adviser, demonstrated an understanding of the complexity of change in an ever-changing world—one that requires balancing risk and interest, cost and achievability, and temperance together with readiness to engage. Although Berger's opinion called for judgment appropriate to the situation—indicating he did not have all the answers—he clearly demonstrated an understanding of the new situation and where it would potentially take the nation in the context of world relations (Lippman, 2000).

Although Berger's description called for judgment appropriate to the situation (indicating that he did not have all the answers), he clearly demonstrated an understanding of the new situation and where it would potentially take the nation in the context of world relations. Similarly, the nurse leader needs to demonstrate an understanding of the fact that health care is becoming more diverse and more emotionally demanding, and put constituents at ease by acknowledging these facts and stating the vision clearly in this context.

Apply Present Activities to the Future Vision. When present activities can be applied to the vision of the future, they should be. Despite the fact that one rarely changes while clinging to the old way of doing things, the old way of doing things is still there and must be dealt with. This is one action that helps translate a desire to change into an actual change, but it can be difficult. People must be prepared to transfer their old habits into a new way of performing or acting.

At times, retaining the old way of doing things is impossible and even absurd. If a new policy is put in place, the boss is not beholden to allow employees to wean off the old policy. If we are going to start filing charts over here versus over there, that change can take place immediately without a transition period. However, if we are going to restructure priorities or paradigms, the situation is vastly different (Kouzes and Posner, 1995).

Begin by understanding the natural need of followers to be successful, which may underlie their reluctance to change. Settle for small victories that build to larger ones (Kouzes and Posner, 1995). Talk about what will *not* change. Speak of the transition from the present way to the new way in terms of a bridge, not a menace. The old way is not an outlaw, but it is an opportunity to improve.

Second, allow what *will* change to become an extension of the old way, if possible. There may be a radical change coming, but help followers to view old patterns as intersections or jumping-off points for the new vision. This natural progression is more comfortable than the implication that things are just being done wrong (even if they are). The suggestion is not that leaders downplay the need for improvement but rather that they recognize that the old way of doing things had its place and still does in the minds of followers and that finesse is sometimes required to change mind-sets and habits.

SELF-MANAGING TEAMS ARE INSTRUMENTAL. Self-managing teams can be instrumental in converting a vision to action. These teams can be given authority over the process of converting the vision to action because they are close to the area where the action needs to be taken. They take ownership of what they do because they will be accountable for it and responsible for working with it later. Self-managed teams have been successful in increasing value, quality, and reliability of institutional processes (Feifer, Nocella, DeArtola, Rowden, and Morrison, 2003). Self-managing teams will be discussed further in Chapter Six.

Summary

This chapter has described six actions of leaders who share a vision: they are known as visionaries; they hold a vision of the ideal; they communicate the ideal to others; they convince others that they can contribute to success; they inspire others to partner with them; and they demonstrate how the activities of the present can translate into fulfillment of the vision. These actions have been described in that order in part because they mirror the building block model of emotional intelligence constructed by Mayer, Salovey, and Caruso (1999, 2000, 2002). The first three actions demonstrate identification and facilitation abilities: the ability to identify one's own vision and that of others, and use emotions to facilitate thought. The second three demonstrate understanding and management abilities: a keen understanding of emotion's effect on individual and team success and the ability to help constituents manage their own emotional abilities. The contribution of emotional acuity to leadership capability becomes more evident.

TEN CRITERIA FOR LEADERS WHO SHARE A VISION

1. They envision what the future can be and seize every possible opportunity to discuss it.

2. They work and support selected processes to ensure that their vision materializes.

3. They know exactly what their vision is and what it will mean to the organization.

4. They articulate their vision in understandable terms.

5. They realize that a vision does not have to be mystical to be ideal; some visions return us to simple principles.

6. They relate their vision to the present and to ideas familiar to their constituents.

7. They understand what motivates people and use this knowledge to convince others that they can contribute to the success of the vision.

8. They know how to tell others what they need to do.

9. They realize the value of their vision, nurture it, and follow through.

10. They understand how to translate present activities into future ideals.

6

LEADERS WHO SET
AN EXAMPLE

A NURSE LEADER'S ROLE would be incomplete if she were extraordinarily creative and able to line up people all around her to accomplish an ideal, yet did not know how, or did not want, to show constituents how to carry out the vision themselves. The third critical action of a leader is setting the example, which involves paving the way for others to lead in a constant renewal of the create-vision-example cycle within the organization.

Setting an Example by Allowing Others to Lead

During World War II, General Douglas MacArthur had a penchant for consulting with the lower ranks of his staff before making a decision. Although he usually knew what his decision would ultimately be, he asked his followers, usually starting with the lowest-ranking ones, for their opinion. He realized that ultimately his decision making would be better if he was listening to everyone on his team, even though he himself possessed remarkable decision-making ability (Wall, Solum, and Sobol, 1992).

Setting an example conjures up all sorts of images: thoughts of those impeccable qualities many leaders desire to pass on to followers, the realization that others are looking on and that misuse of leadership is highly visible, or the understanding that imitation is a natural tendency of many. With these views in mind, consulting with one's followers about a leadership action may seem, in the purest sense of what it means to set an example, counterintuitive.

However, let us examine more closely the relationship between sharing the leadership and setting an example. Let us consider the difference between walking in with the answer and letting constituents mold the initial clay that forms what the decision and, ultimately, the example will be. In doing so, we will attempt to break down the notion that example following should be a one-way upward activity and that example setting is strictly a downward activity.

In their book *Executive EQ*, Cooper and Sawaf (1997) describe "secretive decision making" as a perceived put-down of colleagues. By secretive, they mean decisions that are made behind closed doors, perhaps, or without open consultation with others. Note that this "secrecy" may be an act of omission, not necessarily one of commission. In other words, there may not be a great deal of noticeable whispering or avoidance of others in the process of coming to a decision, but there may be an absence of inclusion and openness.

No Secret Decision Making

Some managers may lead by making secret decisions. While the outcome and direction of their decisions may be clear, the precursors and qualifications are not. Often the whispering begins after the directive is handed down, because team members have no idea where the idea came from or how it corresponds to the welfare of the team, unit, or organization. The leader may think that if team members accept his decision as the right thing to do and follow his example in carrying it out, they cannot go astray. After all, he has made the right decisions before.

However, excluding followers in this way, say Cooper and Sawaf (1997), sends the wrong message—an emotionally damaging one. In addition, says Press (2001), a sign that an organization is in trouble is that consensus on decisions gives way to the need for unanimous decision making. How better to obtain unanimity than to make the decision oneself, with no opportunity for other input? Repeated regularly, this type of decisiveness can cause team members to feel unimportant, unintelligent, useless, and uptight. Over time, faith and confidence in the leader may begin to break down.

Shared Leadership in Health Care

Porter-O'Grady, Hawkins, and Parker (1997) applied the concept of shared leadership to health care. This model encourages health care staff to affect the decisions made about health care organizations and patient care. The model is applied in several areas, from community health (Restall, Ripat, and Stern, 2003) to primary care (Brazill, 2002).

Although leadership has long been primarily a function of management, shared leadership allows management to receive advice from staff in an organized, documented fashion. With fiscal, political, and organizational considerations ever present, managers retain the final say on decisions. Shared leadership committees make recommendations that often become reality as long as they do not conflict with strategic or fiscal priorities. In addition, managers often attend staff council meetings in advisory roles. As such, managers have no voting rights but can provide insight where needed.

Thus, the latitude for decision making at the staff level can be high when it is allowed to be. Staff decisions need not be costly or send the organization into a tailspin: in fact, some changes they make may be relatively minor in scale but far-reaching in scope. Staff decisions can have a large impact, because they are coming from those closest to the issue. There is usually very little fluff or need for motivational, visionary rationale in a staff council's recommendation. They make the recommendation because the need is already perceived, and sometimes the change is adopted in practice before the recommendation reaches management. When they are involved in this way, staff members are truly the people who are carrying the organization where it needs to go.

A disease management organization's quality council participates in program enhancements, and the nursing staff gives input into the implications of program changes. The assessment tools, which the nurses use to telephonically monitor patients with specific diseases, underwent a fifteen-month rewrite, with the nursing staff applying their knowledge and experience with the current assessment tool. In this case, senior management recognized the value of shared leadership: they asked that the nurses who were closest to the tool actually do the work of redesigning it.

In this same organization, the principle of shared leadership is integral to all aspects of developing patient care programs. Its staff education council regularly provides feedback to the company medical director related to educational needs of the staff and reviews and approves new patient educational materials on a monthly basis. Its staff practice council is instrumental in developing care plans and documentation standards for the organization. Nurses have worked with the medical director to implement quality initiatives surrounding disease-specific needs. The people who know the patients best are influencing change that ultimately improves patient outcomes. This is a mark of effective shared leadership.

Seeking the Truth from Those Who Know It

Nonmanagers (often called frontline employees) have the uncanny ability to come forward with the truth. Collins (2001a) indicates that shared decision making is about creating a culture in which people can be heard, because that is how the truth will be heard. In creating such a culture, the leader should use questions to gain understanding ("What bothers you the most about the new process?"), not as a form of getting others to see the leader's view ("Can you see how this new process will save time in the long run?"). The leader should always realize that she does not understand everything. Depending on her level of expertise or time with the organization, she may understand many things and perhaps more than anyone else may in the field; however, she does not understand *everything*.

Dialogue, Not Coercion

In addition, says Collins (2001a), leaders should engage in dialogue, not coercion. At the bowling alley, a certain behavior is almost predictable in some people. The ball will be rolled toward the perfect space between the pins, then mysteriously curve slightly to the right as it approaches the opportunity for a strike or spare. The bowler, holding her breath as the ball makes its way down the lane, may start to make whisking leftward gestures with her right hand, as though magically waving the ball back slightly toward the left so that it will go straight into the pocket for which it was intended. As the ball veers more predominantly toward the right (and the gutter or, at best, the ten pin) the hand movement intended to wave the ball back toward the left becomes more frantic, simulating the amount of force needed to get the ball back to where it was supposed to go. As the bowler and anyone even intuitively familiar with the natural laws of the universe knows, the ball is not likely to be coerced out of its true direction in this manner.

Unfortunately, coercion of team members' ideas is quite a bit simpler than changing the preordained track of a fourteen-pound bowling ball. Yet managers try to do this repeatedly in the guise of healthy dialogue with team members. They will do almost anything to keep from seeing that the ball is veering from the intended course. The team sees a problem; right away, the manager discounts it, countering with arguments that are untested, untried, and maybe even untrue. The problem that the team sees could be a serious right curve in the plan. Hearing the truth, just like seeing the results of an unintentional spin on the ball, often takes us in directions we had not intended to go. Leaders may try frantically to wave the ball back in what they deem the appropriate direction. Many, many succeed, and the resulting decisions may have inherent flaws.

Arguments from the team may be construed as dissident attitudes. They may or may not be. Some team members seem to have a passion for seeing the dark side. Their arguments must be weighed for what they are worth and evaluated for validity. The leader must be incredibly cautious that she does not prejudge arguments based on their source.

Alcock, Berter, Hawkins, Madsen, and McCall (2002) recommend that productive dialogue be encouraged by asking basic questions addressing what the areas of concern actually are, who is accountable for decisions, how the team can accomplish goals together and what, specifically, can be done. An understanding of why things have been done the way they have can also be helpful for group dialogue. The open-ended nature of these types of discussion-starters will serve to discourage the use of coercion by the leader.

Use of these types of questions will spur productive dialogue that allows team input into the situation at hand; the open-ended questions will discourage the use of coercion by the leader.

Who Is Not to Blame?

Collins also says we must "conduct autopsies, without blame" (Collins, 2001a, p. 77). Now, there is an analogy that piques the health care professional's interest. No one would want to be found guilty of causing, intentionally or otherwise, an autopsy to be necessary in the first place. However, Collins refers to the dissection (if one will) of a situation after it has occurred (and gone wrong) as an autopsy of sorts. Why did it go wrong? The emphasis is on "why" and not "who." We all know that in an autopsy, the coroner's report may say, "the patient died of an apparent gunshot wound to the chest" but never "Mr. X shot the patient in the chest during a brawl over a few dollars." Later, that fact may be revealed and dealt with, but it is not the coroner's responsibility to do so.

When people are sharing in the decision making in an organization, someone somewhere is going to be responsible for spearheading or merely suggesting a chosen path. Remember that the autopsy report should only show what happened and not whose idea it was. The autopsy may say "Medication incidents with x, y, or z drugs increased in the first quarter by almost 50 percent because these medications were packaged differently beginning in this quarter." What the autopsy should *not* report is who in the organization originally suggested this change. At that point, it does not matter. Let us assume that the idea was not ill intended; that type of behavior is dealt with in another way. The idea was a bad one. What matters is that the problem should be corrected now.

This is an ideal time to discuss the value of failure, a concept that is explored more thoroughly in Chapter Four. Although risk taking is often thought of as a defining characteristic of good leadership, failure does not receive the value or the applause that it deserves in most businesses. The leader must constantly guard against the double standard of allowing the team to take risks but not fail. The problem with this standard is that it implies that all risks must result in positive outcomes, and that is simply not possible (Chaffee and Arthur, 2002). Besides being a valuable learning experience, failing allows team members to note the insufficiency of failure alone to crumble their career and their practice. Many are afraid to fail because they have never tried to fail or have never risked anything for fear of failure. This cycle must be broken if organizations want to encourage the learning that comes with taking risks.

Having acknowledged that failure is a necessary part of discovery, let us move away from the corpse analogy to examine an idea gone right. If medication incidents declined by 50 percent in the first quarter and a change is seen as the reason, the leader and the team have every reason to commend, laud, and compliment the person or group who came up with the idea to change. This is especially true if the leader did not fully appreciate the prescience of the team members in the first place. If an argument was not acknowledged and was subsequently proved right, it is the leader's responsibility to make that admission. If an argument was heard despite the attempted coercion of a leader, the leader should also admit that. Imagine the gain within the team that occurs and the effectiveness that ensues when right decisions are applauded and wrong ones are examined for what they are and not who was responsible. Some hold the perception that managers do what it takes to make them look good, regardless of what is right, and that they fail to accept accountability or responsibility for their mistakes. Employees, however, can sort actions from words and discern authentic leadership from its unauthentic counterpart (Johnson, 2002).

We have just explored, in perhaps unconventional ways, the age-old principle of expecting constituents to do as one does, not just as one says. Those leaders fostering teams (such as shared leadership committees) that make an impact should be displaying the types of behaviors, attention to priorities, and work ethic that they expect their team members to follow.

Setting an Example Through Mentoring

There are two extremes on the spectrum from leading by example to leading by directive, between which shared leadership falls with a combination of the two. One pole, which has been discussed already, involves the handing down of instructions to staff without staff input or understanding of the rationale. "Please start counting all the narcotics at midshift" is an example of such a directive. The whispering begins: Why, suddenly, must the narcotics be accounted for at midshift? Is a particular employee suspect? Have there been incidents on other units? Was the fact that the majority of the medication distribution occurs at midshift taken into consideration? The recipients of these orders may feel unimportant and uptight, according to Cooper and Sawaf (1997).

The other end of the spectrum is leading purely by example, anticipating that followers will imitate the leader in the absence of coaching, direction, teaching, or explanation of the rationale for actions and procedures. The leader expects that team members will learn, solely from observing her actions, the right thing to do when situations arise. There is little teaching or explanation to back up the on-the-job example the leader is setting. For example, a nurse manager may expect the nurses in her charge to observe interactions with patients and to deal with patients similarly. In addition, the same manager may expect that observing the manager's behavior in a crisis will enable a young nurse to handle a similar situation down the road. While such observation may benefit the new nurse, it is easy to see how the nurse might misinterpret the manager's rationale or judgment call at the moment and apply similar actions inappropriately in another situation.

Many of us number among our most valuable learning experiences the times we spent observing experienced professionals in our work setting; no doubt those observation experiences are more valued than the information-packed lectures during our initial training. It is hoped that the reader will not misconstrue the previous paragraph to mean that one cannot learn from the example of others; indeed, one can. The factor that makes on-the-job observations even more helpful is the explanation, where necessary, of steps taken in a situation (for example, why the nurse manager performed that particular procedure during that code) or the rationale or theory behind the leader's day-to-day interactive style with patients, families, or staff members. The sum of an on-the-job example plus an explanation is mentorship, which lays a beautiful foundation for shared leadership.

The Invaluable Effects of Mentoring

Mentoring encourages development of leadership and advances not only the mentored individual but also the nursing profession as a whole (Owens and Patton, 2003). McKinsey & Company is a consulting firm that specializes in knowledge transfer, among other areas. McKinsey's managing director, Rajat Gupta, underscores the value of learning together and learning with someone who has done it before: mentorship and apprenticeship. In a world where distance learning is increasingly in vogue and where members of large corporations might just as easily train via video or Web conference as in side-by-side interactions, are we setting ourselves up to miss the most valuable method of knowledge transfer: knowing by doing? (Pfeffer and Sutton, 2000).

Mentoring is probably one of the least cost-effective means of sharing knowledge, which means that many organizations may be tempted to opt for other, more efficient means of learning for new and existing employees (Pfeffer and Sutton, 2000). Morrison (2000) and Duff (1999) describe mentoring as a time-consuming two-way transaction. It has at its core a requirement of personal commitment that most forms of education do not have. It is important to note, however, that more technologically advanced and standardized methods of training, although they have their place, cannot equal the added value of solid coaching or mentoring.

Goleman, Boyatzis, and McKee, in their book *Primal Leadership* (2002), state:

> Coaching exemplifies the EI competence of developing others, which lets a leader act as a counselor, exploring employees' goals and values and helping them expand their own repertoire of abilities. It works hand in hand with two other competencies that research shows exemplify the best counselors: emotional self-awareness and empathy.
>
> Emotional self-awareness creates leaders who are authentic, able to give advice that is genuinely in the employee's best interest rather than advice that leaves the person feeling manipulated or even attacked. In addition, empathy means leaders listen first before reacting or giving feedback, which allows the interaction to stay on target. Good coaches, therefore, often ask themselves: Is this about my issue or goal, or theirs? [p. 62].

Goleman, Boyatzis, and McKee's thoughts mirror those of Collins and others referred to earlier in this chapter: listening first, avoiding manipulative dialogue, and focusing on the goals of the team. Although these earlier references were not tied specifically to coaching and mentoring but more to leadership in general, they run strikingly parallel to Goleman's thoughts.

Also confronting us is the reality that complex ethical situations are becoming more and more the norm. Says Johnson (2002) of this dilemma, "Those who lead in health care must do so by their own example and through actions ensuring that core ethical principles—beneficence, honesty, justice, and nonmalfeasance—are embedded in the daily work of our health care institutions" (p. 5).

Socratic Coaching

Fisher (1993) refers to what is known as Socratic coaching. This type of coaching involves helping a staff member understand the reasons for his or her proposed or actual actions by asking questions. Socratic coaching is not an element of the traditional nursing curriculum (Clarke, 2003). Johnson (2002) reinforces the need for Socratic learning, indicating that "strong, ethical leaders can be counted on in their organizations to make the invisible visible by asking the difficult questions and creating forums in which these ethical dilemmas can be discussed honestly" (p. 7). Again, these would not be the types of manipulative questions designed to help the individual latch onto the leader's point of view. Instead, they would be constructed to help the person think through his or her own actions. The assumption is that by doing this, the individual either will understand the appropriate action based on foundational teaching or coaching or will build a belief system to support behaviors and actions that go beyond mere routinization of actions. A mentor who is using Socratic coaching, therefore, does not simply say "No, don't do it that way, because . . ." but guides the coached individual to think through his or her actions.

Difficult, yes. This kind of mentoring activity is also costly, in terms of time, energy, and efficiency. How much easier is it to say to an employee once, twice, maybe five times daily, "We do it this way because . . ." instead of "What options are you considering, and why?" First, the hospital floor is not a simulation or even a formal classroom. Most of the time there are deadlines, tight patient loads, crises, shift changes, and even absent colleagues and no one to fill in. Time is tight, and efficiency is key. The leader must recognize the long-term and not just the short-term benefits to the employee, the patient, and ultimately the organization that will be derived from a nurse who can think through problems critically and independently. That is the long-term judgment call involved in careful mentoring.

A Meeting of the Minds Takes Time

We need to be able to balance everything we have learned about emotionally competent leadership with the development of the skills and experience needed by mentors. This will be covered further in Chapter Seven. It takes a delicate balance of the art of emotional competence and the hard expertise of experience to be a successful mentor or coach. Now, take that balance and apply it realistically to everyday life at work. It sounds as though it contains all the ingredients necessary to produce stellar teams who are following a great example in their leader. What, though, are the core competencies that get us there? What do we do, since we do not have time to walk dozens of direct and indirect reports through every move we make and why? How do we set the example the way we should and still get the job done ourselves?

Brian Pitman, who was CEO at Lloyd's of London for nearly a decade, describing his approach, said, most picturesquely, that if he were asked to start over again with Lloyd's (the scenario of knowing then what one knows now) he would "toss out the cookie cutters" (p. 46). More specifically, he said, "What's important is getting people to arrive at a meeting of the minds around a small number of central beliefs, which will determine their behavior and ultimately the company's performance" (p. 46). In other words, do not just show, create beliefs; do not just tell, but also tell why. If patient education is paramount to the nurse leader, that unit will be about patient education, as long as the leader is setting the example by verbally promoting its value as well as demonstrating it on a daily basis (Pitman, 2003).

A CEO of a Catholic health care facility was interviewing a candidate for the position of mission leader. "When I walk the halls in this hospital," said the CEO, "I expect to feel the soul of what we are all about in our staff work and patient relations. If I hire you, I'll expect you to make that happen" (Broccolo, 2002, p. 38).

Sometimes cultivating beliefs in others takes time. Badaracco (2002) says that one of the actions that sets an effective leader apart is buying time, by which he means taking as much time as needed to arrive at a final solution rather than rushing in with the answer. This, he says, allows constituents to observe and learn from the way people and events interact. We explored this concept of mutual learning at the very beginning of the chapter, but for a slightly different reason. There, it was to highlight the role that constituents can play in decision making and how part of the example the leader sets comes from his own enlightenment by the people closest to the work. Here, it is to underscore the fact that such interaction takes time, which is valuable for its essence, not just in terms of its loss.

Resisting the Urge to Fix Things

Some young leaders feel that the ability to make quick decisions and to avert crises of any magnitude is what sets them apart as qualified management material. Ask any member of the team and see whether decisiveness does not come forth as a characteristic of a leader. Even Mayer and Salovey (1997) mention that decision-making ability is bolstered by emotional intelligence. However, in mentoring and training, sometimes a decision is not required on the spot, as it is in a truly emergent situation. Time, when available, can be used to evaluate potential courses of action. Most situations are not emergencies, argues Badaracco, and this paves the way for experiential opportunities.

The ability to distinguish between emergencies and teaching opportunities determines whether a leader will hasten to fix things that do not need to be fixed or will allow the staff working with him to explore solutions (to discover for themselves that, alas, a solution is needed). This is by no means easy. Imagine that you are a mother watching your child bake a cake for the first time. The child adds flour, eggs, and sugar, all in the wrong order; some of the batter even escapes the bowl boundaries. Will this truly affect the cake baking? Only time and experience will tell. It is knowing when this time and experience is available that is key. Aside from adding motor oil in lieu of molasses, there are few fatal mistakes in mixing a cake; however, there are countless opportunities to improve. Even leaving out an ingredient leads to better judgment next time, since the cake will likely be flat, dry, crisp, gooey, or otherwise less than perfect.

More than likely, there are few mothers who would actually allow their children even this kind of small failure, unless they were out to prove a major point. By nature, we are not like that at all. We do not like to stand by and intentionally watch people goof up, when we have the answer right there in our back pocket. We especially shudder at letting those in our charge make the same mistakes we made: a feeling nags at us that our job as leaders (parents, if you will) is to keep consequences from happening to those who are not as experienced. If the child forgets eggs, why in the world would the mom not remind the child to put in eggs? Does it not seem cruel to stand by and watch the child make a mistake?

That is where we reach the dividing line between opportunities for intervention and opportunities for learning. Let us pretend that we are a dad this time, watching a young son ride a bicycle for the first time. There are so many things we could tell that kid about what not to do on a bike: do not ride standing up, with no hands, without a helmet, or out in the center of traffic. Indeed we should tell the child these things; they are basic principles of safety, which uninformed children (and even some informed ones) are bound to attempt to violate.

To go even further, we could try to prevent accidents altogether by attaching permanent training wheels, running alongside the child with our hands on the handlebars forever, and only allowing the child to ride on the grass and never on the pavement so as to avoid bleeding in the event that our fundamental efforts to stabilize the bicycle failed. However, most readers know the end of the story: training wheels have to come off, parents cannot forever trot alongside, and backyards do not make very good cycling tracks. Thus, there remain lessons to be learned, and most kids who grew up with bicycles learned them sooner or later. The lessons are about balance, speed, distance, and mechanics, those irresistible laws of physics we start learning from the time we take our first steps. There is no way to ingrain these lessons in a child's mind other than by experience. Do not ride too fast? Absolutely critical to teach ahead of time. However, the real lesson that force equals mass times acceleration awaits, and is well known by the time most kids are ten or twelve years old.

Badaracco (2002) says that the majority of situations do not require heroic, on-the-spot decision making but rather happen in a time frame that allows learning. In these more relaxed situations, we can encourage leaders to provide advice when an ingredient is clearly missing but let go of the handlebars. A teaching leader knows how to walk this fine line.

A Three-Step Process to Mentorship

Author and speaker Shirley Peddy, in the introductory phases of her book (Peddy, 1998), emphasizes that concurrent mentor and supervisory roles may present conflicts of interest that are best avoided. These conflicts may arise because supervisors are responsible for group performance, which involves the whole group, not just one or two mentored individuals. Peddy recommends that a formal mentoring relationship be fashioned outside of a direct reporting relationship if possible, although she is very clear that supervisors should provide coaching, support, and evaluation of performance for their subordinates.

Earlier in this chapter, mentorship was discussed as an integral, needed factor in leadership, not an art form in and of itself. There is a certain variety of mentoring that can occur more effectively apart from the supervisory relationship. In the clinical health care setting, this may evolve from a formal preceptorial situation where the preceptor has no real supervisory authority but is charged with short-term intense guidance of and long-term availability to the mentee without any formal attachment or reporting responsibility. In other administrative settings, mentorship may take the form of an intentional or naturally occurring pairing for guidance based on the experience of one individual and the career path or goals of the other. These opportunities are indeed valuable to the developing professional but should not be expected to replace the mentoring component of the leadership role any more than the school system or educational programs (which both have their place) replace the guidance and instruction of a parent or guardian. The supervisor (or manager or director) is the one who is in a position every day to either develop employees or ignore their developmental needs and focus only on what it takes to get the job done.

Peddy (1998) delineates a three-step process to mentorship, which can also be applied to mentorship within the role of supervisory leadership. The three steps of the process, which she has copyrighted, are lead, follow, and get out of the way. Leading refers to the coaching, teaching, and training that occur in the early stages of the mentoring relationship. Following essentially means following up, being available in the later stages of the mentoring relationship but not as intensely involved or as needed as in the leading phase of mentorship. This too is important; applied to the supervisory role, it means that if the mentoring portion of the role is effective, the intensity of the guidance will decrease over time as the subordinate or team member becomes more independent and effective in his or her role. It does not mean that supervisory bonds are interrupted: the employee still reports to the manager, who is ultimately responsible for the employee's contribution to the departmental goals. What it does mean is that the mentor-leader has helped to create a more self-sufficient individual who can more effectively contribute to achieving the goals of the department and the organization. The supervisor continues the formal supervisory component of the relationship but simply does not need to maintain the intensity that mentorship once required with that individual. The supervisory component should become much less taxing as the leader's example is ingrained in and lived through the team.

Getting out of the way is the third component of Peddy's process, and she uses the analogy of getting out of the house or leaving home. Formally structured mentoring relationships often result in collegial relationships after the process is over; sometimes, they dissolve completely. The mentor's role at that point is to assume the role of *past* mentor and understand that the mentee is now on his or her own (Peddy, 1998).

The mentoring aspect of supervisory leadership contains some but not all of the components of getting out of the way. For example, once a nurse is experienced or a team is well organized and functioning well, each is self-directed and independent. Having benefited from appropriate mentoring, these individuals or groups ideally are carrying out the mission and vision of the leader not because they are being guided systematically but because they know and believe it is the right thing to do. As part of the mentoring process, the leader has established core beliefs that guide constituents in the decision process. While it may be impossible for a person in a supervisory position to get out of the way completely, it is possible for managers to step back and allow the results of their mentoring efforts to flourish. In this way, we set the example, then set it free.

Environmental Factors and Leadership Skills Related to Example Setting

The remainder of this chapter will be devoted to specific environments, and competencies, and emotional concepts that are related to the elements of example setting that were discussed earlier. For starters, in a mentoring situation, we should not overlook the emphasis on developing the staff member's emotional abilities. Second, people learn better in an environment that promotes their all-around growth, both cognitively and emotionally. In addition, the emotional competencies that leaders possess and to what degree affects their ability to make the kind of impact that has been discussed throughout this chapter. This is especially true as the leader seeks to transfer this knowledge to others.

I will start by discussing the environment, then move to the mentor and finally the mentee. Chapters Seven and Eight will give much more detailed descriptions of competencies to be developed in the learner; therefore, that topic will only be introduced here.

Environmental Factors

Just as children's growth and development can be influenced by environment, so can that of those being mentored. An environment ripe for setting an example includes social support, structural support, and evaluation.

SOCIAL SUPPORT. "To be a self, to have an identity, is to be involved with others," writes Raingruber (2000, p. 42). For this reason, the environment in which constituents are expected to assimilate and reproduce a leader's example needs, primarily, to include social support. Mentoring in its essence provides an element of social support; however, the learner should also have available the support of other groups or team members who are also learning. This support can come from team members who are more experienced or those who are less so. The key factor is the promotion of independent thought that is consistent with the mission of the department or unit. For most, the very fact that a mentoring situation is present means that change is occurring. After all, mentoring would not be needed if an employee had already reached the milestones the mentoring is designed to accomplish. Several studies indicate that support groups are effective in maintaining change (Cherniss, 2000).

STRUCTURAL SUPPORT. A finer point is that the environment itself must be supportive. There is an element of implied support when a group of people is working together to accomplish something or when two people are talking through a problem, but this may be only a façade. If the organizational structure or philosophy does not foster emotionally intelligent behaviors or any other behaviors the leader is trying to instill, there is a much smaller likelihood that these behaviors will take off within the team. Departmental or organizational policies should promote team development that is consistent with what leadership is trying to accomplish. If they do not, the leader faces an uphill battle and change will be more difficult to solidify (Cherniss, 2000).

EVALUATION. A third environmental factor that is important in effective example setting is evaluation. By their nature, supportive groups and doctrines help to reinforce new competencies, and they aid in self-evaluation when the learner measures himself against them. However, it should not be taken for granted that the social structure of the environment will complete the feedback that is needed so desperately by learners. Hard skills and competencies are typically evaluated as a matter of performance; elements of emotional competence are less frequently evaluated, although they should be. Tools for this purpose include the Mayer-Salovey-Caruso Emotional Intelligence Test (Mayer, Salovey, and Caruso, 2000, 2002) and the Bar-On Emotional Quotient Inventory (EQ-I) scales (Bar-On, 2000); these will be discussed in more detail in Chapters Seven and Eight.

Real-time evaluation can be called reinforcement. Often, we refer to this as coaching, which involves development of skills and knowledge to enhance professional growth (Daddario, 2003). Whether positive or negative, reinforcement aids the individual in understanding changes that are needed or desired behaviors that should be repeated. Annual or even probationary period performance reviews do not provide the opportunity for growth that reinforcement offers. Perhaps more important, they do not provide the opportunity to correct behavior that is on the way to habituation long before the evaluation is due. Unfortunately, many managers and leaders rely on the mandatory evaluation tool as their sole mechanism for providing feedback to staff. This kind of closed-door feedback, which the manager comes forth with after almost a year of coming up with it in isolation, probably has the same effect on individuals as decisions made in the same manner. Staff are not included in the process, are handed down a determination, and are advised to do better after certain behaviors have continued unacknowledged for up to a year or are finally advised that their skills actually do measure up to expectations after being left to wonder about it all year.

This type of isolated, once-a-year feedback should not happen. In fact, there should not be anything significant on an employee's evaluation that he or she was not aware of throughout the course of the evaluation period. The leader should be forthright enough to bring these discussions to bear during the mentoring process, not just when the evaluation tool makes them officially necessary. If reinforcement has been provided throughout the year, employees should be able to look forward to their performance reviews, and so should managers. Often they do not, because of the respective elements of discovering the unknown and broaching something uncomfortable.

Weisinger (1998) provides several pointers for reinforcement. First, it should be consistent. This means that the behavior is reinforced on a regular basis and every time it is observed. (Weisinger refers to reinforcement in the positive sense, but it can also be applied in the area of redirection or corrective coaching.) Suppose an individual is told once that he did a great job in an area where change was a goal but never hears about future endeavors in the same area. Such haphazard reinforcement can be detrimental and confusing to a learner, who does not completely understand the desired outcomes and needs consistent feedback to implement mutually agreed goals.

Second, reinforcement should be as much in real time as possible (Weisinger, 1998). Waiting until three months has passed and then generalizing that "you've been doing an excellent job with coming to work on time lately" or "you still need to pay more attention to your punctuality" robs both learner and mentor of the opportunity to promote a specific behavior throughout that critical three months. By the same principle, if a person is observed to be out of line in a meeting or in a particular patient interaction, she should be advised of this as directly after the interaction as possible. She should not be allowed to believe that her behavior is acceptable and then have a bomb dropped on her days later, telling her that it is not. ("By the way, you have a habit of interrupting. Remember the other day when you were talking with Mrs. Overby's family? They could not get a word in edgewise.") Over time, employees develop a level of trust in their leaders that corresponds to whether they think their leader is telling them the truth. Leaders must keep in mind that at times, the truth is surmised from what the leader does not say as much as from what the leader says.

Finally, reinforcement should determine and reinforce a cause-and-effect relationship. Weisinger (1998) focuses on the expectation of reward as the effect of behavior, but cause and effect also means that an employee needs to know what effect his behavior, either positive or negative, has on individual performance, team goals, and departmental efforts. These can be motivating factors as well.

Essential Leadership Skills for Setting an Example

Besides creating a reinforcement-rich environment, a mentor can foster emotional growth in employees and implant a lasting example in the team in other capacities.

ESTABLISHING PRIORITIES. First, leaders should make it a practice to establish what the priorities really are (LaFasto and Larson, 2001). Establishment of priorities is a basic step and is a key factor in clinical governance (Campbell, Roland, and Wilkin, 2001). Even after she has set a good example for others to follow and established a supportive venue, this is one of the continuing contributions of the leader, one that she may be called on to make numerous times even when a team or individual is functioning independently. People need a framework of priorities or ground rules to prevent the fear that they are going in the wrong direction. Establishing priorities includes clarification and promotion of departmental or organizational goals as often as needed, consistency in direction, and continual feedback and follow-up by management. This is important because organizational goals set the framework for the decision-making process of a team or an employee, and more often than not, teams and employees do not have a practical understanding of the goals or visions set forth by senior leadership. Therefore, it is management's responsibility to clarify and promote their goals and vision, instilling them in every team member (LaFasto and Larson, 2001) and providing support so that this knowledge can be transformed into sustained action (Fontaine, 1998).

BALANCING RESOURCES AND DEMANDS. In a study of physicians and their responses to ethical issues, physicians rated their confidence low in regard to balancing demands and allocating resources (Kenny, Sargeant, and Allen, 2001). Yet balancing resources and increasing demands is expected of most nurse managers. Managers should do everything possible to avoid the frustration that ensues when resources and demands are not sufficiently balanced. "Part of human happiness depends on not feeling overburdened," say LaFasto and Larson (2001). While skimpy resources are a fact of life in many industries, including health care, it is management's responsibility to balance demands against the resources that are available. This may include discussions with staff to get their input on the need for more resources, increased education and training, or additional team members (LaFasto and Larson, 2001). After all, nurses, when asked, identified staffing shortages as one of the drivers of their worry about their job and, more important, their license. When staff was short, the nurses felt care was compromised and their ability to provide competent care was at risk (Cline, Reilly, and Moore, 2003).

Still, there will be times when a resource crunch is unavoidable, just as there are times when an unexpected invoice arrives right after expenses for a major home repair have been incurred. Typically, employees do not expect these types of resource crises to be entirely absent, but they do need them to be the exception rather than the rule. As LaFasto and Larson (2001) put it, "It's okay to have limited resources as long as priorities are pruned and the deadlines are achievable. In other words, over the long term, the equation needs to be balanced. That can be done by scaling back demands or by increasing resources." When a leader becomes aware of a resource imbalance, it is the leader's responsibility to correct it within the framework of what is available and what can be scaled back. Failure to do so over time will impede progress as well as emotional well-being.

SELECTING THE RIGHT TALENT. Selecting the right talent is a skill that is often taken for granted or ignored. However, failing to select the person with the right talent for a team role or a specific position is much akin to selecting the wrong shoe size. A person may be able to wear a shoe that is the wrong size, but after a while, the poor fit will manifest itself in blisters, pain, or even joint problems. Yet repeatedly, managers select the wrong person for a significant role. They may do so because the individual appears confident, verbose, or opinionated (characteristics that remind us, sometimes ironically, of success) or because the person is notably intelligent or professional in appearance. Many employees have a combination of these and other similar traits that overshadow groomable material in other, less prominent individuals. When choosing people to fill key roles, the leader needs to be absolutely certain she has not overlooked potential in less obvious candidates and that the selection criteria go deeper than superficial traits.

Another factor to take into consideration is that talent and skill are multiplied as the group or team grows larger. In other words, larger teams have a larger talent bank. Leaders need to be able to recognize the talent in these groups and effectively utilize it to help the team achieve its objectives (Bennett, 2003).

FOSTERING ACCOUNTABLE, AUTHORITATIVE INDIVIDUALS AND TEAMS. In setting an example, leaders must always aim for the goal of accountable, authoritative individuals and teams. Team outcomes are improved by substantive participation in decision making, and higher performance is an outcome of team autonomy, Cohen and Bailey (1997) remind us. Teams become accountable by claiming responsibility for their own actions and bearing at least some part of the consequences for outcomes. As their accountability grows, their authority grows. The more a team is willing to bear the risk of its own decisions, the more it will be respected and heard by others in the organization.

Leaders must ever be aware of the need to cut the apron strings when teams are ready to flourish in accountability and authority. As leaders cut their team loose, they must tailor their mentoring to provide clear operating principles that include taking action toward goals, being accountable for results, working together as a team, and being aware of but not being fully directed by organizational politics, especially when those politics sap the team of the energy needed to accomplish goals (LaFasto and Larson, 2001).

DEVELOPING EMOTIONAL INTELLIGENCE. A study on predictors of success in leaders investigated three factors in three possible combinations of two. These factors were EQ (emotional intelligence), IQ (what we think of as traditional cognitive intelligence), and experience. The factor combinations were ranked in terms of which combination most predicted success in leaders. The combination found most likely to predict success was experience and EQ, followed by EQ and IQ. The traditional predictor, experience and IQ, was dead last. This demonstrates a difference between EQ and IQ as components of leadership ability, one that supports development of emotional intelligence skills over traditional intelligence in today's leaders. When paired with experience, emotional intelligence is an especially strong predictor of success, but without it, it still has unquestionable merit (Fernandez-Araoz, 2001). With a rich environment for learning and the right example set by the leader, we are ready to pursue the development of finer emotional skills in employees and teams. We will explore that in the two chapters that follow.

Summary

Leaders who set an example do so by allowing others to lead. This includes not only sharing the leadership with staff but also appreciating the input of even the least experienced employee. Leaders should practice an open, not secretive form of leadership that allows followers to learn from what they are doing and encourages them to practice under the same implicit and explicit guidelines modeled by the leader. In doing so, leaders will seek the truth from those on the front lines, practice dialogue rather than coercion, and refrain from laying blame when a problem or failure arises.

Mentorship provides a solid foundation for sharing leadership. An environment that is socially supportive and well structured and that provides continual feedback further contributes to a leader's ability to set an example. It is also important for the leader to establish priorities, balance resources and demands, select the best personnel for each role, establish accountable, authoritative teams, and develop emotional intelligence.

TEN CRITERIA FOR LEADERS WHO SET AN EXAMPLE

1. They share the leadership with their followers.
2. They avoid secret decision making, choosing to include staff in the reasoning behind their decisions.
3. They seek the truth first from those who really know it: the staff.
4. They engage in dialogue rather than coercing staff to agree with them.
5. They lead teams to a few core beliefs that will affect their decision making later on.
6. They resist the urge to fix things when staff can learn from the situation.
7. They provide individualized coaching and mentoring to staff members.
8. They promote and foster an evaluative, well-structured, and socially supportive environment.
9. They place the right talent in the positions for which they have hiring capacity.
10. They establish priorities, balance demands and resources, promote accountability and responsibility of teams, and develop emotional intelligence skills.

PART THREE

INTELLIGENT TRANSFER OF INFORMATION

7

DOWNLOADING

HONING EMOTIONAL INTELLIGENCE

THAT WE NEED TEAMS to function in a multidisciplinary field like nursing is probably not a new concept to most readers. But many may not know that teams need to be intelligent emotionally to function well. How can the team garner emotional skills from its leader and function as an emotionally intelligent unit?

The Team Approach to Leadership and Its Reliance on Emotional Intelligence

In a seminar several years ago, the observation was made that many sports-related analogies are used to describe workplace activities. Phrases such as *coaching, dropping the ball, pinch hitting,* and *running interference* were, anecdotally, said to be used frequently in the business world to describe common interactions between colleagues. The use of these terms was said to imply that the business world was in many ways like a playing field, with players competing and interacting in the game of business as they would in a football or baseball confrontation, playing by specific rules that govern the game.

The Team Concept in the Workplace Today

Just a few years before this seminar was held, the team concept of leadership had caught on. While teams and teamwork had been positive concepts for a while, books and articles fully devoted to studying team dynamics and advantages began emerging in the 1990s (Montebello,

1994; Fisher, 1993; LaFasto and Larson, 2001; Barker, Cegala, Kibler, and Wahlers, 1979). The business world had provided a large venue for this concept, which historically had been reserved for sports and competitions.

Teamwork and *teams* are terms that we take for granted, because they have become so popular in the business world. We must be careful, however, to recognize the differences between teams and groups working on a project. Not every group is a team. In fact, several factors are needed to make a team. Katzenbach and Smith (1993) outline these quite nicely in their book *The Wisdom of Teams*. Differentiating between working groups and teams, they say that working groups focus on individual accountability and sometimes delegate work to others outside the group. One example of a working group is a sales force with members assigned to individual regions. These salespeople are accountable to customers and the company, but not to one another. Teams, on the other hand, have mutual as well as individual accountability. Teams also rely on more than mere debate and information sharing: their members rely on one another. Their products are direct products of the collaborative contributions of members. It is not the individual who is credited with an idea—a sale, project, or policy change—but rather the team.

Why are teams so important in the workplace today? "Much of the work in organizations is done in teams," says Druskat (2001, p. 81). An increasing number of important functions are handled by teams rather than by individual workers. For example, in many nursing units, nurses and nursing assistants care for the same patients. For that reason, this chapter will focus on building the emotional intelligence not only of individuals, but also of entire teams.

Why the Study of Emotional Intelligence in Teams Is So Important

In a 1989 strategic management text, teams were only mentioned twice, and briefly at that. Once, project teams were acknowledged as groups within a business that might dissolve as soon as their project was completed or might go on to form a complete business unit. Little more was said about their development or characteristics. In an earlier section, the authors presented a grid to outline the personality types of effective management team members. For example, there were certain personality traits that the team leader, resource investigator, team worker, and finisher needed to have. In creating this grid, the authors credited earlier works dating back to the mid-1970s that were specifically dedicated to management teams and the traits of team members (Johnson, Scholes, and Sexty, 1989).

One factor that was desirable for some but not necessarily all members of the team was a high IQ. Introversion and extroversion were also defining characteristics for those in various team roles, as were a tendency toward anxiety, a sense of urgency, and emotionality. If a person were an emotional, dominant, impulsive extrovert, for example, he might best be placed in the role of shaper for the team. Finishers were anxious, introverted individuals who might worry excessively about follow-through. Team leaders were described as "stable, dominant extroverts" who concentrated on objectives and made sure people were focused on their areas of greatest ability (Johnson, Scholes, and Sexty, 1989, p. 123). Attempts such as these to define teams and the personalities or abilities of team members continued well into the 1990s. Such delineations as "supervisors work *in* the system and team leaders work *on* the system" (Fisher, 1993, p. 126) and relationship roles such as "encourager, harmonizer and gatekeeper" (Montebello, 1994, p. 128) began to pop up in texts devoted strictly to the formation and management of teams.

There is a marked shift in recent literature to the characteristics of the team itself, not just of the individual team members. The explosion of books and articles dedicated to teams appears to support this thought. What is this entity called a team? the writings ask. What are its characteristics?

Group effectiveness includes a focus on contribution, says Drucker (2001). He points out that hospitals, probably the most complex of modern-day knowledge organizations, require multiple disciplines to work together as a matter of course. Their working together requires that they communicate as professionals with the same goal in mind. Cooper and Sawaf (1997) characterize teams themselves as "building closer connections, experiencing each other as more real, unique humans" (p. 33). Weisinger (1998) says that teams experience additional challenges in communication that are not encountered on the individual level. Also, Fisher (1993) describes teams as being "jointly responsible for whole work processes" (p. 15).

These descriptions represent only a few of the ways that teams have been characterized. The key point is that teams have taken on a life of their own. The individuals who populate teams are of ultimate importance, but the team has become a new entity—a conglomerate that has its own culture and character, much like a corporation or a family. This complexity makes it necessary to study the nature of team dynamics and the emotional dynamics that drive behaviors within teams, influence their decision making, and lead to results.

Why Emotional Aptitude Is Needed for Teams to Work Smoothly: Downloading the Essentials

Another group of analogies that are frequently used in the business world come from the technical sector. Many people are required to understand basic computer terminology in order to do their job. Further, there are some things we are required to do in order to efficiently obtain the information we need. Any of us who have ever visited the Internet or received e-mail has probably been prompted to download something. Downloading, in its most basic sense, has to do with getting a piece of information from somewhere and putting it in a usable form on our own computer. We can visit a Web site, click on a link, download something, and save it to a file on our own personal drive or hard drive. We might download a program to help us view a certain file or download software that will assist with filing tax returns or protecting our computer from harmful viruses. With some e-mail services, incoming attachments from others must be scanned for viruses before they can be downloaded to the subscriber's personal computer.

In a similar way, the team downloads material from its leader. Downloading in this sense simply refers to gathering and using information. Teams do this every day, whether they are conscious of it or not, and the material is of utmost importance. Which abilities must teams garner from their leaders in order to perform effectively? In the next chapter, we will focus on coaching and developing that information; in this one, we will focus on what that information is.

Because people are working on teams, they have the opportunity to learn from one another. The ways in which other team members handle situations and interactions can be learned, both through description and through observation. In this learning process, members of the team have the chance to collectively and individually review the emotional components and management styles present during the interactions (Kram and Cherniss, 2001). In addition, teams promote the sharing of feedback and advice (Kram and Cherniss, 2001, LaFasto and Larson, 2001), which provides additional opportunities for reflection by the individual members. In other words, each team member can look at a situation from his or her own perspective, recognize his or her own emotional reactions, and acknowledge how those reactions are affecting his or her thoughts on the situation. Each team member can also recall how he or she handled a similar situation (Kram and Cherniss, 2001).

One thing that is important to remember is that while we think of teams as organized to accomplish certain work tasks, there is also an element of emotional work that they must accomplish. Katzenbach and Smith (1993) point out that teamwork is risky because it involves overcoming a normal reluctance to trust someone else with one's fate. Whether the team's primary objective is to solve problems, successfully pursue accreditation, suggest quality improvements, or just operate and monitor the day-to-day, an amount of emotional labor will be necessary. Emotional labor involves regulating feelings and expressions in order to meet organizational goals (Grandey, 2000). Morris and Feldman (1996, p. 987) say that emotional labor is "the effort, planning and control needed to express organizationally desired emotion during interpersonal transactions." Ashforth and Humphrey (1993) supported this by indicating that individuals can modify their emotions in order to fit into a broader social setting. The implication from each of these sources is that emotions are not effective in and of themselves in accomplishing goals and facilitating productive relationships; some kind of intense regulation or management of them must occur.

We can imagine how this can be challenging. A variety of people, all with individual motivations and goals, come together as a team, which now has its own characteristics and goals. The goals are perhaps obvious; the characteristics less so. The team is made up of different *individuals*. Suppose someone does not like something that someone else has suggested (and that everyone else has agreed to) and knows that he must modify that reaction to be appropriate within the culture of the team and the organization. First, what exactly defines what is appropriate, and how do other team members interpret that definition? What specific reaction would the team define as appropriate? Do the unwritten rules governing this group's interaction allow feelings to be expressed as they occur, or must they be packaged a certain way? Can the person be blatant about his disagreement, diplomatic about his disagreement, or should he not dare to disagree at all? Once an opinion is expressed, is it heard or is it ignored against the backdrop of the prevailing group opinion? In addition, does this reaction to the opinion lead to further emotional conflict in the team member? Between team members? Would there be those who disdained a negative feeling toward the group's momentum so highly that either unbridled debate would ensue or members of the team would sit seething in their own emotional stew? Would this emotional conflict consequently impede progress? Would the team member become isolated and nonparticipative because his feelings are not heard? Would other team members isolate the team member who tried to express himself?

It sounds like work, and it is. The possible outcomes could be numerous, depending on the emotional capabilities of the team and its members.

As far back as the early 1980s, Hochschild (1983, p. 7) described emotional labor as "the management of feeling to create a publicly observable facial and bodily display." Management of emotions requires effort and often involves a form of acting, especially in a workplace that tends to encourage positive expressions over negative ones (Staw, Sutton, and Pelled, 1994; Elfenbein and Ambady, 2002; Hochschild, 1983; Grandey, 2000). Elfenbein and Ambady (2002) cited Swann, Stein-Seroussi, and McNulty (1992), Tesser and Rosen, (1975), and DePaulo (1992) in observing that emotions are often masked in order to conform to standards, but in social situations, negative interpersonal feelings are apt to show up through poorly controlled media such as vocal tone. Even in a group setting where everyone is trying to agree, there is the potential for vocal tone to break through the façade and create conflict. In situations of conflict, the offended is often heard to say, "It's not what you said; it's how you said it."

Downloadable Emotional Aptitudes Needed for Effective Teamwork

With the emotional potential of teams being so volatile, how can we assist team members in understanding and incorporating the principles of emotional intelligence in their interactions? What we want to accomplish is not playacting but rather continual learning about the meanings that emotions convey about relationships, how emotions progress and change, and their overall function (Vitello-Cicciu, 2002; Mayer, Salovey, and Caruso, 2000, 2002). There are several competencies that sound emotional aptitude may produce and that the team should be able to download from its leader.

Downloadable Competency 1: Perceiving Strengths, Weaknesses, and Issues

Job interviews and performance evaluations are notorious for focusing on our strengths and weaknesses. In job interviews, we are usually asked to describe our own perspective; a performance evaluation may be our manager's perception of our talents and foibles or an agreement that is arrived at jointly about our areas of focus for the following year. Somewhere in the middle, during our years of employment, comes the manifestation of what our strengths and weaknesses truly are, as they relate to the job and the specific challenges it places before us. "Unfortunately," say Marcus Buckingham and Donald Clifton (2001) in their book *Now, Discover*

Your Strengths, "most of us have little sense of our talents and strengths, much less the ability to build our lives around them." The goal of their publication is to help readers determine what the themes of their specific strengths are and then build on those aspects of themselves.

When Mayer, Salovey, and Caruso (2000, 2002) defined perception of emotion, they placed it at the most foundational level of their hierarchy, indicating that one cannot advance to the levels of using, understanding, or managing emotion unless one first has the ability to recognize emotions accurately. Not surprisingly, there are emotional capabilities and tendencies that may be seen as strengths or weaknesses (or both). One of our jobs as leaders is to make sure that we recognize those capacities in team members, as well as within ourselves. In addition, we should be able to recognize when an emotional issue is present.

Recognizing emotion, however, is not always the easiest thing to do. An emotional state may or may not be as obvious as a coffee stain on someone's white shirt. In a meeting or team effort, an emotional state may be masked, suppressed, or so well controlled that it can barely be noticed (Swann, Stein-Seroussi, and McNulty, 1992; Tesser and Rosen, 1975; DePaulo, 1992; Staw, Sutton, and Pelled, 1994—all cited in Elfenbein and Ambady, 2002; Hochschild, 1983; Grandey, 2000). Therein lies the trouble. Not only are these emotions often less than obvious in others, but they are also often unrecognized by the person who has them. This further complicates issues, because team members may experience escalations of their own feelings without even knowing that a specific feeling is at the root. "Teams are cauldrons of bubbling emotions," observes Goleman. "They are often charged with reaching a consensus—hard enough with two people and much more difficult as the numbers increase" (1998a, p. 101).

Boyatzis (2001) outlines the importance of understanding one's own strengths and weaknesses in examination of oneself. This foundation is imperative for a team to be emotionally well equipped. The team must understand its strengths and weaknesses so that it can capitalize on the strengths and address the weaknesses, just as an individual would. Buckingham and Clifton (2001) describe themes such as empathy and positivity as strength themes. The ability to organize people toward a common goal has connections with motivation to achieve, as can the strength of commitment to an organization. Social skills, including empathy, may qualify people for a management role within a team (Goleman, 1998a). Executives who select leadership solely based on technical skills may face disaster as the appointee's lack of interpersonal skills becomes apparent (Edmondson, Bohmer, and Pisano, 2001). As we look for these and other strengths in team members and help them to realize them within themselves, we are laying the foundation for a well-functioning team. This is very similar to selecting the right talent for the job, which was discussed in Chapter Six.

Team leaders and managers must keep an eye on the emotional barometer of the team and of its individuals. Consider the example of a customer service representative who sits in a meeting of a newly formed team and rolls her eyes at every idea, even countering with reasons why each idea will not work. Everyone just assumes she is acting out of character; she is certainly unlike the star performer they have heard about. Some may even dislike her for her bad attitude. What is really happening is that she is unhappy and downright insulted that a team of people has been formed to discuss something she was known as quite capable of handling. The team, and especially the team leader, needs to notice the defensiveness that she is displaying in order to understand the issue and begin to resolve it (Druskat, 2001).

Team members and team leaders need to be constantly vigilant for emotions that may cause dissident behaviors and not just automatically assume that they are the result of someone having a bad day (although they could be) or that the person is a bad fit for the team (although they may be). Finding out what the issues and emotions really are and their underlying causes will enhance the productivity of the team and enable the team members to move on to using emotions to keep the team's momentum going in the right direction.

Downloadable Competency 2: Facilitation of Decision Making

"To make sound decisions, examine the issue in a methodical way" (Kinsella, 2001, p. 53).

"Complex decision making goes hand in hand with critical thinking" (Martin, 2002, p. 243).

"The physician must look elsewhere for guidance when basic principles alone are inadequate to resolve an ethical conflict" (Garrison, 2003, p. 1217).

Obviously, decision making is not an exact science. Yet decision making is what teams, made up of individuals, are usually tasked with doing. Managers and leaders make decisions almost daily, and they often struggle with it themselves. When teams come together to make a decision, the entire process takes place in the "emotional cauldron" (Goleman, 1998a). Therein, a methodical process, critical thinking, or basic principles are certain not to fully suffice. The emotional element must be considered.

Rather than impeding rational thought, emotions handled properly can actually facilitate thought processes, according to Mayer, Salovey, and Caruso (2000). It is essential that we stay aware of what we are feeling and that we use that awareness wisely to affect our mental processes.

In the health care setting, decisions often involve ethical considerations. While some issues are minor and can be resolved quickly, others require team input (Hughes, 2002). There may not be an obvious right or wrong answer, and choosing between principles may be required. Each person on the team may place emphasis on a different principle. Each team member should possess an understanding of how his or her own emotions play into a particular espoused principle.

In the health care setting, uncertainty often arises about the outcome of a decision. In all fields, admittedly, there may be uncertainty about the outcome, but in health care, customers' lives and health states can be affected by our decisions. Although decisions in the corporate world are termed *business decisions* in order to emphasize that they are made based on the objective realities of doing business and not based on emotional considerations, the truth remains that business decisions affect people (Kerfoot, 2002). A business decision to reduce staff may, for example, compromise patient outcomes. In order to keep staff on track, the emotions triggered by the inherent uncertainty in decisions and even crises must often be absorbed by an empathetic leader (Citrin, 2002); the leader must also understand that he cannot keep absorbing this type of stress unless his own emotional stores are routinely recharged.

A decision for or against something often involves change. One challenge of team leadership is that new processes must be implemented often (Edmondson, Bohmer, and Pisano, 2001). Change of any kind implies loss for some, if not all, affected by the change. Team members who would be affected by the change inevitably experience emotional reactions to the prospect of the transition. Potential loss of identity, of belonging, or of job meaning can stir up undesirable emotions that may affect the decision to change (Strickland, 2000). Team members and their leaders should be aware of the potential impact of these emotions and do everything possible to bring them to the table and understand how they are affecting the decision.

Consider the situation of a team meeting among medical office administrative personnel to discuss a proposal that would improve efficiency in the billing process. The group is deciding on recommendations for a new coding system that is said to cut the work of billing almost in half. The new system is said to require only 60 percent of the time that the current system takes to bill insurance payers and patients. Management is, of course, excited about the prospects of such a cost savings, but the future users of the new system have varying views. One member of the team is so swamped with other responsibilities that he is thrilled about such a system. However, someone else is fearful that the increased efficiency will ultimately mean decreased personnel, and because she was the last to be hired, she fears she will be the first to go. Another has spent a great amount of time building, improving, and training others to use the current system and feels a certain affinity for the status quo. You can see how the emotions at the moment might have a great impact on the decision-making process and the decision itself. While in theory, everyone should agree that efficiency is positive, their emotions may affect thought processes, resulting in much different attitudes toward the change.

The team leader should make sure that all of these feelings are recognized. Often this involves careful consideration beforehand of what the feelings might be. The leader can expect the swamped associate to be relatively excited about the prospect of relief and very much for the proposal in the absence of other factors. Excitement about the change might be evident on this person's face. However, the person who is afraid for her job may be afraid to admit it, fearing that her peers will think she is whining when the improvement is supposed to be such a great thing. If she feels strongly enough about this and her concerns are not addressed, she may come up with other, more objective reasons for rejecting the change. So might the person who feels the strong relationship with the old system. He may know the system so well that he is able to point out its benefits, as well as the corners cut by the new system. He, too, may not want his fellow team members to know that he feels like griping or mourning the loss of something very meaningful to him. Acknowledging these feelings (or, if they are not verbalized, the potential for these feelings) might promote freer dialogue and also might encourage team members to put their feelings in perspective when considering what is best for the organization. None of this can be done without understanding how emotions facilitate thought.

Downloadable Competency 3: Evaluating Emotional Components of Communication Transactions

Several principles of emotional intelligence involve relations with others (Mayer, Salovey, and Caruso, 2000, 2002; Goleman, 1998a; Kram and Cherniss, 2001). Recently, there has been increased focus on relationship-centered care, which has been shown to improve patient satisfaction and outcomes (Marvel, Bailey, Pfaffly, Gunn, and Beckman, 2003). *Relationship-centered* means having awareness of interpersonal process, listening carefully, and responding to clues during interactions (Levinson, Gorawam-Bhat, and Lamb, 2000).

Marvel, Bailey, Pfaffly, Gunn, and Beckman (2003) conducted a study of forty-five meetings in health care settings in order to study the type and frequency of relationship-centered actions in meetings. The preliminary results of this study showed that the leaders involved, especially female leaders, used relationship-centered communication techniques such as praising group members for effort and encouraging input. Other techniques that were less frequently used included verbally summarizing a discussion, setting clear agendas, and responding to the feelings of the team members.

The researchers found that participants in 84 percent of the meetings expressed emotions but that leaders only responded to the emotions in 42 percent of the meetings. More frequent relationship-centered interactions were acknowledging opinions (71 percent) and recognizing contributions of participants (96 percent) (Marvel, Bailey, Pfaffly, Gunn, and Beckman, 2003).

This is only one study, but it points out that a group of key skills are necessary for relationship-centered team interactions. Many of us think of good communication skills as those skills that assure our words and intentions are clear, our message understood, and desired results obtained. Skillful, relationship-centered communication takes it a step further. Leaders who practice this type of communication are focused on the team. They acknowledge contributions as well as concerns; they value opinions and backgrounds. They look for the emotional element. The goal of their communication is not just to be understood but also to understand.

Leaders who recognize the emotional potential inherent in group communications will pay particular attention to relationship-centered transactions, for the following reason: as discussed earlier in this book, emotions have a way of building on themselves and progressing to other emotions that can be either more productive or more harmful than the ones from which they originated (Mayer, Salovey, and Caruso, 2000). The ability to understand how this occurs is critical for a team leader and ultimately for all members of the team.

The study participants who failed to give credence to the feelings expressed by meeting attendees (Marvel, Bailey, Pfaffly, Gunn, and Beckman, 2003) did the team a disservice not only because they may have avoided the issue at hand and prevented uninhibited communication but also because they might have missed an opportunity to manage a negative feeling that had the potential to escalate into something much worse. Expression of a negative feeling may indicate the need for clarification or for feedback, both of which indicate that clear communication is not taking place. Further, negative emotions can provide warning that an uglier, more counterproductive emotion may be just around the corner. An expression of a negative emotion in a team setting is actually a benefit in that way, although many leaders prefer not to acknowledge it because they would rather press on with a particular agenda.

By applying emotional understanding to group communication, team members and leaders can consciously avoid the pitfalls of ignoring emotions that are not going to go away, and present themselves with the opportunities to manage them through building alliances, negotiating, strengthening morale, and carrying the team's banner to others within the organization.

Downloadable Competency 4: Managing Emotions Through Negotiation

The preceding competencies reflected the first three branches of the Mayer, Salovey, and Caruso (2000, 2002) model of emotional intelligence, and the next four competencies will emphasize the aptitude of emotion management, which Mayer, Salovey, and Caruso define as modulating feelings in oneself and others in order to promote growth. This level of emotional intelligence is explored in greater depth because it is often the desired outcome of emotional transactions. While recognizing, using, and understanding emotions are all essential building blocks, they are but foundational to the effective management of emotions, which leads to desired results. Team members who have mastered the first three elements can also achieve the ability to manage emotions to accomplish goals.

One important emotion management skill is negotiation of conflict. "Conflict," say Smith, Tutor, and Phillips, "is a natural part of life, an ordinary part of human interaction, and like all other interactions, may be constructive or destructive" (2001, p. 37). A particular conflict may be exhibited in intrapersonal, interpersonal, intergroup, or even all three spheres. "Teamwork can also be a source of conflict," says Sessa (1998, p. 41).

The need for negotiation of conflict or of group decisions may arise when feelings are acknowledged and understood. As Chapter Nine will emphasize, many leaders are afraid of conflict, and this may be one reason that emotions are not acknowledged: they bring the threat of conflict. This book devotes an entire chapter (Chapter Nine) to conflict resolution and the emotional principles behind it, but we will touch on a few points here.

First, negotiation needs to occur with emotions under control. The most important emotion to control is anger. Anger can progress from mild irritation to explosive rage (Smith, Tutor, and Phillips, 2001). Anger is a secondary emotion that may have roots in unexpressed jealousy, hurt, or fear (Kaye, 1994).

The emphasis must be resolution, not who is right (Smith, Tutor, and Phillips, 2001). This is the same principle that was reflected in the discussion of performing autopsies of situations in Chapter Six.

Benton (1999) describes seven types of power that many people use to effect desired results. For example, a certain amount of power is present in our position or resource availability. If we have the title or the staff to get something done, it is more likely that we can make it happen. Perceived position is very important. How do the team members see you? Do they see you as trustworthy or as manipulative? Benton warns against using coercive power, which can actually generate hostility, although it appears on the surface to garner rapid results. As leaders, we must remember that negotiation should take into account team members' feelings, the mental processes that arise from those feelings, and the potential for escalation of those feelings.

Smith, Tutor, and Phillips (2001) further explain that our methods of communication affect the way we negotiate conflict as well. Passive avoidance behavior often results from low self-esteem, while responding passively involves going along with what others decide to avoid making a choice of one's own. Aggressive reactive behavior may leave others feeling attacked when their ideas are shot down. Assertive proactive communication is the type that is truly focused on resolving issues (Covey, 1990). Note how emotions play a part in the various methods of communication and how they may affect the leader's or the team's ability to negotiate conflict. When the leader recognizes one of the maladaptive behaviors, he should work with the team member to overcome it and become more assertive and proactive in his approach to conflict.

Downloadable Competency 5: Building Alliances Through Attention to Emotional Needs

Trends in the workplace such as shift work, long hours, harassment, low wages, downsizing, and the burdens imposed by technology contribute to more anger and anxiety in employees than ever before (Helge, 2001). Stress, job dissatisfaction, and anxiety disorders cost employers, collectively, billions of dollars per year in health care. Other costly factors that may not be as easy to measure include absenteeism, poor productivity and performance, and undesirable behaviors at work, such as theft, aggression, and hostility (Chen and Spector, 1992; Lundberg and Tulczak, 1997).

Unfortunately, most of these stress-producing culprits are present in health care. Nurses cite patients, understaffing, administration, and coworkers as the top four categories of stressors at work (Humphrey, 1998). Shift work is expected: hospitals never close, not even in horrible weather; unlike those of industrial and white-collar concerns, their doors remain open, with staff expected to report in any way possible. Long hours may be common, especially if downsizing reduces the available staff per unit, and technological advances keep coming in spite of it all. Our colleagues are in no way protected from the consequences of the corporate drive toward efficiency. Even worse, loyal performance no longer guarantees job security, as it might have several decades ago (Helge, 2001). Poor relationships with coworkers also are associated with feelings of threat (Ross and Altmaier, 1994). When we are working in a team situation, any or all of these organizational factors may be present. The team may be on the receiving end of the consequences of an individual's stress, lack of sleep, or feelings of being overwhelmed. Undoubtedly, many team members bring similar stress factors to the table.

While it is difficult to modify the nature of the health care environment—for example, the long hours, shift work, or downsizing—it is possible for the team leader to modify the emotional environment wherein team members practice and share dialogue. The team leader can build alliances with team members and encourage them to share their feelings openly. It is very important that plans and processes take into account the emotional needs of the team members and not just the task at hand (Gustafson, 2003). This means encouraging employees to express their feelings and to develop their emotional strength so that they can cope with the stressors that are relentlessly thrown their way (Helge, 2001). Effective management of the environment of the team helps to create an atmosphere of trust and alliance within the team.

Downloadable Competency 6: Building Team Morale

Low morale is said to contribute to poor productivity, yet it may be one of the least talked-about phenomena in business. Least talked about, that is, in the venue where it can be resolved. Reluctant to share their feelings with the boss, workers with low morale will typically discuss their feelings with colleagues, friends, and family members. In these situations, an us-versus-them mind-set may encroach on the team environment (Fuller, 1990). Obviously, this is not the kind of mind-set we want to foster among teams. Yet when morale is low, enthusiasm can be sapped to such a degree that nothing gets accomplished. On the other hand, too much enthusiasm can result in mismanaged hopes and eventual discouragement when an idea fails (Egan, 1994).

If morale problems are sapping a team, empathy can be part of the antidote. Right off the bat, it helps to dispel the notion that the leader and the team members are on opposite sides. Empathy, according to McLeod (1999), is used in situations in which the ability of someone to understand someone else's feelings or experience has become problematic. Because we are each defined by our own unique blend of culture, background, work experience, education, position, and socioeconomic circumstances, we must invoke empathy in order to be able to understand or appreciate the views of others whose life experiences differ from ours. We need empathy to relate to those around us who come from diverse perspectives. Empathy allows and encourages us to look deep into the inner self of the other person (McLeod, 1999).

The empathic leader can apply this ability as he or she identifies and manages morale problems. Managers do not enjoy admitting that teams have sagging morale. We certainly would never intentionally try to ruin morale, but we can if we fail to consider the impact of our decisions on team members, act consistently, or give timely feedback in the appropriate setting (Fuller, 1990).

These are basic supervisory principles, but they are included here because they contain so many relational principles that are basic to maintaining high morale. Many of them have been discussed in previous chapters in more detail. How do we, as leaders in a challenging, technologically complex, and sometimes stress-laden environment, go beyond day-to-day supervisory responsiveness to stay attuned to and manage the morale of our associates?

Silversin and Kornacki (2003) give some excellent pointers in their article on implementing change. Sagging morale can foster resistance to change. People feel more included, more a part of the process, when leaders acknowledge their constituents' diverse contributions to their department, unit, or project. It is all about centering the thought process on the team. Studies have, in fact, shown strong relationships between high morale and employee involvement (Lundberg and Tulczak, 1997).

Each team member should be allowed to share how he or she envisions the results of the team's efforts. Openness, as well as divergent points of view, should be encouraged. The vision should be something meaningful to the team. The team members should feel that they will benefit from the work of the team, because it is very likely that they are giving something up to work on the project or effect the change. (Emotional responses to change were discussed earlier in this chapter under Downloadable Competency 2.) Expectations should be clear; staff should be treated fairly; and negative, morale-sapping emotions should be acknowledged and managed (Silversin and Kornacki, 2003).

Change management goes far beyond these simple principles; it was addressed much more fully in Chapter Four. But these principles are fundamental to maintaining the group spirit and morale needed to effect positive change. The team leader skilled in emotion management will be better equipped to apply these principles to their intrateam interactions.

Downloadable Competency 7: Acting as Ambassadors

Most of us are familiar with what an ambassador does. Loosely defined, he or she is someone who represents a group to an entirely different group. Ambassadors are the spokespeople for the group they represent.

Speaking of health care leaders in general, Tyler (2003) remarks that times have changed for organizations. Leaders who were accustomed to being ambassadors who represented their organization to the outside world and maintained visibility in the community and in the industry have been swept into the morass of financial, staffing, and other issues. One might rightly argue that nurse leaders have time to do little other than put out fires at home.

But the role of ambassador is extremely important within the organization and the community. Birrer (2002), for example, describes physician leaders as ambassadors of sorts. Specifically, the physician is a diplomat who acts as a liaison between a provider organization and the medical community. He or she is often in a position to conduct business with managed care organizations, other specialists, and the hospital, and must do so to effectively treat patients. Nurse leaders have similar responsibilities. Diplomacy is key to interaction with multiple hospital departments, physicians who must be awakened at 2:00 A.M. to secure a medication order, and a variety of staff members. The nurse leader must represent strength, tact, and understanding.

Tyler (2003) relates that leadership should be redefined to be consistent with the changes in the health care environment. The term *team builder* is perhaps more central to being a nurse leader than ever before. In addition to building the team, the team leader should support and applaud the team's efforts and contributions within the organization, which may be so large that the efforts of the individual might go unnoticed. In this way, the nurse leader is an ambassador not only for her team, but for her profession as well.

There are certain characteristics that the physician or nurse leader needs to have that may not have been necessary centuries ago, including courage, focus, energy, and vision. Physicians and nurses do have distinct roles in the delivery of patient care, but the nurse role is particularly unique. He or she must often coordinate the services that the physician deems medically appropriate for the patient, and also must ascertain that the services are rendered properly and on time. The nurse represents the face of health care, and must advocate for the patient with physicians, other disciplines, and sometimes insurers. The nurse leader takes this role a step further in working with the team. In much the same way that the nurse advocates for the patient and is the face of the health care system to the patient, the nurse leader advocates for the team and serves as a window for nurses to look into when they want to understand the organization that the leader represents.

Nurse leaders should also be ambassadors, for the team, to the organization. In a memorial written about a talented colleague who passed away in early 2003, the decedent was described as "an outstanding ambassador for nurses" ("Colleagues remember talented leader," 2003). Further, this individual was described as someone who was "down to earth, approachable and full of fun, but never lost sight of her role as a nurse leader." Interestingly, twenty years earlier, she had "helped to ease tension among midwives annoyed that their profession was to be regulated alongside nursing for the first time."

Here was a nurse leader who, in a very brief memorial tribute, was remembered not only for her leadership and character but also for her role as an ambassador for the profession. Most significantly, the act she was most remembered for was her success in easing tension among a group of midwives who were experiencing emotional conflict over a change. In her long career, there could have been dozens of other outstanding acts, but the writer chose that one to exemplify her many contributions to the field. She was remembered most because she represented the nursing staff in a way that eased conflict and helped the profession. This is what is meant by serving as ambassador for nursing to the organization. The nurses who had known the decedent no doubt cherished the memories of her attempting to represent them in making the hospital a better, more peaceful place to work. One might imagine that she was a problem solver and someone you could go to when you did not know how to handle a situation. Then, because she was on your side, she would help you come to a conclusion about your course of action while preserving your dignity and accountability. That is being an ambassador for nursing and nurses within the team itself: respecting each staff nurse and promoting their value continually, while representing a standard of nursing that nurses should want to achieve.

Leader Support Capabilities for Leading Effective Teams

Thus far, this chapter has focused on teams—specifically, on competencies of group leaders and members that foster effective teamwork. In addition, effective team leaders need to cultivate some specific capabilities in order to support the transfer and development of the team-building competencies. Much like the capacity of the Internet to support downloading of files, leaders must have the capacity to allow their teams to effectively download and use the information and skills that have just been discussed. The remainder of this chapter will present three of these support capabilities and explain why they are so important to teams.

Support Capability 1: Acceptance and Recognition of Experimentation

Someone once quipped that it was paradoxical that physicians and dentists claim to *practice*. If they are only practicing, why in the world are they working on patients? While this remark was made lightly, it reflects a common attitude in business. If you are constantly experimenting or you make many mistakes, what in the world are you doing in management or even in a line position? Shouldn't people in a job know what they are doing well enough to make keen judgments about change and good decisions about next steps?

The theoretical answer is no. There are indeed managers who cringe at the thought of a mistake being made or of being used as an example of what not to do, and often their anxiety is justified. On the other hand, there is a pervasive idea in the literature that effective and wise leaders are those who encourage experimentation, expect mistakes, and have a practical understanding of which experiments and mistakes can be made without undue consequence to the organization (Chaffee and Arthur, 2002; Grazier, 2003; Christensen and Raynor, 2003). The emotionally astute leader masters this kind of weighing of risks versus benefits and builds his followers' comfort level with this mind-set.

Stories about experimentation and failure in industry, invention, and even government are romanticized so much that we almost forget that the failures even happened. The rough advent of air travel is one example. Today we whisk around the country or across the sea with little effort and remarkable precision and speed. But decades ago, aviators were struggling to understand why their application of flight principles worked some of the time but not all of the time. Today, that standard would be unacceptable: we must have an assurance that, barring outside incident or malfunction, the airplane is made to stay in the air and to compensate for external forces that may challenge that ability. There was a time, however, when every successful flight was a victory (Christensen and Raynor, 2003). It is hard to imagine that air travel was ever so experimental, but that stage was a necessary though long and hard first step to what we now take for granted.

"That wasn't so bad," we are able to say today. But put potential failure in front of someone, and chances are good that he will want to run and hide. "While companies are beginning to accept the value of failure in the abstract—at the level of corporate policies, processes, and practices," write Farson and Keyes, "it's an entirely different matter at the personal level." Everyone hates to fail. We assume that we will suffer embarrassment and a loss of esteem and stature. Perhaps nowhere is the fear of failure more intense than in the competitive world of business, where a mistake can mean losing a bonus, a promotion, or even a job" (2002, p. 65).

Leaders who encourage experimentation realize that failure is possible, but they further realize that failure is necessary to achieve just about anything substantial. However, until recently, the value of failure has received little attention in the literature. The leader who prizes, studies, and treasures failure is definitely swimming against the current of a modern business environment that prizes success.

The effective leader will be able to manage the emotional conflicts (fear, anxiety, embarrassment) arising from an aversion to risk taking and find it possible to promote experimentation within their team. Grazier (2003) describes a hospital training program that seeks to integrate the ideas of innovation, idea flow, and creativity into organizational culture. The president of the organization that runs the program says that one can reduce risk by improving the ability to prototype and experiment. Experimentation is a skill that we can get better at.

By accepting the fact that experimentation is a skill, we can move toward the concept of organizational or group learning. Organizations learn from experience just as individuals do (O'Sullivan, 1999). How can we pretend to always see clearly what we should do when the environment before us is so full of clouds? To do so would be unfair to ourselves as leaders and especially to our followers. To help guide your steps, encourage experimentation, and encourage learning when failure has occurred. "That's the key to coming up with breakthrough products and processes:

viewing mistakes for the educational tools they are and as signposts on the road to success," according to Farson and Keyes (2002, p. 71).

Support Capability 2: Problem Solving

"I have excellent problem-solving skills," boast many job applicants. Problem solving, unlike failure, is not something we tend to avoid. We do not want to cause problems, certainly, but we love to be known as being able to solve them.

Our jobs are laden with problems. Some problems are good problems, such as how to grow an organization or how to manage a high-profile project that has been handed off to us. We sometimes refer to these as "exciting challenges." Other problems are not as desirable—for example, physician complaints, declining patient status, or absenteeism. The first thing that comes to the mind of most nurses is likely to be the negative aspect of the word *problem*.

An emotionally capable nurse leader views problem solving from the perspective of one who has accepted that problems will arise. If the health care consumer did not have or anticipate the potential of a problem, she would not show up for treatment. Problems do not devastate the seasoned leader; rather, they represent focal points for the leader's emotional energy.

Broad-scale problem solving often occurs through restructuring an organization or a process. When a problem has become thematic or pervasive, organizational leaders begin to discuss what kind of overall change (such as restructuring) might eliminate the problem. For example, in response to a plethora of nurse complaints and reports of job dissatisfaction, leaders may decide that that nurses need education in new skills and that patients should be taught more self-management (Porter-O'Grady and Afable, 2002). The types of problems that we cannot restructure away—conflicts between people, personal issues, situational crises—tend to hit us in the face when we are getting ready to leave for the day or just when we think things are going smoothly. These are the types of problems that nurse leaders must have the emotional wisdom to recognize, process, and assist the team in solving. Since many problems have an emotional element (either an emotional root or an emotional reaction), one of the key functions of the nurse leader is to recognize emotion as one of the factors in either the problem or the fallout caused by the problem. As the leader develops in emotional ability and helps team members to do the same, she can guide employees through the thought processes and the understanding and managing of their own emotions in order to come up with a satisfactory solution to the problem (Mayer, Salovey, and Caruso,

2000, 2002). If nurse leaders don't consider the emotional component of a situation and address it, they limit themselves to a logical and rational approach to a problem that may not be solely logical and rational.

Support Capability 3: The Ability to Let Go

Letting go comes more easily to some leaders than to others, but it is a necessary skill for the effective leader. Letting go means allowing team members to take over tasks, management of processes, and responsibility for decision making once they have developed sufficient skills to do so. Letting go also involves allowing the team to experiment and solve problems before it has developed sufficiently to be independent.

The clear opposite of letting go is micromanagement. "The administrator who is able to let go can enjoy the role of facilitator and mentor to subordinates" (Davidhizar and Shearer, 2002, p. 34). Letting go goes hand in hand with encouraging experimentation. Often a manager will fear letting go and letting team members try something new because she fears that they will fail to handle the situation. Failure on a team is thought to reflect poorly on the leader's performance. The leader who has become skilled at letting go can truthfully say that she trusts her team members as competent professionals. She doesn't supervise constantly, but she encourages her constituents to ask for assistance if they need it (Davidhizar and Shearer, 2002).

Peddy (1998) describes how in mentorship there comes a time to let go. However, letting go as a mentor means maintaining loose ties that are never broken; the same is somewhat true for team leaders who are empowering and delegating to their teams, although their formal ties remain intact. Business as a whole is still struggling with the concept of having team members and nonmanagement personnel accept responsibility for problem solving (which used to be strictly the responsibility of management) while management focuses on facilitating and supporting the teams that are getting the job done (Fisher, 1993). The emotionally intelligent leader will grasp the concept of delegation as an empowering and enlightening tool.

Summary

The concept of teams in business and in health care is not a new one, but it has gained increasing recognition in the past two decades. Emotional intelligence is important not only for team members individually but for the team as a functional unit. Through emotional learning, whole teams can be aware of and fully utilize emotions to facilitate the best possible solution to problems. Teams that are emotionally intelligent evaluate communication transactions for emotional components and are skilled at negotiation, building interteam and intrateam alliances, and building morale through empathy. With high team morale, leaders and members of a team are able to be ambassadors for the team to other areas of the organization.

Because leaders lead teams, not just individuals, leaders must be especially careful to promote emotionally healthy teamwork through encouragement of experimentation, acute problem-solving abilities, and a willingness to let go and empower the team when the time is right.

TEN CRITERIA FOR AN EMOTIONALLY COMPETENT TEAM

1. Team members and leaders can recognize emotional issues and the strengths and weaknesses of team members.

2. Team members and leaders can effectively use emotion to assist, not impede, decision making.

3. Team members and leaders are able to evaluate emotional components of communication transactions.

4. Team members and leaders are able to build alliances within the team.

5. Team members and leaders are able to negotiate in times of conflict.

6. Team members and leaders maintain high morale.

7. Team members and leaders can act as ambassadors to other organizational groups and to individuals outside of the team.

8. Team leaders promote and recognize the value of experimentation.

9. Team leaders are skilled at recognizing and solving problems.

10. Team leaders are able to let go when the team is ready for independence, empowering the team and its members to carry out the work with the assurance that they will still have guidance when they need it.

8

UPLOADING

COACHING EMOTIONAL
INTELLIGENCE

IN 1987, THE SAN FRANCISCO 49ERS were losing a football game to the Cincinnati Bengals, score 26–20, with two seconds left on the clock.

"It could have been a hopeless situation," head coach Bill Walsh recounted to an interviewer as he described the play used in the last seconds of the game to achieve the comeback touchdown (Rapaport, 1993, p. 116). The team's consistent preparation and practice of six desperation plays had allowed them to execute the one that would win the game for them. "You need to have a plan for even the worst scenario," said Walsh. "It doesn't mean that it will always work; it doesn't mean that you will always be successful. But you will always be prepared and at your best" (Rapaport, 1993, p. 116).

Emotional coaching is an aspect of leadership that requires an enormous amount of skill on the part of the leader. While it can help in preparing for crises both physical and emotional, it goes far beyond that. Emotional coaching involves helping the people whom we lead to identify, use, understand, and manage their emotions in any situation, from the routine to the unreal. We will find as this chapter progresses that we must use these same four emotional skills not only to encourage appropriate team behavior but also to make sure that beliefs and behavior align. These are two distinct but interdependent skills of the emotionally intelligent team or organization.

Aligning Beliefs with Behavior

"Behavior is guided by personally held principles, beliefs and values" (Martin, Yarbrough, and Alfred, 2003, p. 291). What exactly does it mean to align beliefs with behavior? Let us look at it fairly simply. There are many behaviors that one might practice, for example, that are not aligned with beliefs. Performing a task or routinizing a behavior because one is asked to by one's superior or expected to by one's organization or peer group may at times be difficult, but transforming one's own belief system to incorporate the behavior or need for the behavior can be even more challenging. How many of us, for example, perform day-to-day tasks without really appreciating the value of what we are doing or without feeling motivated or driven by the process that is supported by the task?

When emotional elements are involved, belief-behavior alignment becomes essential. The reader may notice that the concept of changing one's emotions has not been mentioned thus far in this book. There has been discussion of knowing what they are, of knowing how they affect thoughts, of understanding where they can lead, and of managing them but never of changing or obliterating them. Emotion, like rain, occurs whether invited or not. Our management of that emotion, like opening an umbrella, determines how wet or uncomfortable the situation will get. Aligning our beliefs with appropriate behavior, or causing our behavior to align with our beliefs, often requires a great deal of skill in managing emotion. In this context, *beliefs* refer to those internal values and professional responsibilities that nurses and nurse leaders "own," in a sense; for example, the belief that patients have a right to quality care or that compassion is a key ingredient in the delivery of care. *Behavior* refers to the outward expression and inward processing of emotion: the way a nurse reacts to and manages threats to or challenges brought about by particular beliefs or responsibilities. When beliefs and behavior are at odds, there is high potential for failure to carry out a personal or organizational mission.

"The goal of professional development is improved practice through change—changes in ways of doing or thinking about one's work," states Eisen (2001, p. 30). As professionals, we should be thinking about developing ourselves professionally; however, as leaders, we should also be thinking about developing our organization professionally. Cranton (1996) and Mezirow and Associates (2000) describe the phenomenon of transformative learning, in which "learners become more critically reflective, participate more fully and freely in rational discourse and action, and advance developmentally by moving toward meaning perspectives that are more inclusive, discriminating, permeable, and integrative of experience" (Mezirow, 1991, pp. 224–225). Those transformations essentially take us beyond task-centered learning to a deeper, more integrated and holistic learning that can occur only through communication and discourse. These transformations of our habits "may be epochal, a sudden, dramatic, reorienting insight, or incremental, involving a progressive series of transformations in related points of view that culminate in a transformation in habit of mind" (Mezirow and Associates, 2000, p. 21). Standard orientation curriculum alone cannot prepare new staff for competence, especially in areas such as critical care where indeterminate and complex situations are ever present. An ongoing program to promote and expand nursing knowledge should include reflective practice, experiential learning, and transformative learning (Rashotte and Thomas, 2002). The leader should be on the lookout for complaints and feedback from learners, for they are key to facilitating this type of learning (Schreiber and Bannister, 2003).

Other recent authors emphasize coaching and mentorship in various settings and at various levels (Daddario, 2003; Hutton, 2003; Tanner, 2003). There is no shortage of literature promoting the art and skill of coaching as it relates to specific job behaviors and reactions to individual situations and categories of situations.

Mezirow's descriptions of how people learn (Mezirow, 1991; Mezirow and Associates, 2000) parallel the kind of emotional coaching that aligns beliefs with behavior. Emotional coaching sometimes involves a frank discussion of why a reaction to a situation could have been better, or it can involve a gradual transformation of the learner's emotional ability over time. Rashotte and Thomas's (2002) insights about reflective practice can apply to emotional coaching as much as they do to other nursing skills: allowing a team member to reflect on the influence her emotions have on others and the situation at hand—use and understanding of emotions— paves the way for emotion management.

Behavior-Belief Alignment Requires Mutual Effort

Emotional coaching requires a mutual effort on the part of the learner as well as the coach. Emotional skills are defined groups of abilities (Mayer, Salovey, and Caruso, 1999, 2000, 2002) that the teacher and learner must develop integrally with each other. For example, the leader needs to be skilled emotionally and must actually use these skills in order to coach his constituent in emotional skills. The learning individual, who is growing in emotional skill, provides feedback to the coach through interaction and through actions that are observed by the coach. The coach and the learner must work together to polish the emotional skill of the learner.

In the preceding chapter, the analogy of downloading was used: the effective leader was said to download information—that is, make essential elements available for the team as a whole to garner and use. In this chapter, the dominant analogy is uploading. A common example of uploading is placing ads or messages on a Web site bulletin board. If a person is interested in sharing or communicating with a group of people, he or she can upload the individual submission to the larger system so that it will be visible to all. This is different from downloading, of course, because the sender is tasked with the action in uploading, whereas the receiver is tasked with downloading necessary materials. Emotional coaching is more similar to uploading, wherein the leader is providing specific, customized materials to the learner as they are required. Coaching requires a more targeted effort on the part of the leader than does example setting, vision sharing, or team leadership in general. Coaching requires identification of the elements that must be uploaded to an individual or team and specific efforts to transfer these skills to the appropriate receivers.

Tanner (2003) refers to cultivating compassion in nurses. Clancy (2003) speaks of maintaining courage over time, not just in situations in which it is tapped. Florence Nightingale is quoted as saying that there should be no difference between "men of thought" and "men of action": in other words, philosophies should be innate to everyday actions (Jacobs, 2001, p. 17). For the receiver or learner, the uploading of specific emotional skills requires an acceptance of the skills the coach is seeking to impart. For many, this requires not only a change in action but also a change in attitude or behavior.

The Rewards of Belief-Behavior Alignment Are Often Subtle or Intrinsic

Throughout history, people have most often been rewarded for behaviors rather than beliefs. A behavior is an outward expression that may or may not correspond to an internalized belief. For example, one might attend religious services or civic functions without feeling strongly about the purpose or group. Students may turn in incredibly accurate papers on subjects that are not particularly their favorites and receive an A. Individuals may receive a tax credit for contributing to a charity whose mission holds no specific passion for them. The display of appropriate behavior in a group setting may be rewarded by group acceptance or the absence of group disapproval. In all of these scenarios, the individual appears to believe, have an interest in, or uphold something that he or she may not actually care anything about.

Society as a whole tends to extrinsically reward specific behaviors through salaries, high grades, promotions, financial incentives, and job status (Joshua-Amadi, 2002; Feinstein, 2003). Society, cannot, however, delve into the vast resources of heart and mind and survey a person's actual beliefs and principles. Only through overt or covert expression do these beliefs manifest themselves, and these expressions are all we have by which to judge a person's inner beliefs or values.

Intrinsic rewards include personal growth and development, interest in one's job, or satisfaction with helping others (Joshua-Amadi, 2002). Those who are more motivated by external factors may find it more difficult to see the necessity of belief-behavior alignment than those who feel an intrinsic reward for this alignment.

For example, increased pressures in today's health care system may decrease the value of intrinsic rewards garnered by both preceptors (Wright, 2002) and learners. In the absence of extrinsic rewards—like additional compensation or professional advances—the stress involved in delivering and teaching patient care can ultimately lead to anger and dissatisfaction with the preceptor-preceptee relationship. These feelings, if left unmanaged, can have an incredibly negative impact on the learner's ability to learn and the teacher's ability to teach. In this instance, belief-behavior alignment involves identifying the problematic emotion (anger or feelings of unfair reward for additional work), acknowledging how it affects thought processes and actions (negative attitude toward preceptee or subversive thoughts), and recognizing what the consequences might be (resentment, ineffective interpersonal relations, or ineffective patient care). Managing these emotions and their potential consequences allows the preceptor to align the emotionally based behavior with what she fundamentally believes: that her ability to teach the novice staff member benefits the learner, the organization, the patient, and the profession as a whole. Once emotions are managed, the intrinsic rewards—satisfaction with the resulting benefits—are more apparent.

Beglinger (2003) theorizes that for nurses, the challenge of reaping adequate rewards in the face of the frustration and stress inherent in health care may be lessened because "nurses' top priority has always been excellent patient care and the intrinsic rewards associated with the practice. Certainly, they want to be well compensated for their professional services, but few have ever gone into nursing primarily to make money. Nurses are knowledge workers who are drawn to nursing because it is one of the few professions that allows one the opportunity to make an incredible difference in people's lives" (p. 31). Obviously, this motivation may be true for some nurses more than others. For example, Kubsch, Henniges, Lorenzoni, Eckardt, and Oleniczak (2003) found that nurses had specific motivating factors for obtaining continuing education. Nurses whose states or employers did not require such education had varying reasons for attending educational opportunities. Some did it for personal growth, curiosity, or desire for knowledge; others did not attend because they did not see the benefit in attending such sessions.

Coaching Emotional Intelligence

Our challenge as leaders is to identify factors that will motivate staff not only to behave in emotionally intelligent ways but also to incorporate these behaviors into their own belief patterns. Effective emotional coaching will allow this to happen.

A Brief History of Nurse Training, Coaching, and Mentoring

Emotional coaching has its roots in traditional mentoring. Nurses and nurse leaders have been mentors and coaches for almost the lifetime of the profession. The concept of mentoring itself dates at least as far back as Greek mythology, in which Odysseus, upon leaving to fight in the Trojan War, trusts the care and training of his son, Telemachus, to his friend Mentor. Mentor is said to have supported, protected, affirmed, and nurtured Telemachus, as well as to have established goals and plans for the youngster (Haack and Smith, 2000).

The profession of nursing was born in the context of war and evolved from its hierarchical practices. In ancient Egypt, ages before Florence Nightingale began her revolutionary efforts, slaves filled nursing roles, and anyone choosing such a role no doubt carried that stigma (Savage, 2003).

Nursing education and professionalism have their roots in the efforts of pioneers such as Florence Nightingale, who founded the Nightingale Training School for Nurses at St Thomas's Hospital in London and based her training on goals of better patient care (Savage, 2003). The rudimentary training the nurses received there focused on the patient's moral and educational good, and instruction in theory was provided primarily by physicians. Pfeill (2003) cites South's (1857) text, which indicates that nurses require little teaching beyond how to make poultices and tend to the patient's wants. In 1854, Charles West (cited in Pfeill, 2003) reminded nurses that they were quite inferior to physicians and that they should follow physicians' orders explicitly. West is also quoted as saying that nursing primarily required kindness, a love of children, and "humbleness of mind, cleanliness, neatness and diligence and order" and that little factual knowledge was required for the profession (Pfeill, 2003, p. 33).

In 1864, a delegation visited St. Thomas's Hospital in order to summarize the skills that needed to be learned in Nightingale's training program. In addition to domestic skills, this list included custodial activities (feeding and hygiene), bed making and convalescent care, and basic wound and injury care. Most of these skills were said to be learned on the job and not specifically taught (Pfeill, 2003).

In the early part of the twentieth century, the first nurse instructors were instituted, and formal training programs were implemented at St. Thomas's Hospital. Not until 1927 was there a course that prepared nurses for teaching. By the 1930s, hospitals were evolving more rapidly than the nursing profession, and turnover and dropout rates of nurses were increasing. Work conditions declined, and women sought other types of work. By the World War II era, student nurses spent large increments of their nursing education performing domestic functions in a nursing education culture that tended to ignore the potential of bright, promising young professionals (Pfeill, 2003).

It is perhaps not surprising that nurses historically have not seized opportunities for autonomy and independence. The clinical setting has long lent itself to practicing under rules and orders given by others. Many nurses leave the clinical setting for administrative or academic roles because they seek freedom or autonomy (Campbell, 2003). This may relate to disempowering attitudes, behaviors and beliefs that have continued into the present (Ashley, 1997; Campbell, 2003).

Traditionally, mentoring relationships in nursing have taken place at the master's level or above (Owens and Patton, 2003), but mentoring and coaching principles can and should be applied at all levels of nursing. Conditions essential for mentoring in nursing differ little from those in other professions (Byrne and Keefe, 2002). A North Carolina hospital instituted a formal mentorship program, and within one year, turnover rates among nurses dropped from 34 percent to 8 percent. Many nurses attributed this to the increased self-confidence, support, and skills provided by the mentoring relationship (Verdejo, 2002, p. 16). The focus on mentoring in nursing continues to grow and change (Byrne and Keefe, 2002). Today, emotional mentoring should be an expected element of formal mentorship programs and preceptor-preceptee relationships.

Our challenge as nursing leaders is to develop emotional skills and integrate them into traditional teaching (Dearborn, 2002). Western schools continue to focus on mathematics, literature, and language and not on emotional skills (Mayer, Salovey, Caruso, and Sitarenios, 2001). For nursing practice and team interactions to achieve maximum effectiveness, nurse leaders must take the responsibility to educate constituents in emotional abilities.

What Is Involved in Emotional Coaching

Coaching, unlike classroom or seminar training, has an ill-defined end. In fact, coaching is often said to have no end, but to be a perpetual activity that continues with each new level of achievement. A goal, once attained, lays the groundwork for the next goal, which is focused upon through another cycle of coaching (Eaton and Johnson, 2001). The continual development of skills and abilities is elsewhere referred to as professional development (Haack and Smith, 2000) and mentoring (Haack and Smith, 2000; Hutton, 2003). Mentoring is distinguished from coaching in some literature as being more personal or individualized (Morrison, 2000) than coaching. A mentor, for example, may be a more experienced colleague but not a supervisor, while a coach is presumed to have some authority over the individual. Although this is a valid distinction, individualized mentoring can involve coaching elements, and many of the same principles apply in either coaching or mentoring. Even outside of direct supervisory bounds, emotional coaching combines the roles of mentor and coach. The emotional coach takes explicit responsibility for helping the constituent develop emotional skills while serving as an experienced guide and reference to the learner.

Results of Emotional Coaching

Nurses want to be valued. They want to participate in decision making and to be appreciated and respected. Simply increasing salaries or adding benefits are not enough to prevent a crisis in filling the need for competent nurses. Unit leaders, executives, recruiters, and retention planners must take emotional factors into account (Upenieks, 2003). As they do, strong emphasis must be given to emotional coaching. On top of the skills and nursing judgment imparted by traditional education and mentoring, emotional coaching takes into account the emotional and social roots of nurse and team behavior, passes on specific elements of emotional knowledge, and results in a vision that is not only followed but believed.

BELIEF THAT DRIVES BEHAVIOR. "'Ownership' of an organization's services, by those who provide them, has been demonstrated to be the most significant driver of the organization's success," asserts Beglinger (2003, p. 25). "Ownership, in this context, can be understood by contemplating the behaviors and attitudes of a partner in any business. The partner is intellectually and emotionally committed to acting in a way that will best advance the purposes of the enterprise at all times. The partner not only feels free to act in a way that will be right for the organization; he or she feels obligated to do so. Belief and investment in the organization's mission is characteristic of ownership. A sense of ownership, on the part of those who do the organization's work, is an essential characteristic of success" (Beglinger, 2003, p. 25).

This statement presents the key terms involved in belief-behavior alignment. "Emotionally committed to acting" is one central principle of this statement, as is "belief and investment in the organization's mission." One way to organize this belief is through reflection on actual and intended actions. Because what we do on the job shapes the environment of the organization, it is critical that action be balanced with reflection.

Earlier in the chapter, the personal rewards of belief-behavior alignment were described as primarily intrinsic in nature. The result of this alignment, however, is a stronger organization or group, which increases the potential for extrinsic reward. One health care executive kept a sign on his desk that both he and all who entered his office could read. Its imperative was, simply, "If you're not serving the customer, you'd better be serving someone who is" (Savage, 2003, p. 14). This is just one outward method of aligning belief and behavior: allowing our everyday actions to be driven by a constant belief. Whether this occurrence is subtle or demonstrative, conscious or subconscious, it needs to be present. It was likely this executive's demonstration of his commitment to customer service that gained him extrinsic recognition within the organization, but the underlying philosophy that he chose to visibly adopt also drove him intrinsically and was a key contributor to his portion of the organization's success.

In striving to act out his belief consistently, the executive would have needed to exercise understanding and management of his emotions at times. Certainly, there were days when he did not *feel* like serving the customer. Maybe there were times when the customer frustrated or angered him or he would have been happier at home with his family or more relaxed if he had time to resolve a personal issue. On these days, his appropriate *behavior* was probably the product of discipline, and the discipline a product of emotional skill.

Of course, we do not know this man, nor can we say with certainty that he ever had any problems with emotions getting in the way. Unless he was superhuman, however, it is likely that he did. On the days when he felt happy or positive it was probably much easier to take a customer-centric view than on the days when he did not. Likewise, it is easier for a nurse to take a patient-centric view when she is comfortable emotionally and not struggling with negative feelings. She needs to identify, understand, and manage those feelings to align her behavior with her core beliefs. Emotional coaching can help sharpen that ability in the nurse.

INCREASED EMOTIONAL KNOWLEDGE. Coaching is defined by Daddario (2003) as encouraging development of skills, professional growth, and knowledge. Self-directed learning plans are key to emotional coaching and ultimately lead to behavioral change (Dearborn, 2002). The growth of knowledge is foundational to any skill or expertise we obtain, and in team members, this growth should be facilitated by continual feedback. Whenever a learning experience is unsuccessful, every attempt should be made to identify the issues that contributed. In any case, the learner should have the gift of honest feedback about his or her strengths, weaknesses, and factors that contributed to the performance (Hom, 2003).

Especially when emotions are involved, this can be some of the most difficult feedback to give. Such feedback may involve explaining why emotions were inappropriately managed or allowed to facilitate a line of thinking that led to an unsatisfactory behavior. Because of the intimate relationship between a person and his or her emotions, this can be more challenging than evaluating efficiency and quality. Discussing another person's emotions can seem overly personal, even invasive. An individual might acknowledge that a behavior was inappropriate but claim that the feeling that contributed to it was unavoidable. Perhaps one of the most difficult coaching sessions that a leader can deliver, then, involves pointing out negative emotions and how they affected a circumstance. This requires a clear distinction between discussing the root emotion itself and how it was managed under the circumstances. It was the action on the emotion (behavior), not the emotion itself (feeling), that caused the problem or contributed to the lack of success.

SHARED VISION. The culmination of effective emotional knowledge sharing and alignment of beliefs and behaviors is the ability, of both individuals and teams, to share and act on a vision as a unified whole. "Developing effective, visionary leaders who motivate, engage, spur and retain employees, as well as tapping into the potential for leadership within our current employee base, is a key accountability listed in many of our personal performance objectives," writes Dearborn (2002, p. 523). This would be an excellent personal performance objective for all leaders who are seeking to move an organization, team, or department forward. How effective, after all, can leadership be, when either the path is unclear or the people are unwilling, unmotivated, and unbelieving?

Skills Learned from Emotional Coaching

Turning again to and Mayer, Salovey, and Caruso's (1999, 2000, 2002) four-branch model of emotional intelligence, let us examine the emotional competencies that can be strengthened through effective emotional coaching.

Perceiving Emotion

The emotional aspects of behavior, like other aspects, can be acknowledged and recognized through benchmarking an employee's self-perception against others' perceptions. In this way, approaches or actions can be changed and developed over time as the employee grows professionally. In this way, we can actually coach ourselves: as our relationships and conditions improve because of changed behaviors, we record the experience psychologically; consequently, our emotional intelligence grows. The leader who has already experienced this self-assessment can coach others in it as well, encouraging them to look at their own experiences as tools for self-development (Dearborn, 2002).

The emotional coach will continue to point out, whenever appropriate, observed and acknowledged emotions in the learner. Although this may be uncomfortable at times, it is imperative, especially in situations where emotional display is inappropriate. An inappropriate outburst in a meeting, for example, should be met with coaching that is as timely but as private as possible. During this coaching, the individual should be asked to recall the emotion, define how it could affect group dynamics, and describe how similar feelings might be better handled in the future.

Not all emotions are negative or require personal coaching after the audience has cleared. Many emotions are apparent or recognizable, whether positive or negative, and appropriately displayed. For example, a coach should actively seek opportunities to say things such as "Brenda, I can see that you are not sure about these alternatives" or "Randy, what don't you like about the proposal?" Doing so not only bolsters the coach's personal recognition mind-set but also stimulates the group or individual to consider the fact that emotions are indeed visible and recognizable.

Using Emotion

Introspective ability has much to do with the self-assessment defined above and is key to using emotion to facilitate thought and action. How are emotions related to our beliefs and actions? Why do I (or you) as a manager act a certain way under certain conditions? How can we change our thinking about a situation in spite of or aided by our emotions?

Affective and emotional learning stimulates critical thinking, which is so vital to medical and nursing practice. In addition, this type of learning enhances the caring perspective espoused by the nursing profession (Zimmerman and Phillips, 2000).

Understanding Emotion

In a book review of Martha Nussbaum's (2001) book *Upheavals of Thought: The Intelligence of Emotions*, Hoffmaster (2003) points out that emotions are more than just happenings that overtake us and sweep us toward particular thoughts or actions. Rather, they are responses that can be rationally assessed, contrary to the metaphors we are so accustomed to hearing: swamped by grief, paralyzed by fear, blinded by love, and the like.

Understanding emotion involves knowing how emotional states progress and interact to form new emotional states (Mayer, Salovey, and Caruso, 2000, 2002). Much of what we observe in group or team emotions can be referred to as *dynamics*, a term often used to describe the interactions between members of a family or group. Waldroop and Butler (1996) put it this way: behavior never takes place in isolation. To know what is really happening, one must observe the dynamics between a manager and the people around her. Continual observation with an eye on dynamics can enhance understanding of how emotions interact to form new emotions and how they can be used as catalysts to help groups solve problems and move forward.

Managing Emotion

Understanding the emotions that are at hand as well as those that may arise from a particular situation can lead to decision making and problem solving based on emotional as well as rational fact. For example, disagreeable work schedules, cumbersome processes, or shaky team interactions must first be understood in terms of their emotional underpinning. Stayer (1990) described how weekend work was disliked by a group of delivery personnel. Careful study of the issue revealed the root of the problem: worker inefficiency and lateness, slow start-ups, and absences were causing equipment downtime. Once the workers discovered and acknowledged that they could affect the problem by changes in behavior, they improved their punctuality and efficiency, downtime decreased, and so did the necessity of weekend work.

Although we will probably never succeed in eliminating weekend work schedules from the health care environment, we can use this example as a starting point for other situations more relevant to nursing. Emotion management and problem solving have similarities: they both require assessment of a situation and thoughtful efforts to correct it. A shortfall occurs when we as leaders fail to recognize the emotion that a problem is generating or we fail to consider the emotional element in solving it. The success of emotion management is demonstrated in the ability to process negative energies into positive outcomes (Staring, 1999).

Leadership Skills Needed to Be an Effective Emotional Coach

Just as there are skills that improve teaching effectiveness, there are skills that enhance emotional coaching. These are the ability to share knowledge, the ability to align beliefs with behavior, and the ability to share a vision.

Ability to Share Knowledge

The sharing of emotional knowledge is the foundation skill of the emotional coach. The coach identifies the emotions present in a situation, how they were used, and how they could have been better managed. This is emotional training at its most basic, and it often occurs in a real-time situation. However, there are ways to impart this emotional knowledge other than reactively.

IMPLEMENT AN EFFECTIVE TRAINING PROGRAM AND NETWORKING OPPORTUNITIES. An effective training program, along with appropriate testing, is essential for proactive establishment of emotional awareness. Departments or teams can use one of many tests, including the Mayer-Salovey-Caruso Emotional Intelligence Test (Mayer, Salovey, and Caruso, 2002) and those provided by Weisinger (1998) and Bar-On (2000). Benner's (1984) novice to expert model, which models nursing competency at five levels, might also be applied to development of emotional awareness.

When emotional knowledge is heralded in the organization, networking opportunities with other learners can provide nurses with more foundational knowledge of the topic. Others learning emotional skills can serve as supportive resources for one another, just as others learning about a new procedure can.

PROVIDE AN UNDERSTANDING OF THE COACHING PROCESS. Learners should be consciously aware of coaching activities as such, no matter how subtle or integral to day-to-day procedures they may be. Simply put, it is important that learners have an understanding of their leader's interest in their growth and development. Young and Perrewe (2000) outline five factors that influence a mentoring relationship: individual characteristics, relationship factors, environmental factors, career factors, and relationship type. The leader must keenly understand all of these as they relate to coaching his staff. Some of these factors, such as individual characteristics, must be applied to each learner, while others, such as environmental factors, can be more broadly applied. Learners should also be aware of how each of these factors may affect their learning experience. The fact that coaching is occurring should be no secret; rather, it should provide active opportunities for growth and clarification.

ENGAGE INTRINSIC RATHER THAN EXTRINSIC MOTIVATION. Earlier in this chapter, the differences between extrinsic and intrinsic rewards were discussed briefly. It was noted that the rewards garnered from belief-behavior alignment are often intrinsic in nature, because behavior alone is often what is most recognized extrinsically. Ideally, the leader will engage the intrinsic motivation of his constituents as much as possible, encouraging them from the perspective of personal growth and integrity. In fact, when these become valued components of an organization's culture, they are likely to be rewarded through peer recognition and greater job satisfaction as well.

CULTIVATE EMOTIONAL INTELLIGENCE AS A GARDEN. When we hear the word *cultivate,* our thoughts turn to small gardens or to large fields capable of producing nourishment for thousands. This analogy has been used numerous times and can also be applied to the emotional intelligence context. Tanner (2003, p. 287) asks the question "How can we cultivate the compassionate and inquisitive nurse within each student?" In this context, we should ask, "how can we cultivate the emotionally competent nurse and nurse team?" There are several seeds to plant, including interpretive skills, practical knowledge gained from experience, and best practice or evidence-based practice. Other seeds planted for us might be experiences with others or experiences from childhood (Tanner, 2003; Campbell, 2003).

Campbell (2003) explains how exchanges that occur between individuals are very similar to what happens when a garden is grafted. Grafting is a process that causes plants to propagate. A plant graft is a cutting obtained from an existing plant that establishes its own roots and is planted to grow as a separate plant. Successful learning and empowerment occurs as a mutual exchange between individuals that causes growth in one individual without draining the other. The learner, in a sense, is a "cutting" of the teacher. Grounding, likewise, occurs when individuals make decisions about how to respond or be involved in situations. People will ground themselves in a direction that affects their behaviors and take root in that direction. Each of these analogies can be applied in the arena of emotional management, but the sequence of events involved in cultivating a garden can also be applied to emotional learning itself. Suppose we recognized, for example, our root emotions as seeds that grow either healthily or not. Campbell's analogy of grafting might apply in the scenario of using emotions to facilitate thought (Mayer, Salovey, and Caruso, 2000, 2002), while grounding is more closely related to understanding how emotions progress. These and similar analogies can be used to teach emotional knowledge to learners in the organization and kept in mind as leaders seek to filter appropriate skills and points about the emotional management process to each learner.

ESTABLISH AN EMOTIONAL INTELLIGENCE PRECEPTOR. The importance of emotional competence in nursing underscores the need for an expert organizational leader in the field. Department heads should focus on establishing one or two key individuals whose role includes transferring emotional knowledge to other staff members. These individuals can support and consult with leaders as new information related to emotional intelligence becomes available.

Ability to Impart Belief That Underlies Specific Behavior

The emotional coach must also be able to assist learners in ownership of the beliefs they portray through their actions. This lays the groundwork for a shared vision and actions that wholesomely support team effectiveness, not just rote behaviors carried out because they should be. When team members are acting out of expectation or obligation but they lack the enthusiasm to back it up, there may be something wrong with their core belief. Just as there are times when the behavior does not exemplify the belief—for example, when a nurse believes that patients are her priority but dawdles and does not give them her complete attention because she feels unappreciated and undervalued—there are also situations where seemingly appropriate behavior belies a lack of ownership of the belief. In other words, a team member may go along with the team just because he is supposed to, when in fact he is resentful of the team's mission because it encroaches on some personal desire of his own. It takes emotional skill on the part of the leader to identify the true emotional makeup of the individual's belief and to help him understand it. He can then be encouraged to examine his feelings in the light of how his personal concerns now may affect his willing participation later, and encouraged to talk through his concerns with the group or seek ways to manage the feelings that are causing him difficulty.

TEACH THE TEAM TO BACK INTO GOALS AND BELIEFS. Back planning involves starting with a goal and planning actions around reaching that goal. It is difficult to get started with something or even to know where or when to start, if one is unsure of the steps involved. Savage (2003) recommends approaching complex tasks or changes as one would approach dinner preparation: determine the end result (for example, serve dinner at 6 P.M.) and then work backward to formulate desired steps (for example, carve the turkey at 5:45 P.M., roast the turkey at 2 P.M.). Similarly, nurses can be taught to back into beliefs that support behaviors by acknowledging the desired behavior or goal, then planning the changes needed to bring it about, including acknowledgment of any beliefs or feelings surrounding the change.

USE RESPECT, INTEGRITY, AND COMPASSION. Along with emotion management, professional empowerment, and empowerment by values, Staring (1999) identifies respect, integrity, and compassion as mutual core values that affect a team's success. Aligning belief with behavior certainly must involve having core values that are synchronized with those of other team members if the team is to work together for the good of the unit or department. As the leader guides individuals to align their beliefs with their behaviors and establish common goals, she should ask whether appropriate respect and compassion is demonstrated for each team member and whether integrity underlies her interactions with the team.

UNDERSTAND EMOTIONS' RELATIONSHIP WITH CULTURE AND MORALITY. Emotions are very personal parts of our being, partly because emotions have much to do with culture and morality. Hoffmaster (2003) points out how some emotions may compel people to harm others (for example, hatred may result in murder), while others, such as gratitude, might spur benevolent actions. While not all actions can be generalized as related to one specific emotion, the leader should be aware and make others aware of the relationship between an action and an emotion or even between potential actions and emotions. When individuals can understand emotions, they are more able to relate emotions to thought patterns and specific transitions that might lead to an action (Mayer, Salovey, and Caruso, 2000, 2002).

A more specific application of this principle is that understanding emotions' relationships with culture allows the nurse leader to have a more nuanced understanding of cultural patterns that may affect a person's reactions. Consider the phrase "How are you?" In the United States and perhaps in other cultures, when "How are you?" is said to a nonacquaintance, it is often interpreted and responded to as a greeting. For most of us, being asked "How are you?" by the teller at the bank or the cashier at the supermarket would not result in an outpouring of our feelings about the day's events. However, visitors from Europe and Asia have anecdotally reported being taken aback by the brusque "How are you?" offered on their initial contacts with U.S. citizens. Many of the visitors interpreted it as a genuine inquiry, not merely a greeting. In their countries, a question such as "How are you?" would be interpreted as genuine interest, so they felt frustration and hurt at the clipping of the greeting in the United States. This is only one example of the many ways in which culture affects our social expectations, including those that may influence our emotions. Therefore, when beliefs and behavior seem misaligned, the astute nurse leader should also consider any cultural or background experiences that may be affecting the constituent's beliefs or actions. These might include social background, religious or moral principles, or ethnic and regional influences. It is important, if the leader does sense a problem that she has difficulty understanding, that she approach the constituent with genuine willingness to understand, and to help the constituent better understand, the root causes of the issue.

PROMOTE SELF-DIRECTED LEARNING. Merely teaching emotional competencies is insufficient to translate beliefs into behavior. Behavioral changes are best ingrained through self-directed learning in which the learner practices different behaviors and receives feedback from a coach or mentor (Dearborn, 2002). Traditional nursing training does not provide the opportunity for this kind of learning, partly because it focuses on providing vast amounts of critical knowledge in a short amount of time. Nonetheless, experimentation and follow-up are key to developing emotional memory and competence; we learn to be more effective emotionally only through learning which emotional behaviors are most and least supportive of effective practice. As we learn, we integrate our learning into our belief system.

Self-directed learning also contains an element of self-assessment, the same fundamental tool espoused by Mayer, Salovey, and Caruso (1999, 2000, 2002) and Goleman (1998a). Dearborn (2002) recommends tools for self-assessment that allow learners to understand where they are with emotional skills, how they are perceived by others, and what changes in belief or behavior are needed to reach a desired goal.

FACILITATE SYSTEM CHANGE. Often, an entire system needs to be changed in order to optimize practice or to accommodate new organizational realities. Unit and organizational structures, which may affect a nurse's beliefs about practice, are usually established by leaders above the nurse level. The shared leadership model does allow nurses to have input into change processes and can be powerful in the unit setting. Feinstein (2003) promotes care dictated by patient need, not medical supply. We might apply the same to nursing systems and cultures. When the unit or team culture is dictated by the needs of the patients or of the staff itself, beliefs become more naturally aligned with the behaviors of the group. Feinstein's recommendations for health care as a whole include investment in an infrastructure capable of supporting system improvement, relaxation of counterproductive policies, and measures that would introduce the appropriate sequences or processes. The nurse leader should apply similar approaches in areas where system change appears to be needed.

PRACTICE AND PROMOTE ETHICAL BEHAVIOR. Of course, we cannot overlook ethical behavior and beliefs in coaching emotional fitness. In situations involving ethical issues, it is most important that belief and behavior be aligned. As leaders and health care professionals face ethical challenges, whether due to technology, business decisions, or staffing issues, they should continually strive to advance the ethical development of both themselves and their team (Clancy, 2003). The ethical fitness of the team and its members will play a large role in their decision making, and certainly as leaders, we want their decisions to be ethical ones! Continuing education courses in ethics or review of the profession's code of ethics may also help learners understand their own ethical positions and undertake any reconsideration of their positions that they deem appropriate.

ALLOW REPRESENTATION TO OTHER ORGANIZATIONAL GROUPS. When a group is self-contained, it is much easier for individual members to act out of line with beliefs by going along with the crowd, especially if there is peer pressure to conform. Promoting a belief to another group, the organization, or a department head, however, is more challenging if beliefs are not aligned with behavior. For example, if a team member did not truly endorse a group decision, it would be more difficult for him or her to approach the CEO with the rationale for the decision than it would be to silently not approve in the group setting. For this reason among many, team members should be aware that they are potential liaisons to other organizational constituencies and that their work will be recognized at higher levels of leadership (Druskat, 2001). The nursing staff at a disease management organization, who were rewriting and updating each disease-specific assessment tool, were constantly aware that their work would be presented to senior management and incorporated into their daily practice. Knowing this, their belief in their work product was enhanced and emboldened, and they were able to produce a product that they firmly believed in.

Ability to Share Vision

The leadership skill of sharing a vision, which is treated in detail in Chapter Five, is imperative for effective emotional coaching. Specifically, the visionary leader must be able not only to pass the vision to others, but also, through coaching, to strengthen their belief in and mutual agreement with the vision. Or the leader may collaborate with team members to form a vision for their practice. The leader then extends the sharing of the vision into the action surrounding it. Fundamentally, the leader must have shared a vision and belief, but as the vision is shared, the leader then assists constituents in managing their own emotions so as to carry out the vision and align their behavior with that belief. It is not, after all, enough to strongly support a course of action if actions themselves are contrary to that belief.

ENCOURAGE A VISION FOR NURSING AS A PROFESSION OR FOR THE ORGANIZATION. Have you ever been hungry without knowing what you want to eat? Some nurses certainly understand that they want change, but they are not able to pinpoint their ideal. Instead of stipulating what the vision should be, it is helpful if the leader encourages his team members to formulate their own visionary goals for the nursing profession or for their unit. Teams may create their own vision by brainstorming, or they may adopt guiding principles from an organization such as Sigma Theta Tau International. Their initiatives include repositioning the entire nursing profession as more versatile and educational, promoting a more attractive image, creating models that encourage autonomy, providing career enhancement incentives, and developing retention strategies (Sigma Theta Tau International, 2001).

These types of ideas or ideas more specific to the unit or department can form a vision for nursing at the staff level that team members can carry far, especially in a culture of shared leadership. Perhaps a vision for greater understanding of emotions and their impact on patient care or the nursing profession could also be part of the team's vision. A concrete goal to use emotional skills to improve practice and teamwork may lay the groundwork for further emotional learning.

POINT OUT THE BURNING DECK. Often, leaders try to impart a vision that they firmly believe in by glorifying the vision, but that tactic may only work if people are already on board with the need for change, especially when changing a comfortable status quo is involved. True, there are some visions that involve spectacular solutions to a pressing need, and everyone seems happy to accommodate and adopt those. But what about visions for betterment that require investment beyond the scope of what appears to be needed?

One CEO described vision sharing this way: When an oil rig foreman yells, "Jump into the water!" those who do not actually recognize the fact that the platform is burning are less likely to jump than those who do. Why? Because they anticipate the risks of jumping more than they realize the need to jump. For those who see the licking flames, the need to change location or position is obvious. For those who cannot, it is the foreman's responsibility to make them aware of the need to move. This is best accomplished by making them see the present situation, not by attempting to convince them of the glories of the new situation (Tichy and Charan, 1995). Likewise, if a team member needs emotional coaching, he must be able to see how his emotions can be used to facilitate undesirable outcomes. If he sees a need to change his behaviors in this context, the path to emotion management can begin.

CHANGE THE INPUT INTO THE VAST FLOODPLAIN. Perhaps the most basic of principles for sharing vision and knowledge via coaching is that we must rely on the fact that the brain can change (Holloway, 2003). The perception held by someone can change as their brain forms new connections based on new information or emotional learning. The coach's responsibility is to change the flow of information into what Holloway refers to as a "vast floodplain" (Holloway, 2003, p. 78), wherein water might cut shallow channels one year and deep ones the next, all the time changing the surface map of the brain. As leaders, we must remember that, contrary to earlier thought, the brain is not hardwired and our coaching can go a long way. Coach, coach, coach, believing in the ability of faithful guidance to affect and mold the vision of the organization.

Summary

Coaching is not a new concept, nor is mentoring. However, principles from both have implications for the changing face of nursing practice. As nursing becomes more reliant on emotionally intelligent behavior and mindful judgment in critical situations, effective coaching is of paramount importance in creating mind-sets and beliefs that will produce effective behaviors at the appropriate times.

The nurse leader as coach will share knowledge, help align team beliefs with behaviors, and share a vision that can be carried to the organization or the profession as a whole. As this occurs, learners will improve their emotional skills through leaders' sharing of knowledge and feedback on their effectiveness. Ultimately, organizational culture will be influenced through this emotional development at the team and department level.

TEN CRITERIA FOR EFFECTIVE EMOTIONAL COACHING

1. Emotional knowledge is shared through structured learning and situational feedback.
2. Learners understand that they are being coached and are aware of the expectations of the coaching.
3. Learner improvement is based on intrinsic rewards, but their effectiveness may be extrinsically rewarded.
4. Emotional competence is cultivated in individuals and teams as needed.
5. Learners are taught to model their beliefs through effective behaviors.
6. Learners are encouraged to learn in a self-directed manner.
7. Learners are liaisons to the organization, able to herald their beliefs at higher levels.
8. Learners and leaders practice ethical behaviors that align with ethical beliefs.
9. Leaders promote and encourage a self-directed vision for the organization or the profession.
10. Leaders translate a vision to learners via realization of the need for change.

9

WEATHERING A CRASH

CONFLICT RESOLUTION IN THE
HEALTH CARE ENVIRONMENT

NO MATTER HOW SKILLED we are as leaders, we will never avoid conflict in our work environment. As long as we work with different people holding different values, there will be conflicts to resolve. The underlying reasons for conflicts are as varied as the issues that spark them, but most conflicts can be resolved by using a straightforward and systematic process while applying emotional knowledge and skill.

Why We Cannot Ignore Conflict

Wind, like the other elements, can be constructive or destructive. Despite the damage that wind has inflicted through tornadoes, downbursts, and hurricanes, its powerful forces have been used for centuries to generate power and are often sufficient to transform a hot day into a pleasant one. Heating, cooling, and the earth's rotation combine to produce wind.

Like wind, conflict is an inevitable part of life, both in personal settings and in the workplace. Also like wind, it can be constructive or destructive, depending on how it is managed (Smith, Tutor, and Phillips, 2001). It is generated, simply, from the different strengths and weaknesses inherent in human nature. Because we cannot obliterate these strengths and weaknesses but only work with them to improve ourselves, it is likely that we will not be able to eliminate conflict. However, many will try to avoid it, manipulate it, or ignore it at all costs. The cost to effective health care management is great when conflict is not addressed appropriately.

Workplace transition, corporate downsizing and restructuring, and the change to managed care have created conflict in the health care arena. The change to managed care immediately created the potential for conflict in determining what constitutes ethical nursing practice in a cost-conscious setting. For example, two nurses may have strong but divergent convictions regarding discontinuance of care for a terminally ill patient. One nurse may see the discontinuance of care as an unpleasant but humane decision; another may view such discontinuance as immoral health care rationing. Another impact of managed care is that nurse administrators must confront differences about the methodology for meeting managed care goals—for example, which type of patient care delivery system best balances quality and cost factors.

Conflict itself must be differentiated from the events that appear to cause it. Conflict does not equal the need to accept things that are not likely to change. Wishing it were warmer outside, for instance, is not a conflict, even though there seems to be a conflict between what is and what is desired. Similarly, although a lack of storage space or a patient's condition may appear to engender conflict, these situations do not represent conflict in and of themselves: they are existing facts that cannot be wished away. Conflict may arise from such concerns, however, if the condition of conflicting values or desires is present. For example, a lack of storage space may represent an inconvenience to some staff members, but correcting the problem may cause inconvenience to someone else. A patient's declining condition may create conflicting views on whether life-sustaining treatment should be continued. Threat lies at the core of almost every conflict, and at the core of every threat lies fear. These emotions may result in either aggressive attempts to resolve the issue or avoidance in hopes that the issue will resolve itself (Truby, 2000).

If health care is to move in positive, innovative directions, conflict must be resolved in ways that promote the growth of cost-effective, high-quality patient care practices. Thus, improving performance as a team requires nurses at all levels of practice to use conflict management and conflict resolution skills to help direct this growth (Kaye, 1994). Traditionally, nurses are masters of negotiation; however, they usually have not been trained to use their negotiation skills in conflict situations (Evans, 1991). Conflict management and conflict resolution abilities result from an attitude that is more "us-centered" than "me-centered." In other words, nurses who are skilled in conflict resolution are more concerned about the feelings and beliefs of the whole group than they are with getting their own agenda pushed through (Halm and Penque, 1999).

The goal of this chapter is to explain the relationship between conflict management skills and emotional intelligence, emphasizing the ways in which emotional know-how comes into play in day-to-day conflict resolution. This chapter also includes a case study in which the skills defined in this chapter are applied to an actual health care situation.

Conflict and Its Relationship to Health Care

Although the word *conflict* usually engenders a negative response, not all conflict has negative results. In fact, out of conflict have come some of the greatest ideas in history. One obvious example is the founding of the United States, which was born out of conflict with England. Students of literature and drama are taught that a story or dramatic sequence is empty, essentially meaningless, without some form of conflict that needs to be resolved. It is conflict, in addition to character development and setting, that keeps plays, action films, fast-paced novels, and even comedies interesting. In literary or dramatic contexts, the conflict may be a problem or situation that needs resolution and not necessarily a clash of ideas or philosophies. Closer to home, the conflict between two health care systems, fee-for-service and managed care, grew out of the need to provide more accessible, more cost-effective health care coverage for more Americans. The evolution of managed care has undoubtedly been painful, but the outcome may be a change in the focus of health care from illness to prevention and wellness as well as acute care that is more accessible to a greater portion of the population.

Out of differences come innovative ideas. When handled creatively, conflict in the health care workplace can provide the basis for the enhanced teamwork necessary to achieve excellence in care delivery. Katzenbach and Smith (1993) relate that teams should have "open conflict and debate that are supportive and constructive" (p. 229). They propose that teams must have conflict to move forward, rather than discouraging conflict. Kaye (1994) describes conflict as "the opportunity to learn" (p. 2). The key is conflict resolution, which transforms disputes into new directions in care. In essence, conflict is not the problem itself, but a means to resolve an existing problem. Truly, there are times when a lack of conflict would indicate an even bigger problem, such as purposeful ignoring of an issue that might cause serious problems if allowed to continue without resolution. Leaders must actually seek out the origin, cause, and motivation behind the conflict in order to avoid this (Miskell and Miskell, 1994). Emotional skill, including the ability to deal with different temperaments, is a key ingredient in making conflict supportive and productive (Kaye, 1994), thereby leading to solutions that address the source of the conflict.

Definition and Explanation of Conflict

The Random House Dictionary defines *conflict* as a mental struggle arising from opposing demands or impulses. For this discussion, we will more narrowly define conflict as a dispute between two or more individuals that arises in a health care setting and has the potential to negatively affect care delivery. Because conflict can never be totally eradicated, a realistic goal for nurses from executive to staff levels is to use conflict resolution as a means of transforming differences into shared goals that promote the departmental and organizational vision and mission.

Conflict, as we intuitively know, varies in its intensity. In negotiations, there may be accepted differences of view, such as how much time or money should be allotted to a certain project. This type of conflict seems natural and is for the most part expected. More intense and more extreme conflict may result from the desire to annihilate the point of view of the other party and "win" by whatever means necessary (Truby, 2000).

Three Stages of Conflict Resolution

Transforming conflict into shared goals requires knowledge of three stages of conflict resolution: promoting effective dialogue, analyzing the elements of the conflict, and facilitating resolution. Conflict resolution requires one-on-one communication that empowers a disputant to help find a solution. The first stage, promoting effective dialogue, may include breaking through emotion so that communication can focus on the actual issues at hand, as well as listening to the views of others and stating one's own (Truby, 2000). The analysis stage involves reflection, through which the facilitator determines the sources of conflict as well as the part that personalities and emotions play in communications about the conflict. This stage may occur either concurrently with or separate from the actual dialogue. In the facilitation stage, the facilitator works with the disputants as a group in order to develop or negotiate a workable solution. The purpose of facilitation is not to issue ultimatums but to create a structured flow of communications through which disputants can resolve differences and commit to a solution. Often, agreement must be solicited and an agreement reached in order for disputants to let go of the conflict and move past it (Truby, 2000).

The stages of conflict resolution bear some similarity to the stages of emotional intelligence that have been discussed throughout this book. In effective emotional processing, there is always identification of either one's own emotions or those of others, followed by analysis of those emotions, and then usually some form of moderation, facilitation, or management of the emotions in order to clear the way for effective work with other team members. Often, our description of someone's conflict resolution skills includes references to their emotional acuity. "She doesn't have much patience for others' point of view," or "He really stops to consider how the other person is feeling when there is a disagreement" are just two examples of emotional credentials we might assign to an individual when discussing this ability. Emotions, though they tend to muddy our black-and-white problem-solving scenarios with many shades of gray, cannot be ignored in conflict or as causes of conflict (Kaye, 1994). Ignoring emotions and their ramifications puts us in grave danger of missing the opportunity to bring about positive change through the conflict. Indeed, some of our most disliked emotions, such as fear, anger, and jealousy, at times may be the source of a conflict that leads to productive change (Kaye, 1994).

How to Effectively Enact the Stages of Conflict Resolution

To assist team members in effectively negotiating and resolving conflict, the leader can follow three stages of conflict resolution: promoting effective dialogue, analyzing the elements of the conflict, and facilitating conflict resolution.

Stage 1: Promoting Effective Dialogue

"The ability to read the feelings of the opposition during a negotiation is critical to success," asserts Goleman (1998b, p. 179). This key principle also applies to all stages of conflict resolution; in the first stage, the ability to read emotions is essential in order to structure the discussion so that it has the best chance for success.

When there is a conflict, it is not enough just to talk to colleagues. In a professional workplace where everyone is pressed for time, any dialogue surrounding a conflict must produce outcomes that lead to a resolution. By mastering specific techniques of communication, nurses can conduct dialogues that lead to resolution. Inherent in this first stage is the need to master tools that facilitate the identification and understanding of emotions.

Of course, open, honest communications that reflect how we really feel should be encouraged (Grossman, 2000), but the fact is that emotions do not always come packaged neatly so that we can identify them without effort. The parties may be intentionally or unintentionally masking their emotions. How, then, do we read the feelings of the "opposition"—who, after all, may merely be a colleague who is working for the same goal but using a different approach (Wall, Solum, and Sobol, 1992)—in a way that allows us to work appropriately with these feelings? The answer is simple: active listening.

SKILLS REQUIRED FOR ACTIVE LISTENING. In their book *The Art of Managing People,* Hunsaker and Alessandra (1986) divide listeners into four categories: nonlisteners, marginal listeners, evaluative listeners, and active listeners. The nonlistener, as the name implies, is more concerned with speaking than listening and may be characterized by blank stares, nervous mannerisms, and her continual interruptions when others are speaking. The nonlistener seems to have little regard for what the speaker is saying, perhaps appearing to be out of touch with the entire conversation but purporting that a valid communication is actually occurring (after all, someone is doing the talking to someone else). In reality, a complete communication is *not* occurring, and most of us would not want to emulate this person's listening skills. Emotional skill required: zero. Dividends: zero, maybe even negative if walls are built and further conflict develops because of breached understanding.

The marginal listener hears the sounds and words of the speaker but does not focus on the meaning of what the speaker is communicating. This essentially describes the "Yes, dear" syndrome, in which the listener is easily distracted by his own thinking as well as by outside occurrences. As with the nonlistener, there is little cognitive involvement and even more negligible emotional involvement. While there may be attention to sounds and syllables, the ability to accurately read the meaning is significantly impaired by the failure to attend emotionally.

The evaluative listener hears the speaker's words but is emotionally detached, making no effort to understand the intent of what is said. This type of listener focuses on content and can parrot back facts but rarely exhibits empathy or understanding of the feelings underlying a conversation. Despite the fact that some of the speaker's material is absorbed, this style of listening can be more damaging to conflict resolution than the previous two, because an attempt to understand is present, but the understanding of intents and meanings, which make up the emotional meat of the conversation, goes uncaptured. Therefore, the individual who listens in this way may appear to have digested the intent of the speaker but may have interpreted the message of the speaker very differently by giving no credence to the emotional cues the speaker was exuding.

The active listener is by far the most effective, seeking to understand the person as well as the spoken words. Active listening involves suspending one's own thoughts and giving total attention to the speaker, listening for feelings and asking questions. This is the key to reading the feelings of the other person.

Conversation, which is a thoughtful and interactive rather than a careless one-way process (Qubein, 1997), requires active listening. The active listener has three skills. The first skill is sensing, which is the ability to recognize the speaker's silent messages of body language, vocal intonation, and facial expressions. The second skill is attending, in which the listener provides visual, vocal, and verbal messages that encourage the speaker, such as eye contact, affirmative head nods, or verbally encouraging expressions ("uh-huh," "yes," "I see"). The third skill is responding, an attempt to make the speaker feel understood through a mutual dialogue (Hunsaker and Alessandra, 1986). The response part of listening includes validation (acknowledging the personal feelings of the speaker), questioning (clarifying points the speaker made or asking about the feelings involved), and summarization (repeating the speaker's story to ensure that it has been correctly interpreted).

Like any other skill, active listening requires effort to develop. Notice how Hunsaker and Alessandra's outline of the skills of active listening mirrors the construct of emotional intelligence proposed by Mayer and Salovey years later (Mayer and Salovey, 1997). In active listening, sensing involves identification of the feelings and emotions woven through a speaker's verbal and nonverbal communication. Attending corresponds to the facilitation and understanding levels of emotional ability and involves understanding the interaction of emotions and the responses that certain actions and reactions will evoke. Finally, responding invokes the skill of emotion management. The three active listening skills of sensing, attending, and responding are also present in caring behaviors and selflessness, which, according to Halm and Penque (1999), are two elements of having one's spirit at work (p. 35).

Because the other types of listeners described earlier lack the most basic level of emotional skill, emotional identification, they would not be able to use the more advanced emotional skills (see the discussion of emotional intelligence in Chapter Three). The nonlistener and the marginal listener do not identify emotions in communications because they do not hear them. The evaluative listener ignores them. Only the active listener combines emotional cues and facts to lay the foundation for effective conflict resolution.

There are several cues that someone is not listening well: jumping to conclusions, excessive talking, or blatant inattention (Qubein, 1997), all of which may dampen the effectiveness of a communication to varying degrees. At times, bad listening manifests itself in extreme ways, and as a result, communication breaks down in more serious ways than just the misinterpretation of meanings and cues.

Take, for example, the department manager who attended a meeting with other members of his health care organization, some of whom were involved in structuring a quality initiative for the facility. Although the primary reason for the meeting was dissemination of information (a common reason for many meetings that makes listening skills extremely important), the manager entered the room with his usual evaluative stance: he had little time for such a meeting but was attending so that he would not miss anything that might have an adverse impact on his bottom line.

The speakers presented the project with earnest enthusiasm, and most of the attendees asked questions when appropriate. Most of the questions were for the purpose of understanding the initiative further or understanding how the initiative would affect the area the attendee represented. Because the project was in its early stages, some showed mild skepticism at first, which softened during the course of the speakers' presentation. The body language of a few others reflected nonlistening or listening marginally.

The department manager, however, boldly and harshly manifested his cynicism. He interrupted constantly with reasons that the project was unimportant and irrelevant. He insisted that the initiative would be a financial drain without even questioning the cost of the project. Attempts at explanation on the part of the speakers were met with intensifying criticism. As a result, the presenters left the meeting feeling embarrassed and demoralized.

Although this is an extreme example, it represents the negative potential of faulty listening. The department manager was inappropriate in the way he addressed the presenters, but even leaving interpersonal skills aside, the manager boiled during the meeting because he was not *listening*. Others in the room took advantage of the opportunity to explore the initiative further, even though they had questions about the project and its impact on their areas. The department manager completely slammed the door on this opportunity, because he determined its impact based on his own prejudices and shut the speakers out. Unfortunately, the manager's actions had a trickle-down effect on all involved: the presenters lost confidence in their own ability to make a valuable contribution to the organization, others in the room felt embarrassed for the presenters and lost respect for the manager, and a well-thought-out initiative never got off the ground.

Fortunately for purposes of this illustration, the department manager was bold in demonstrating his faulty listening ability. Many times, the same phenomenon occurs without being as abundantly obvious. Nonlistening, marginal listening, and evaluative listening all may occur because the listener does not feel she needs to hear more or to understand the meanings behind the words she is hearing. She has made up her mind already not to absorb valuable information.

These types of ineffective listening can be just as detrimental as, if not more than, the explicit kind of nonlistening exemplified by the department manager in the previous example. When someone listens only marginally, or pretends to listen but has his mind already made up, the consequences of nonlistening are still present. In situations where conflict is present, this type of covert nonlistening hampers the conflict resolution process.

For example, imagine that a supervisor is attempting to help two nurses resolve a conflict related to the development of a unit policy, but sees personal advantage to herself in one possible solution. She may pretend to listen to both individuals' thoughts about what the policy should contain, but she may already have her mind made up. Because she does not effectively listen, she not only misses significant information but she actually resolves the conflict unfairly based on her own predisposition toward a solution.

Often conflicts go unaddressed because leaders choose to ignore the emotional aspect of a communication. Consider this example of marginal listening. A unit supervisor asks a nurse to care for the patient in room 603, a room outside his normal assignment. The staff nurse complies with the request, but it is obvious in his response that he is uncomfortable with the assignment. If the supervisor is listening marginally, she will choose not to explore the reason for the nurse's hesitation and will miss an opportunity to resolve the issue with the staff member.

UNDERSTANDING DIFFERENCES IN COMMUNICATION STYLES. Another important tool for promoting effective dialogue is understanding differences in communication styles that stem from different personality types. These differences were researched and defined by the psychiatrist Carl Jung, who divided the human personality into four types: the thinker, the feeler, the sensor, and the intuitor (imaginer). According to Jung, thinkers are typically organized, structured, accurate, and research-oriented, while feelers are emotional, spontaneous, and introspective. Sensors tend to be goal-oriented, active, and concerned with results. Intuitors, or imaginers, are often imaginative, impetuous, and visionary (Hunsaker and Alessandra, 1986).

When categorizing individuals by personality types, it should always be kept in mind that people rarely fall into only one category and that a personality type is not a total personality description. These categories only describe ways in which individuals tend to interact with others. Also, we must remember that personality does not equate to emotional ability in the scientific sense (Mayer, Salovey, and Caruso, 1999), although the two may appear to support each other logically.

Emotional skills are intricately and sensitively woven into effective dialogue, and no less in the ability to use personality types than in active listening. If, for example, I know someone to be a sensor, I may tailor my communication by keeping in mind his desire to achieve goals and results as I work through conflict with him. This does not mean that I will use what I know about his personality to sell him a point of view but rather that I understand his motivations and therefore know how he is likely to react to emotional cues within a certain interaction. In other words, I will frame my interaction with him so the resolution process appeals to his results-oriented side and he feels that he is directly involved in finding the solution. I will have skillfully combined emotional identification, facilitation, understanding, and management (Mayer and Salovey, 1997) to help someone resolve a conflict.

Stage 2: Analyzing the Elements of the Conflict

When initiating the analysis stage of conflict resolution, it is important to understand common sources of conflict, frequent responses to conflict, the impact of corporate culture and of personality, as well as how to identify conflicts that are essentially irresolvable.

SOURCES OF CONFLICT. It is obvious that analysis of a conflict involves focusing on the basic source or sources of the conflict. In health care, as in any other field, the primary sources of conflict in an organization generally fall into disputes about professional roles, goals, and procedures. Although people tend to personalize conflict—that is, they ascribe blame to another person who is involved—a majority of workplace conflicts stem from differences regarding what role a particular individual should play in a given situation or structure, what an individual wishes to achieve, or how work should be done (Wall, Solum, and Sobol, 1992). A fourth source of conflict, especially common in health care, concerns values; conflict is often generated by differences in belief systems (Barton, 1991). This type of conflict is particularly significant, since shared values have been shown by research to promote personal vitality (Kouzes and

Posner, 1995) in addition to that of the team or organization. Finally, some conflict is caused by miscommunication or misunderstanding due to differing styles of communication. This is not always caused by a lack of communication; even if you communicate well, the other person may still disagree, especially if the two of you have different communication styles.

In nursing, managed care exacerbates role conflicts in a variety of ways. At a time when care is moving toward a team approach that includes physicians and ancillary personnel, nurses may feel a loss of autonomy in patient care practices. On the other hand, nurses accustomed to following a previously existing care plan are being asked to assume more authority and more accountability for patient care decisions. This may lead to role uncertainty, as any team situation renders roles more ambiguous than does a tightly structured vertical hierarchy (Wall, Solum, and Sobol, 1992).

Another role conflict generated by managed care is perceived by nurses, who traditionally have the role of patient advocate, when they feel that the limited resources of a health care facility force them into the role of organization advocate. A prime example would be a situation in which an elderly DNR-code patient requires constant care. If this patient is in a hospital with limited staff resources and the majority of resources tend to be allotted to patients with a higher potential for recovery, the nurse may experience a value conflict.

For nurse executives and managers, role conflict may be caused by changes in what constitutes nursing leadership. As the traditional vertical hierarchy continues to be replaced by horizontal structures that emphasize staff empowerment, nurse executives may disagree on which fundamental leadership style is most effective within the organizational structure. At the same time, staff nurses may experience conflict in the overlapping roles created by downsizing or in new work assignments that alter traditional areas of nursing responsibilities.

Goals are a second major source of nursing conflict. Nurses may disagree over patient care goals in the unit or department, feeling that the goals are either too ambiguous or too difficult to measure to be a basis for quality care. Other goal disputes may occur over what constitutes a desirable patient care outcome. For example, two nurses may disagree over the indicator used to measure a patient's mastery of the self-care procedures required after discharge (Maher, 1991).

Procedure, or how work should be done, tends to be a major source of conflict in health care facilities. In mapping critical paths for nursing interventions, nurses may have disputes over the sequence and timing of nursing activities or procedural issues such as the relative effectiveness of various patient teaching modalities. In addition, disputes may arise over documentation practices that reduce time for patient care or over performance evaluations, which may be perceived as unfair (Maher, 1991) or inappropriate for a smaller staff. An example might involve a nurse working in case management for an insurance company. She may feel that a certain therapy is appropriate for a patient, but the company's approval criteria do not support the recommendation, so she is unable to substantiate a case for approval. The nurse may experience both role conflict and value conflict in this situation.

Differing communication styles can also be a source of conflict. Although personality is rarely a source of conflict, it dictates how conflict is perceived and communicated—or misperceived and mistakenly communicated. Two individuals may have the same opinion on a given issue but express their opinions so differently that they fail to perceive similarities; they might even perceive conflict. One person, for example, may feel strongly about quality and may make her sense of urgency apparent in her communication; while the other person feels quality is equally as important but refers to it in a matter-of-fact way. In this instance, the first individual may infer that the second individual places a low value on quality, based on her communication style. Because the similarity in their respective feelings toward quality is not perceived, a conflict is perceived. For this reason, a general understanding of personality types can serve as a tool for conflict resolution.

RESPONSES TO CONFLICT. In the past, nurses have frequently used avoidance, or withdrawal, as a means of conflict resolution, based on feelings of powerlessness in their job relationships (Jones, 1992). Although avoidance is a method of conflict resolution, it is effective only in a few limited instances. One instance is a situation in which the conflict will be settled by forthcoming events, such as the retirement of a supervisor. Another example is a value conflict with the organization of such magnitude that the only way of resolving the conflict is to work elsewhere. Avoidance is likely to cause the problem to escalate and result in a negative impact on care delivery. The fact that the problem is not acknowledged does not mean it does not exist, and when the conflict inevitably arises, it is likely to be fraught with frustration and blaming.

Avoidance of conflict may arise from a reluctance to expose underlying emotions that go along with it. Many would rather ignore the problem than pay the emotional price that goes along with it. Unhealthy conflict avoidance in management may stem from the notion that conflict is bad and, more specifically, that someone who has not kept things running smoothly will not be favorably viewed by peers or administration.

What is lacking here is a vision of how to incorporate the emotional skills necessary to manage the conflict, which consist of knowing what feelings are at stake and skillfully managing them to a solution. Goleman (2000) describes extremely affiliative leaders who are so concerned about getting along with people that they ultimately worry themselves into failure. They are unwilling to confront conflict and usually do not know or care to admit that something is wrong.

At the other end of the spectrum is the attack or aggression (Montebello, 1994) mode of response, expressed by aggressive actions such as ultimatums, which are characteristic of a rigid hierarchical authority pyramid. As is the case with avoidance, the aggression mode has very limited applications in the workplace. In a military organization, a direct order or ultimatum is a traditional conflict resolution method; however, in a health care setting, ultimatums tend to be limited to emergency situations in which a patient's life depends on an immediate and particular order or to situations in which an impaired nurse or physician constitutes a danger to patients. Aside from these instances, the aggression mode is largely ineffective, because it results in temporary solutions that create resentment and resistance in colleagues and staff.

As with avoidance, the aggression mode of conflict resolution has its misplaced applications as well. The authoritarian way of dealing with issues fails to take into account the fact that this mode does not always motivate people or resolve situations as one would hope. Why? Because people have emotions that cause them to react in certain ways to aggression—specifically, fear, resentment, and hostility. Perhaps aggression can result in an immediate solution, but it will almost certainly have severe fallout in the long run.

A third mode of response is accommodation, in which the conflict is resolved because one party gives in to the other without deriving any satisfaction from the outcome. Accommodation may be used when an issue is significantly more important to one person than to another (Barton, 1991). For example, a nurse might develop a particular patient teaching modality and have a vested interest in implementing it. A second nurse could feel that a new modality is unnecessary, since patients respond very well to the existing one. However, because the issue is not as important to the second nurse, she can resolve the conflict by accommodating the new modality. Similar to accommodation is compromise (Barton, 1991), in which the issue is equally important to each party, and each party accepts a partial solution. Using the example of the nurse conflict over teaching modalities, a compromise resolution might be that the new teaching modality is implemented, but only as a test case and over a limited period of time. The limitation of accommodation and compromise is that these responses tend to produce short-term solutions, which normally do not promote growth. In addition, similar to the evaluative type of listening, this method may take facts into account but not the underlying issues. It is often a rote, split-the-dividends approach that yields compromise based on equality alone. Each nurse may achieve some of what she wanted without ever considering or working with her own emotions or those of her colleague. A more efficient approach to resolution might be to determine the issues behind the problem, read the situation in terms of emotion, and understand the impact of any solution on all parties involved.

A fourth and generally the most effective response to conflict is collaboration, which involves negotiation among all the disputing parties. Collaboration demonstrates the affiliative leadership style, described by Goleman, Boyatzis, and McKee (2002) as "collaborative competence in action" (p. 64). Collaboration is used when the situation requires that all parties be satisfied with the resolution, because it includes input from different perspectives as well as commitment of all parties to the resolution (Barton, 1991). The conflict resolution model outlined in this chapter is structured to support a collaborative response to conflict, as opposed to a response based on avoidance, aggression, or accommodation. Collaboration invokes the most emotional skill of all the approaches to conflict resolution and comes closest to the practical definition of constructive conflict. The most effective conflict management involves drawing out all parties and understanding their various perspectives (Goleman, 2000). It further entails bringing the conflict to the surface and redirecting group energies toward a collaborative ideal.

Cooper and Sawaf (1997) present approaches to what they call "constructive discontent," or dealing with the disagreement from adversaries, which can also be applied to constructive conflict. They suggest the use of entrainment, or changes in vocal patterns and rhythms, to show that emotions are understood. When things become heated, Cooper and Sawaf recommend remaining open and listening more in order to increase the opportunity to understand. The thinking process should be almost visible as advocacy is balanced with inquiry. Potential points for cooperation should be identified.

In addition, Cooper and Sawaf (1997) recommend speaking from experience while avoiding defensiveness. When the answer is no, say no. Following through and productive management of anger are also key elements in dealing with those who disagree. Perhaps most important, one must understand that even in the face of the most constructive conflict resolution, there will still be cynics and disagreement.

THE EXTERNAL ENVIRONMENT OF CONFLICT: ORGANIZATIONAL CULTURE. In analyzing conflict, an important factor is the organizational culture in which the conflict occurs. Organizational culture is a combination of symbols, language, assumptions, and behaviors that manifest themselves in a setting (Fleeger, 1993). Values form the bedrock of an organization's culture (Kouzes and Posner, 1995). Clues to an organizational culture are both explicit and implicit. Explicit clues are written policies and procedures, organizational charts, levels of authority structure, and communication channels. Implicit clues are found in the informal, unwritten rules and expectations regarding communications, dress, and so on (Fleeger, 1993).

Another factor in corporate culture is the structure through which staff members are managed. For example, in organizations such as the military, the top echelon maintains maximum control through a rigid vertical hierarchy. This is the maximum control organizational structure (Kaye, 1994), in which there is little latitude for self-expression or innovation, and rules dictate procedure to an extreme. Another extreme is the individualistic maximum internal competition structure, in which managers are pitted against one another to compete for the same goal. This structure can create an intensely negative environment in which teamwork is virtually impossible. A third extreme is the maximum trust and internal support structure, which frequently creates a corporate climate so interdependent and undirected that it ceases to be effective. These three extremes form a triangle, with each corner representing an extreme. Typically, organizations fall somewhere near one corner of the triangle, but the ideal corporate environment is a balance, located in the middle of the triangle (Kaye, 1994).

In the 1990s, many organizations, especially health care facilities, were still in transition, moving from vertical to flattened horizontal hierarchies. Due to this transition, organizations tended to contain elements of both new and old cultures, creating an uneven and often unpredictable corporate culture.

Many hospitals and other health care organizations are still organized in a traditional top-down authority structure, with the board and CEO at the top. As such, traditional health care organizational hierarchies limit an institution's ability to deal with conflict (Evans, 1991). There is a tendency in these types of organizations to defer to the opinion of the most senior person, since people at lower levels do not always have the authority to resolve a conflict. Environments that are competitive run counter to collaborative efforts, no matter how strong or well intentioned they might be (Kouzes and Posner, 1995). However, through models such as shared leadership, based on a recognized partnership between the organization and its staff, nurse administrators are attempting to create structures within the nursing service that are governed from the bottom up, with accountability and responsibility delegated to staff colleagues. Within this context, it is possible for nurse executives to implement conflict resolution models that eventually may serve as a model for the rest of the organization.

In the absence of a corporate culture of staff empowerment, it is virtually impossible for those involved in a dispute to openly express their points of view, so avoidance, aggression, or accommodation responses to conflict are frequently used. If nurses are to solve the complex issues arising from the transition to managed care, it is essential that they achieve conflict resolution through collaboration. Rising to that challenge will require a paradigm shift at the highest administrative level.

THE ROLE OF PERSONALITY IN COMMUNICATION. Personality analysis can be a useful tool in both the analysis and facilitation stages of conflict resolution. Basic personality structure tends to dictate styles of communication. In the Jungian model of personality, the thinker will tend to communicate facts, whereas the visionary intuitor (imaginer) may focus on all the possible future ramifications of the situation. The sensor lives in the present, reacting more to immediate input from the environment than from past experience or future possibilities. The feeler reacts to the emotional content of a given situation rather than the external facts. Again, every individual's personality contains elements of all four types; however, one approach to interactions will tend to be dominant (Read, Fordham, Adler, and McGuire, 1971).[1] Differences in personality can mask similarities. Two individuals may have exactly the same goals, but one may express the goal in factual, intellectual terms, while the other is likely to describe the goal in terms of possible outcomes. Knowing these differences enables the administrator to determine the role that miscommunication has played in the conflict and thereby help the disputants come to a better understanding of each other.

RECOGNIZING THE IRRESOLVABLE CONFLICT. While analyzing and before seeking to facilitate a conflict, we must recognize that most conflict is resolvable, as long as the sources of conflict are within the control of the organization or people involved. Some conflicts, however, are unresolvable, and we can save ourselves time and effort if we recognize those situations. In cases where the values of a staff member clash with the values of an organization, the conflict will remain and possibly escalate. One such situation might be a pro-life nurse working in a facility that performs abortions. Another would be a nurse who cannot accept aspects of his organization's care guidelines. In these situations, each individual has the right to his or her own beliefs, and depending on the strength of those beliefs, the only long-term solution may be for the nurse to work elsewhere.

Given this reality, the most effective conflict resolution for these situations is prevention. Part of the interviewing process for any nursing position should be a candid overview of organizational values, as well as questions regarding how the potential candidate relates to these values. In interviewing a desirable candidate, it is only human to present the organization in its best light; however, omitting organizational perspectives that may later produce conflict may have negative effects on both the organization and the job candidate in the long run.

Another conflict that is normally irresolvable through collaboration is one generated by a colleague who is impaired because of substance abuse or other serious personal issues. In such an instance, counseling, referral, or temporary removal from duty may be the only options available to a manager who must put patient welfare above all other considerations.

In situations where conflict is caused by fear of job loss due to staff reductions, resolution in the usual sense is not possible, because the nurse administrator cannot assure the staff that no jobs will be lost. However, in an atmosphere of collaboration and communication, the fear of potential loss can be reduced to some extent.

Stage 3: Facilitating the Resolution

Emotional intelligence, as defined by Mayer, Salovey, and Caruso (1999, 2000, 2002) and measured by a four-branch model, can be called on to assist in the facilitation phase of conflict resolution. There are other aspects of character, such as optimism and tenacity, that have been erroneously equated with emotional intelligence (Jones, 1997), but these are separate contributors to the conflict resolution process.

Once analysis of the conflict has taken place and the conflict has been deemed resolvable, facilitation should begin. This involves invoking the emotional skills needed to arrive at a suitable resolution and move past the conflict.

IDENTIFICATION OF PERSONAL CONFLICT MANAGEMENT STYLE. Conflict resolution mirrors team or group process in that it necessitates collaboration, which is a developmental process for teams (Gardner and Cary, 1999). One of the first steps that team members must take in developing skills in conflict facilitation is to identify each individual's usual conflict management style. This can be done individually or in a group session; any noted areas for improvement should be addressed. Participants may be asked to describe how they typically handle conflict situations. For example, does a team member typically avoid conflict, minimize it, face it head on, hope it will disappear, give in too easily, or tenaciously hold his point of view? Each participant should then evaluate his or her conflict management tendencies as to whether they have been effective or ineffective in resolving the conflict. For teams wanting to make this a more formal exercise, the leader might secure a published conflict management workbook for each team member. Understanding how each team member reacts to conflict not only helps the individual, it helps the team understand its collective conflict management strengths and weaknesses.

Robbins and Hunsaker (1996) contrast characteristics of those unskilled in conflict management with those who are skilled. Those who are unskilled generally avoid conflict with people or situations likely to result in conflict, accommodate so that everyone will get along, get upset or take the conflict personally, and are unable to work under conflict long enough to get a good deal. In other words, these individuals may give in too easily just to avoid continuing conflict.

Successful conflict facilitators know how to overcome destructive emotions that may be at the root of avoidance. Goleman (2003) describes steps to overcome such emotions, and Mayer, Salovey, and Caruso (2000, 2002) provide the framework for emotional skill that can be applied in conflict management. Emotion management, the highest level of their skill set, essentially involves moderating one's own emotions and helping others do the same in order to successfully navigate through situations and be more productive. Conflict is no exception: what better venue is there in which to practice these management skills? Rather than cower behind the hope that some day the "threat" will go away, conflict managers face the threat and are able to manage their emotions about it.

Those who are unskilled in conflict management often fail to notice conflict in time to be proactive. They often stumble into conflict without seeing it coming. When conflict does occur, they tend to allow issues to fester and grow rather than dealing with them, as though they hope the problems will go away. Also, people who are unskilled in conflict management tend to be excessively competitive (Robbins and Hunsaker, 1996). On the other hand, those skilled in conflict management will step up to conflict and view it as an opportunity. They read situations quickly and tend to be very good at focused listening. They reach equitable settlements after hammering out tough agreements. These people tend to find common ground and get cooperation with minimal noise (Robbins and Hunsaker, 1996).

APPLYING THE TOOLS OF CONFLICT RESOLUTION. There are fundamental tools of conflict resolution that can be applied once the conflict has been understood and analyzed. They include giving credence to emotions, avoiding assumptions, active listening (which plays a part in the facilitation stage as well as the earlier stage of promoting effective dialogue), validation, summarization, and questioning. The team member skilled in conflict resolution will often use these tools and apply emotional skill in carrying them out.

Giving Credence to Emotions. Human emotion constitutes a powerful part of any conflict (Vargo, 1997), whether the battleground is a country or a nursing unit. In many instances, individuals become locked into feelings and maintain negative emotions that persist long after the initial issue of the conflict is eliminated. Emotions tend to obscure the real source of conflict, creating roadblocks to resolution. For this reason, feelings must be addressed and emotions controlled before any progress can be made toward a solution (Smith, Tutor, and Phillips, 2001).

Avoiding Assumptions. The second tool for resolving conflict is approaching the situation with a mental and emotional clean slate, avoiding assumptions or prejudgments about what has happened. This is a difficult task, for every individual has personal preferences and past experiences that trigger particular points of view. However, to make assumptions about a conflict is to set up a roadblock to resolution and narrow the options available for problem solving. Perhaps more detrimental to conflict resolution itself, making assumptions without clarifying shows disrespect for the parties involved (Gebelein, Lee, Nelson-Neuhaus, and Sloan, 1999).

Active Listening. As in the first stage of promoting effective dialogue, active listening involves sensing the feelings or intent of the speaker, providing visual and verbal messages that encourage the speaker, and responding to the speaker. The first message that the speaker receives comes from the environment. To create an environment for active listening, it is important to structure a conversational setting that says, "You are just as important as I am." In a manager-subordinate interaction, this might include sitting next to the employee, as opposed to across the desk from him, putting phone calls on hold, and preventing other interruptions.

During active listening in conflict resolution, be especially alert for emotional cues that follow the resolution process. While emotional reactions to the initial conflict may be strong, reactions to an attempted resolution or facilitation may be even stronger, since the outcome of the resolution may not completely satisfy everyone involved. Use the same skills of active listening described in the section on promoting effective dialogue to ensure that all emotional aspects are addressed and managed appropriately during this stage.

Validation. Identifying with others involved, including their emotions, promotes effective communication (Qubein, 1997). Especially in conflict resolution, it is not enough to simply identify or understand feelings: the individual must understand that her feelings are validated as well. The validation technique includes (1) listening for the emotion underlying a speech and (2) mirroring that emotion back to the individual through the use of key phrases. To validate another person's feelings is not to agree with them but to acknowledge that those feelings exist. Some examples of validating statements include "It sounds as if you're feeling very angry" and "That must be a very frightening feeling."

In dealing with a third-party dispute in which you are a neutral party, the use of the word *I* should be avoided. If the "neutral party" says, "I really understand your anger," it may be interpreted by the disputant as an indication that the third-party individual is on her side. Again, validation is the process of acknowledgment, not agreement.

In addition, *You must* or *You should* or *The facts are* should be avoided, since these phrases may be perceived as ultimatums. The goal at this point is to move past emotions by validating them. Even in crisis situations, validation tends to relax the speaker, lower the emotional defenses that have been erected, and allow the individual to move into the cognitive, or rational stage of expression (D. Fenelon, training lecture, Crisis Intervention of Houston, 1992).

In a situation in which an individual must confront a colleague who is angry at the organization or the administrator herself, the use of *I* is appropriate—for example, "I can really understand your anger" or "I can see how that might make a person feel really bad." The difference is that only one person is involved, so there is no risk that the administrator may be perceived as favoring one staff member over another.

Summarization. Once the other party has finished speaking, the listener should summarize what the speaker has said, in order to establish rapport and ensure that the speaker has been heard correctly. A summary generally begins with something like this: "Let me make sure I've understood you correctly. In your view, . . ." A summary or paraphrase is useful both in confirming what has been said and in developing rapport with the individual, who at least feels that he or she has been understood. In addition, a summary provides information that may eventually be used to explore resolution options (Fenelon, 1992; Qubein, 1997).

Particularly in superior-subordinate interactions, once the manager is clear about the employee's view of the conflict, it is important that the manager communicate value to the employee—that is, assure the employee of her importance to the organization. Valuing is assuring an individual that she is appreciated by the organization. Valuing is different from validation, which is to acknowledge feelings. Frequently, valuing eases or eliminates fear of job loss or resentment created by the perception that an employee is unappreciated by management.

Questioning. Effective questioning can greatly simplify the situation by providing the basis for understanding the current circumstances and actively seeking viable solutions. There are two major types of questions: closed and open. The purpose of a closed question is to elicit specific and narrow information, such as "What are the patient's vital signs?" The open question, which is designed to solicit feelings and opinions, typically contains the word *what* or *how*. For example, an open question could begin, "In reviewing this situation, what ideas have you had about . . . ?" or "In your opinion, how could this situation best be resolved?" (Hunsaker and Alessandra, 1986). Although individuals may be overwhelmed by or locked into their emotions regarding the conflict, underneath the emotion they are still functioning at a cognitive, or thinking level. At a cognitive level, individuals tend to mentally review the situation and consider different options for resolution, even if they cannot take action due to emotional roadblocks (Fenelon, 1992).

The tools we have considered for use in the facilitation stage are designed to move disputants beyond feelings and into a mind-set in which they can use their own cognitive processes to help resolve the situation.

Summary

Conflict is inherent in everyday life, and the workplace is no exception to this rule. Although conflict is often avoided, conflict resolution can instead be implemented at all levels of an organization and can result in increased organizational productivity. The three stages of conflict resolution are promoting effective dialogue, analyzing, and facilitating. Sound techniques of conflict resolution, when properly applied at each stage, can result in emotionally intelligent conflict management. As the example in the chapter supplement will demonstrate, conflict resolution skills can aid in solving even the most sensitive problems in an organization.

Emotional acuity is key to successful conflict resolution. The ability to identify and understand emotions, while facilitating change and productive management of those same emotions, is a strong catalyst in the transition from conflict to effective change.

TEN CRITERIA FOR EMOTIONALLY INTELLIGENT CONFLICT RESOLUTION

1. All members of the team practice active listening.
2. There is an understanding of differences in communication styles that may relate to conflict management.
3. There is an analysis of the source of the conflict, the nature of response to the conflict, the encompassing environment, and the effect of personality.
4. There is an analysis of whether the conflict can be resolved.
5. Each team member is aware of his or her own personal conflict resolution style, as well as how emotions influence that style.
6. The crucial role of emotions in conflict and conflict resolution is recognized.
7. The team avoids assumptions while listening for facts and feelings.
8. There is validation of the feelings of each disputant in the conflict.
9. There is summarization of the facts and feelings at hand.
10. Effective questioning is used to gather needed information.

NOTE

1. C. G. Jung's theory of personality is considerably more extensive than the elements outlined in this text. For a complete study of Jung's theory of personality, see Read, Fordham, Adler, and McGuire (1971).

DEMONSTRATION OF A CONFLICT RESOLUTION PROCESS

In the following example, a scenario is presented to allow the reader to walk through the steps of conflict resolution and the rationale for each step of the process.

Scenario

An orthopedic nursing unit was in the process of changing to a team approach to patient care when the unit supervisor resigned. One nurse, Leslie, who had worked on the unit for five years, expected that she would receive a promotion to unit supervisor. The position was instead given to a new nurse, Carol, hired from a different facility. This decision was made because Carol had evidenced innovative thinking in her former position and had played an active role in implementing the team care approach. Leslie, who was well liked and respected on the unit, sabotaged every effort Carol made to implement changes. She also began to create allies among the nursing staff, some of whom were upset by all the changes.

In addition, the two nurses had very different personalities. Carol was a sensor—enthusiastic, bold, and action-oriented, with a tendency to make decisions quickly. Leslie, a thinker, was cautious, reserved, and methodical. The conflict reached such proportions that the unit was disrupted, and Carol brought the matter to the attention of her manager, Suzanne.

Intervention

Suzanne explains to Carol that she will try to help her and Leslie resolve their conflict by using a three-step conflict-resolution process. First she will promote effective dialogue, second she will analyze the elements of the conflict, and finally she will seek to facilitate a resolution.

Stage 1: Promote an Effective Dialogue

To promote a dialogue that will be effective for conflict resolution, Suzanne gathers information, helps Carol and Leslie to explore options, and seeks to discover the individual goals of the nurses involved.

GATHER INFORMATION. Suzanne begins her information gathering with Carol, the new nurse supervisor, using the tools of active listening, validation, summarizing, and questioning.

Carol's story: Carol was aware that she had been hired to make changes and was afraid of losing her job if Leslie continued to block changes on the unit and align the staff nurses against her. In Carol's opinion, Leslie was slow, resistant to change, and jealous of Carol's position.

Leslie's story: Leslie felt, in her own words, "trashed" by having been overlooked for the unit supervisor's position, given her experience on the unit and dedication to her patients. Leslie also was offended by Carol's boldness and rapid approach to problem solving on a unit where she was new, as well as by her tendency to disregard input from experienced staff.

Rationale. Each nurse has the right to air her side of the story. Suzanne's decision to hold one-on-one dialogues with each party is effective; an intimate setting allows each participant to openly express feelings and opinions that would remain private in a collective meeting. In this situation, neither nurse would have been as candid in expressing her feelings if she had had to face the other nurse at the height of the conflict.

EXPLORE OPTIONS. Suzanne asks Carol what ideas she has about resolving the situation. Carol replies that she had hoped to create a unit quality control team headed by Leslie but that she doesn't feel that Leslie will support any ideas that Carol initiates.

When the same question is asked of Leslie, she replies that she has thought of either resigning or confronting Carol about disregarding input from unit staff. However, she confides to Suzanne that confrontation simply is not in her nature, and she feels hopeless about it both because Carol is her supervisor and because Carol does not seem to value the opinions of the staff.

Rationale. Generally, individuals involved in conflict review alternative methods of dealing with it, but the roadblock constituted by emotions prevents them from translating potential solutions into action. By inviting the individual in conflict to share options, the manager empowers that individual and gains his or her commitment to help find a resolution.

ELICIT INDIVIDUAL GOALS. In her one-on-one meetings with Carol and Leslie, Suzanne asks each nurse to list her goals for the unit.

Carol's primary professional goal is to eventually move into nursing administration. Her goal for the unit is to create a cost-effective team approach to patient care that will streamline and enhance current care delivery.

Leslie, who prefers bedside nursing to administrative nursing, wanted to be the unit supervisor while maintaining significant responsibility for patient care. She felt that the team approach would enhance patient care but also felt that a person familiar with current unit personnel and procedures should implement it over a long period of time.

Rationale. Knowing each disputant's professional and organizational (unit) goals provides the manager with a basis for determining whether the primary source of the conflict is in the area of roles, goals, or procedures.

Stage 2: Analyze the Elements of the Conflict

Once dialogue has been established and individual concerns are heard, Suzanne analyzes the elements of the conflict. She seeks to identify its true source and analyzes personality differences that might be significant in the conflict.

IDENTIFY SOURCES OF CONFLICT. Each nurse has the same goal for the unit—enhanced patient care—and their professional goals do not conflict. Carol is more interested in administration than bedside nursing, and Leslie, even in her goal of being unit manager, wishes to remain a bedside provider to the extent possible. This being the case, Suzanne identifies the primary source of conflict as a dispute over roles, with procedures as a secondary source. Each nurse feels that she is qualified to assume the leadership role in the unit—Carol because of her position and background, Leslie on the basis of unit experience. Each nurse favors changes to enhance patient care; however, they differ on the time frame and procedures for implementing change.

Rationale. In conflict resolution, it is essential to separate feelings from the true source of the conflict. In this instance, the conflict is a role dispute, complicated by Carol's fear of losing her new job by not making changes fast enough and by Leslie's disappointment at not having been appointed to the supervisory position. In any conflict, emotions tend to obscure the real issue. To resolve the conflict at its basic level, it is necessary to identify these emotions, reduce them to the extent possible, and isolate them from the real issue.

ANALYZE PERSONALITY DIFFERENCES. Using the Jungian-based personality model, Suzanne determines that Carol is predominantly a sensor: goal-oriented, active, and concerned with immediate results. These characteristics communicate themselves to Leslie and possibly to others on the unit as aggressiveness and disregard of input.

Leslie, on the other hand, is a thinker: organized, structured, and accurate. Her caution and methodical approach to situations are interpreted by Carol as reluctance to change.

Rationale. Since personality shapes communication styles, it is important to understand the primary personality type of each disputant.

Stage 3: Facilitate Resolution of the Conflict

The resolution process is now ready to begin. Suzanne assists the individuals to identify commonalities, identify sources of the conflict in practical terms, discuss areas of miscommunication, and brainstorm options for resolution. She then encourages the two nurses to commit to the resolution of the conflict and to develop a plan for monitoring the outcomes.

IDENTIFY COMMONALITIES. Finally, Suzanne meets with Carol and Leslie. Because each nurse has similar goals for the unit, Suzanne's first step is to compare the goals that each nurse has listed and to point out the ways in which these goals agree with and complement one another.

Rationale. Identifying the common ground among disputants tends to reduce tension and establish a tentative basis for communication.

IDENTIFY SOURCES OF THE CONFLICT IN PRACTICAL TERMS. Suzanne identifies the primary source of conflict as one of roles: which role each nurse will play in the unit. The secondary source of conflict is procedures, or how the transition to team care will be accomplished. Suzanne also shares Carol's idea of developing a unit quality control team headed by Leslie.

Rationale. Identifying the core sources of conflict to each disputant defines the conflict in practical rather than emotional terms, setting the stage for a practical resolution.

DISCUSS AREAS OF MISCOMMUNICATION. Suzanne points out to Carol and Leslie that as individuals, they tend to react and communicate in vastly different ways. She notes that Carol's enthusiasm and rapid approach to issues comes across to Leslie as disinterest in other staff members' input. And Suzanne notes that Leslie's methodical, analytical approach comes across to Carol as reluctance to try new ideas. These differences have created miscommunications that have made the conflict worse and have prevented Carol from mentioning the quality control team idea to Leslie.

Rationale. Pointing out ways in which different personalities perceive and communicate helps the disputants separate intent from style. In many instances, an individual may mean well but may communicate and react in a way that obscures good intentions.

BRAINSTORM OPTIONS FOR RESOLUTION. Suzanne asks each nurse to list at least three changes that will reduce the conflict between them. Carol lists the following: Leslie will assist in making the needed changes on the unit; Leslie will help explain changes to the other staff members; and Leslie will assume the position of head of the quality control team.

Leslie lists the following: Carol will invite the input of staff through weekly staff meetings; Carol will slow the pace of change, so that the staff has time to accustom itself to a new patient care approach; and Carol will take more time to get to know staff members and understand individuals' strengths and weaknesses.

The nurses discuss these options and decide that all of the listed changes are acceptable. Leslie, in keeping with her personality, wants to see how Carol will structure the weekly staff meetings before agreeing to help gain the staff's support.

Carol agrees to slow the pace of change, but to a lesser degree than Leslie wishes. She explains to Leslie that the hospital administration has informally requested that she implement team care as soon as possible.

Rationale. Conflict resolution is most effective when it is based on suggestions by the disputants. Asking the disputants to suggest solutions accomplishes two positive objectives: the disputant is personally and often professionally empowered, and the disputant becomes an active part of the resolution process, rather than merely following orders.

GAIN COMMITMENT TO RESOLUTION. The manager asks both nurses to make a commitment to the changes suggested by working together to develop an action plan. Suzanne requests that the action plan contain a good faith gesture from each nurse: one action that will be taken by each nurse to express belief in the other person's good intentions.

Rationale. Each disputant must actively commit to a resolution in order for it to be effective. Although a verbal commitment is a good beginning, real commitment must be manifested in action. For this reason, it is important to ask that a commitment from each disputant be put in writing. A good faith action encourages the disputants to begin building a trusting relationship.

Monitoring Outcomes

One way to monitor the outcome of conflict between two people is to request a written plan of action. A mutually developed, written action plan empowers each employee to plan an active role in resolving the conflict, crystallizes the resolution on paper, and serves as a guideline for implementing the resolution. In this case, the final action plan developed by Carol and Leslie reads as follows:

1. Carol will initiate weekly staff meetings, beginning the following Monday.
2. In the meeting, Carol will share her plans for changes, as well as the hospital's requested time frame.
3. Leslie will encourage staff members to contribute ideas to the meeting.
4. Carol will announce the development of a unit quality control team headed by Leslie.
5. Leslie will submit a proposal for the quality control team within three weeks.

Follow-Up

At the close of the facilitation meeting, Suzanne schedules a collective follow-up meeting for three weeks from the current date. She explains that at that meeting she will want to know the status of implementation of the action plan.

It is important to determine whether the conflict is resolved. Asking about the "status of the action plan implementation" rather than "Is the conflict resolved?" keeps the focus on action and resolution rather than conflict.

PART FOUR

CHANGING THE CULTURE OF NURSING AND THE ORGANIZATION

10

SHAPING THE WORK
ENVIRONMENT
AND CULTURE

THE ENVIRONMENT in which we work is probably one of the most important factors in job satisfaction, but it is also one of the most difficult to construct. While salary and benefit changes are relatively easy to decide, and schedules and patient loads can be reorganized at a moment's notice, forming a work culture that fosters growth and satisfaction among staff and leadership is a process that requires time, dedication, and careful attention to the emotional element.

Why All the Talk About Emotions and the Work Culture?

Anthropologists define culture as learned behavior (Parvis, 2003). Sometimes, specific behaviors in individuals are attributed to that individual's cultural background. For example, how one celebrates a holiday or one's tendency toward shyness might be explained partially by the fact that one was reared in a particular country or as a member of a particular ethnic group. As a result, culture has become ingrained in many of our minds as a differentiating factor between individuals and groups. In recent times, increasing efforts have been made to cross the implicit boundaries imposed by culture, so that now we have philosophies that promote experiencing other cultures and breaking down cultural barriers. Surely, in the eclectic society that is the United States, we need these principles to communicate with and relate to neighbors and friends who come from diverse origins and experiences.

It is little wonder, then, that the word *culture* has seeped into the language of business. Culture, according to Vestal, Fralicx, and Spreier

(1997), critically links strategy and results, and provides the framework for alignment of everything else, including who the leaders are and what they do. Much like *culture* in the broader sense, *culture* in the business sense can be used to describe the atmosphere in which people work, which imparts to these workers specific traits and work habits. Such habits and traits are more familiarly known as *cultural norms*. Cultural norms define what we can and cannot do (and get away with) in a specific culture. Cultural norms vary between cultures: what is acceptable in one culture may be unacceptable, or at least perceived as odd, in another.

Druskat and Wolff (2001) argue that groups have cultural norms just as societies do and that these influence the processing and expression of emotion within their group settings. For example, in a group whose cultural norm espouses harmony and an "everybody gets along" philosophy, there may be extreme attempts to suppress emotion and decrease conflict. In another group, where the norm is to "duke it out" until a decision is reached, there may be more vivid expression of emotions, both positive and negative, in group interactions. At times, these emotions may be used ineffectively, with little or no regulation, but they are still accepted in the group because that is the norm. As one might suspect, there can be a middle ground between these two extreme examples.

This chapter will focus on work cultures, specifically as they relate to emotional ability. In accord with the preceding chapters of the book, it will point out how the skill sets of identification, use, understanding, and management of emotion described by Mayer, Salovey, and Caruso (2000, 2002) relate to an emotionally relevant work culture. In addition, this chapter will examine the pervasive thread of the emotionally able work culture—empathy—and how it affects team interactions and individual successes, as well as a department or business as a whole.

The Continuum of Emotions in the Workplace

We are all subject to a range of emotions, from what we would consider positive ones to less desirable ones. Because we are involuntarily subject to these feelings, we are hardly immune to their effects on our thought processes, our actions, and our overall outlook on life. Understanding how emotions affect thought and using them to change our thinking are emotional skills that must be learned by individuals throughout their lifetime. People bring their raw abilities in this area to every group meeting they attend. One can see, yet again, why group settings can host a multitude of issues that are undoubtedly related to the use of emotions.

Cooper and Sawaf (1997) describe an emotional continuum that helps to explain the use of emotion and how emotions can affect thought. Along this continuum, they explain, emotions may be interpreted in a context that ranges from engaging or fully participating in the emotion at one end to feeling constricted by or wanting to escape that same emotion at the other end. In other words, the same emotion can be located at different points on the continuum and result in different meanings and impacts on thought and action. "In the spectrum of human feelings," they explain, "each emotion is imbued with its own 'signal' or intelligence. It does not simply *happen* to us; our inner self *generates* it, always for a reason, always to communicate something." They go on to point out that "The ability to experience the heights of enthusiasm and passion, for example, is commensurate with your capacity for experiencing the feelings of— rather than *acting out*—frustration and fury" (Cooper and Sawaf, 1997, p. 37). They also describe how the same basic emotion may generate concern on the participative end of the spectrum and fear on the constrictive end. Similarly, curiosity might engender creativity on the engaged side and jealousy on the constrictive side. The almost boundless possibilities of a context (which we learn) applied to raw emotion (which we experience involuntarily) might encourage us to strengthen our emotional ability so as to field emotions at the appropriate point on the continuum.

How the Continuum Affects Individuals

Every work culture and every individual either knowingly or unwittingly subscribes to a continuum like this one. In other words, the cultural norm of the group encourages the use of emotion in a certain way or context, as does the individual's emotional ability. In a particular setting, dissatisfaction might be channeled into resolve, or it might inhibit the ability to carry out daily tasks. If we take this idea further in an example, we might think of a unit clerk who is disturbed by a feeling of being "stepped on" by doctors and nursing staff, he might channel that feeling into resolve (to become more visible and valuable) or resentment (which may lead to exacerbation of the perceived slight and an increased inability to function). In another scenario, imagine that an angry family member has just bawled out a nurse. That nurse might initially feel anxiety or embarrassment. Depending on that nurse's ability to apply that emotion to thought, she might meet it with a demonstrated desire to understand the family member's root frustrations (an example of engagement with the emotion), or she might retreat in shame and avoid the patient for the next several hours, performing the bare minimum to serve the patient's needs or swapping patients with another nurse in order to avoid the patient entirely (an example of being constricted by the emotion).

The Group's Emotional Culture Is More Than Just Its Ideal

If business leaders hoping to be successful were asked which side of this particular continuum (participative or constrictive) best described the culture of their business, we can comfortably assume that most of them would place their organizational culture in a positive light. Who would want to believe, after all, that emotions—those necessary, uninvited, and often ugly invaders of our psyches—are handled in any way but well? Perhaps no team leader or business owner would describe her group as unable to do their work because they are constantly upset. She is more likely, of course, to say that her workers are eager and enthusiastic about working through issues and solving problems in order to carry out the mission of the company, department, or team.

Unfortunately, many groups are not typified by the more positive processing of emotion. The ideal that the group leader has for the group does not set the culture of the group. Rather, the group's emotional ability shapes that culture and makes it what it is. What that culture becomes will depend on many things, but one key ingredient either will or will not be in the mix and as such, will define the direction of the group's emotional culture. That key ingredient is empathy.

Empathy in the Work Setting

We each have our own conception of what empathy involves. A basic recollection of the term might take us back to a vocabulary lesson or a therapeutic communication class in which empathy and sympathy were differentiated. Some of us were taught that, essentially, sympathy could be bestowed on anyone (such as someone who experienced a death or illness) whether or not the sympathetic person had actually "been there." Empathy, however, required a firsthand knowledge of what the person was going through. If one had not experienced the death of a child, for example, he could not adequately empathize with someone else who had, although he would be very much able to sympathize. Many of us were cautioned, during instruction on therapeutic communication, to avoid assuring clients with "I know what you are going through" if we indeed had no experience on which to base this knowledge.

What Is Empathy, Really?

All of this makes perfect sense until we become aware that empathy (and not just sympathy) is a key ingredient in establishing an emotionally strong work culture. Of course, no one in a group can be expected to understand firsthand the emotions and experiences of everyone else.

Group members can, however, learn to understand emotions and experiences without having actually experienced them. First, we turn to Webster's definition of empathy: "(1) the identification with or vicarious experiencing of the feelings, thoughts, etc., of another" or "(2) the ascribing to an object of one's feelings or attitudes." Thus, we see that empathy involves intentionally putting ourselves in the position to understand someone's feelings and experiencing or even processing those feelings as if they were our own, even when the feelings did not originate within ourselves. Groups rich in empathy are able to do this, and there are several reasons why.

Fundamental, root empathy is said to develop in early childhood. "At 18 months, a toddler becomes aware of himself and his relationships with others" (Poole, 2003, p. 68). Even this early, toddlers are aware of and can identify with the emotions of others. By age four, children begin to understand the results of their behaviors on others' emotions (Miller, 2003) and can usually make choices based on empathic thought by age six (Church, 2003). At each stage of a child's development, educators recommend that empathy be taught to the child and that his manifestations of empathy be encouraged.

The Significance of the Empathic Work Culture

Why are a large number of Americans (some of them nurses) dissatisfied with their work (Helge, 2001)?

One explanation may be that the culture, or environment, of their workplace is oppressive and anxiety-producing. Anxiety disorders related to work contribute to absenteeism and increasing health care costs, and sometimes they manifest themselves in overt misbehavior in the workplace. This subtle yet ever-present emotion probably does more damage than it is credited with. Studies cited by Sauter and others (1999) reveal that between 26 and 40 percent of employees report problematic job stress (p. 99).

We tend to think of stress as something that occurs when our physical, mental, or emotional capabilities do not meet or do not appear to meet the expectations of our job. For example, if a nurse carries a heavy patient load, with high-acuity patients, we may automatically assume her to be more stressed than a nurse with a lighter load. In addition, we would expect an employee's lack of understanding of his job duties to contribute to stress, and we would expect exposure to highly emotional stimuli (which are frequently encountered by health care professionals as they care for sick and sometimes dying patients) to contribute to stress, too.

No job is worry-free. However, problematic stress lies over the line of exhilarating challenge in a job. As leaders, we want to provide employees with sufficient challenges without stretching them to the point of exhaustion. On the other hand, we do not want our departmental or corporate culture to be driven by the need for stress management. In other words, creating an empathic, emotionally relevant culture will alleviate some of the ill effects of stress, but relieving stress should not be the ultimate goal of creating such a culture.

What Are the Objectives of Infusing Empathy into the Work Culture?

Empathy in the work culture accomplishes several results. First, where empathy is present, there will be a sense of collegiality among workers, leading to improved teamwork. Second, empathy allows leaders and other team members to diffuse any negative emotions that may be contributing to ineffectiveness. Third, empathy provides channels for understanding and sharing visions for accomplishment and achievement. In the end, a sense of empathy in the culture is barely noticed, but it is reproduced in very tangible ways. The maturing team will move from clearly defined attempts to see things from another person's viewpoint to unconsciously making that part of its collective thought process.

Overt Manifestations of Empathy at Work

When assessing an environment in terms of its culture, look for manifestations of empathy. The presence of the factors described next are also overt goals to work toward while building an empathic culture.

TEAM COLLEGIALITY. Teams are not together just to have a good time, but team members who cannot relate to one another on at least a basic level are hindered in their collective ability to make decisions or achieve results. Collegial relationships between staff and management are credited, at least partially, with decreasing nurse turnover (Beglinger, 2003) and establishing win-win outcomes (Hagenow, 2001). Suppose this type of relationship does not exist between two or more team members. Because it will be the exception, rather than the rule, that all team members instantly find common ground, the leader in this case is charged with establishing empathic behavior within the team setting. The leader could start by displaying empathy toward both individuals, then outwardly encouraging each to see the issue as the other team member sees it.

MANAGEMENT OF NEGATIVE EMOTIONS. Over time, empathic behaviors evolve into a framework for processing emotions. Using the continuum concept that was proposed by Cooper and Sawaf (1997), we can visualize an empathy continuum, on which emotions are processed at varying levels of empathy. For example, when a team member with low levels of empathy, Sally, offers her opinion, another team member, Jack, with a differing opinion might stir up feelings of contempt, which might ultimately lead to isolating Sally's views as irrelevant. On the other end of the spectrum, a team member with high empathy, Anne, might offer the same opinion as Sally, but Jack will probably process his differing opinion in an entirely different and more productive way.

We learned from the Mayer-Salovey-Caruso Emotional Intelligence Scale that emotional identification is the most basic level of emotional ability (Mayer, Salovey, and Caruso, 2000, 2002). Without empathy, it is difficult to effectively identify, use, understand, or manage emotions. Recall that empathy involves feeling the feelings of another without actually experiencing the event that generates the feeling. The ability to facilitate thought with emotion (use of emotion) can be greatly influenced by empathy or the lack thereof, as can the ability to identify emotions in others.

Without empathy, more advanced emotional skills are hindered as well. If, for example, I have no ability to feel or relate to the emotions of someone else, how will I understand the potential of those emotions to influence their thought process or progress into other emotions? Furthermore, how will I help myself and the other person to manage those emotions if I do not understand them? The nature of the emotional building blocks becomes increasingly clear within the framework of empathy.

SHARED VISIONS AND GOALS. Because it helps teams to vicariously experience the feelings and thoughts of their collective memberships, empathy is a staunch facilitator of shared goals and visions. A shared vision can be viewed as empathy turned outward: it is a kind of external reapplication of the ability to absorb and modulate feelings and emotions within the group. The ultimate sharing of visions and goals can be conceptualized as the projection of group empathy into one complete, concise manifestation of group thought. A shared vision, like an empathic culture, is a manifestation of maturity in the team.

Empathy and Polarities in Team Communications

The term *gray area* is used to describe something that is not cut and dried. Although many would prefer that all decisions and situations had clear-cut solutions, it is abundantly apparent, especially when working with diverse individuals, that this is rarely the case. Often, there are two very different sides of the issue, and both must be taken into consideration. That is where empathy comes in.

WHAT ARE POLARITIES? Polarities, briefly defined, are interdependent values that may appear to be different or in opposition to each other. For example, staff satisfaction and patient satisfaction are two important issues. Neither one, achieved alone, will create a comfortable work culture. Both must be managed together, even though they may appear to be in conflict at times. Other examples of polarities are cost and quality, and work demands and staffing. We cannot totally sacrifice either of these polarities at the expense of the other (Wesorick, 2002).

Many political campaigns operate based on polarities; values that each candidate upholds frequently appear to be in opposition to the values of the opponents. Polarities in political campaigns are easily managed because we expect the candidates to have opposing viewpoints. In actuality, the candidate whose values best represent those of the voting majority will be elected. To simplify this to the present context, if I were running for "president" of a hospital unit and I based my campaign entirely on cutting costs, while my opponent based his campaign entirely on improving quality, the value nearest and dearest to the heart of the majority of voters would determine the election. We accept this as part of the political process. Different values exist no matter which side we are on.

WHY ARE POLARITIES SO DIFFICULT FOR TEAMS? A team interaction is not as clear-cut as a political campaign when it comes to polarities. Team members are supposed to be working together, not in opposing camps. However, team member A, just like team members B through J, usually will possess values that are polarities. The existence of these polarities creates a challenge for communication on the one hand in that they masquerade behind statements and opinions, beliefs, and views. For example, team member A might say, "I believe we should begin discharge teaching earlier," to represent his view that discharge teaching is of utmost importance, while team member B might say, "I think the patient retains more when we begin teaching closer to discharge," to represent her view that patients are not receptive to learning about discharge on admission. Both views are polarities: equally reasonable views about the appropriate place for discharge teaching, but they are represented with statements, not a description of the two views. Because they both refer to teaching, the views at hand here are much easier to decipher than they would be if team member B had said, "I think the early stages of admission should focus on assessment and stabilizing the patient." In that instance, one would have to surmise that she meant, given the context, that she did not agree with early discharge education. In another context, however, she might be pressing for more thorough assessment on admission. For this reason, deciphering the different views that exist in what people say requires careful attention on the part of a leader or facilitator. When team leaders and members acknowledge that there are polarities, they are able to facilitate dialogue that will result in a more solid team decision. For example, the leader could say, to continue the most recent example, "Team member A, I can see that you feel patients need teaching from day 1, and Team member B, you don't seem to see it that way." This identification of feelings is the open door for dialogue to begin. At that point, both team members feel acknowledged and that their views hold equal weight. If a team is doing its job, no one should emerge the political winner: a successful outcome for the group, not a victory for one individual, is the goal of teamwork.

HOW EMPATHY ASSISTS IN MANAGING, NOT FIXING, POLARITIES. "The dominant skill in health care," says Wesorick (2002), "is problem solving or fixing the issue. That approach to a polarity will make things worse over time" (p. 21). Yet it seems to be a natural instinct of nurses to want to fix something, whether it be a patient's dressing or the staffing issues on the unit. If it is not right, we try to fix it.

However, merely taking a "fix it" approach to one of the two or more conflicting issues may make things worse in the end. Polarities are values, not problems. The existence of a perceived conflict is a problem, but simply "fixing" one polarity without consideration of the other is not recommended. For example, simply finding ways to cut staffing costs on the unit will have detrimental effects in that it will probably have unrecognized ill effects on nurse workload or patient care quality.

Team communications are the conduit through which empathy flows. Every spoken word, nonverbal gesture, reflex, and calculated response represents the level of empathy present. Empathy is absolutely critical in managing polarities. Empathy guides us to understand what the values are, understand and identify which emotions are evoked by these values, understand how the values can be integrated, and establish a shared purpose in team communications about the issue at hand. The teams themselves are then equipped to lead (Higgins, 2003).

The Empathic Leader's Contribution to the Empathic Work Culture

Of course, the empathic work culture is not solely a product of one leader, but the empathic leader does contribute to its development. In fact, it would be difficult to establish a culture rich with empathy if the organization's leaders were not skilled in this area. For this reason, it is necessary to develop empathy in leaders as they work with teams and to develop it in such a way that they will be spurred to pass along the skill to team members.

We would expect the empathic leader to be especially skilled in the attributes discussed earlier in the book and for empathy to contribute to each of these skills. For example, creating and motivating for change requires the emotional skill to understand the team's attitudes and feelings about change; empathy enhances the skill of emotional understanding. Sharing a vision requires a great deal of emotion management in relation to others and has a great deal of empathy at its foundations. Setting an example also requires emotional skill as leaders prepare team members to lead themselves. It requires empathy to set an example that others will wish to follow.

Empathy is a key skill to be both downloaded and uploaded, and it is essential in effective conflict management. While the chapters devoted to these skills have discussed empathy in leadership, an entire culture marked by empathy is the ultimate goal of cultivating leader and team emotional skills.

Characteristics of the Empathic Leader

While every leader possesses distinct leadership characteristics that often can be categorized in a particular leadership style, there are certain characteristics that are central to all empathic leaders. These characteristics pervade the interactions between the leader and his constituents regardless of other leader traits.

NONJUDGMENTAL ATTITUDE. A nonjudgmental approach to team members is foundational to empathy. If we enjoyed being judged by others, the prospect of being sued or going to court would not faze us.

Rather, being judged or punished is an event we typically avoid if possible. While consequences for mistakes and inappropriateness are to be expected, leaders who base their actions and opinions on a preconceived notion or judgment of others are displaying low levels of empathy. In some cases, this judgmental attitude is referred to as self-righteousness, which carries with it fear and suspicion on the part of everyone who works with that person (Ryback, 1998). Not only are mistakes not accepted, but, worse, mistakes are expected by leaders who prejudge others.

This is not to say that a leader should not apply caution in dealing with individuals who have a history of inappropriate behavior. On the other end of the spectrum is the all-forgiving leader, who fails to take past patterns into consideration because he feels that doing so would render him harsh or unforgiving. There is certainly cause for considering past behaviors in making decisions or even in working to develop a team member. For example, if chronic tardiness or absence has been an issue, the leader would be naïve to overlook that fact when choosing someone to be a dependable project leader.

However, unfounded judgmental attitudes may stem from a leader's feelings of inferiority or, in unfortunate cases, a predisposition against certain groups or demographic categories such as age or race. Empathy is the antidote for each of these. Leaders who feel threatened or that they must one-up their constituents in order to maintain their position of authority would greatly benefit from taking a hard look at their own feelings and those of the ones around them. Except in rare cases, chances are that no one is out to get the leader's job or to usurp the leader's position of power. Ironically, the very hedge that self-righteousness builds around a leader is the same one that prevents his leadership from flowing outward to the team.

Although laws are clear about overt discrimination in the workplace, legislation alone will never banish all prejudices from the minds of workers. They still exist, and leaders are not immune. Leaders who have predispositions against groups or individuals due to factors such as race, age, disability, or lifestyle can apply their emotional skills to understand their own feelings about the individual or group (What am I feeling? What has occurred that resulted in these feelings? How can I strive to manage my feelings about this individual or group?). Such leaders can also apply empathy to see life from the point of view of the group or individual with whom they are uncomfortable. How might it be, for example, to be a U.S. resident of Middle Eastern descent? A single mom raising three small children and trying to work three jobs to support them? An individual who has hearing loss? Simple exercises in emotional perception and empathy will allow the leader to not only understand the source of her own feelings but also to more closely identify with other team members.

UNDERSTANDING OTHERS' POSITIONS. "Empathy is the function by which we attempt to perceive and understand what is happening in other people," says Greenhalgh (1994, p. 87). While this may seem like a broad definition, it can be directly applied in many situations. It can be applied in a situation such as the one described above, in which the leader attempts to see the difficulties of living in a situation beyond one's control, or it can be applied in evaluating why an employee is not living up to his potential at a given point in time. When applied to a real situation, this understanding translates to sensitivity, in which the leader is aware of how her approach or actions toward an individual may be affecting his emotions and feelings (Weisinger, 1998). In essence, empathy requires remaining in one's own frame of reference while stepping into that of another.

LISTENING. The fact that these manifestations of empathy sound so fundamental to "just being a good leader" helps us to realize just how deep the thread of empathy runs in effective leadership. The importance of listening is a concept that many of us are exposed to from an early age. Listening, after all, provides us with information that we need to avoid trouble, avert mistakes, and produce good results. Just as we got burned with the hot iron when we did not listen to our mother, we sacrifice the gift of guidance when we do not listen to our team members.

Listening in the empathic sense is more complicated than merely heeding important instructions. This type of listening involves emptying of the self (including any previously drawn conclusions) so that there is room for the feelings of the other person. It involves recognition of feelings in oneself that may impede understanding. It involves making sure that what is heard is what was said. Perhaps most important, it involves being able to hear the feelings that go along with the facts (Ryback, 1998). This is the most fruitful, albeit the most painful, consequence of listening to our team members.

Furthermore, as leadership is shared more with team members, listening to them becomes more important. In this scenario, listening is no longer reserved for the captive audience, and getting across ideas is no longer reserved solely for the leader. Team-driven leadership will stall and ultimately stagnate in the absence of effective listening.

WILLINGNESS TO ACT. A leader may truly understand the issues, identify completely with the emotions involved, and be purely nonjudgmental in her approach to staff. When a problem arises, for example, she may feel unthreatened by it and even have a deep sense of understanding as to how it affects the individuals involved. Without action on the problem, however, all attempts to identify and understand are ultimately nonproductive. The empathic leader deals with issues head-on (Ryback, 1998), because problems are not resolved merely by understanding or by letting go of preconceived ideas. Truly, these are prerequisites to problem solving, but they do not actually solve the problem.

Some leaders find this to be the most difficult aspect of empathic leadership. Understanding, listening, and being nonjudgmental are soft skills; action is harder. Action involves direct intervention, for which there may be consequences, either favorable or unfavorable, and in an emotional situation, it is difficult to predict what the consequences will be. However, team members who approach a leader with a concern and come away with understanding must also perceive that the understanding will be followed up with some sort of action or direction from the leader.

The skill of listening in order to discern what is needed is critical when acting based on empathy. Away from the work setting, how many of us have felt absolutely powerless when a friend or family member was experiencing some sort of emotional pain or trauma and all we could do was listen and try to understand? In fact, in many such cases, that is all our loved one really wants from us, unless we actually have the means to eliminate the offending situation from their life. Likewise, action on empathy is really only called for when there is a significant contribution that the leader can make to resolve the issue or lessen the team member's emotional struggle. The leader must use discernment as to what lies in his power to correct. If a nurse is having family problems that are hindering her work, for example, the nurse is not necessarily sharing this with the leader so that the leader can go in and hold therapeutic discussions with her family members. But if the nurse is explaining how her working too many third shifts is causing strain in her family, it is the leader's responsibility to understand how this situation affects that staff member and take steps to explore solutions.

When the leader manifests and uses empathy in dealing with team members, a department, or an organization, the stage is set for the development of an emotionally sound work culture.

Aligning the Work Culture with Philosophies of Empathic Patient Care

Naturally, we want to be empathic with our patients. Our bedside manner is important in how we relate to these individuals and their families. In patient care, as we have seen, emotional intelligence can help facilitate better communication and patient-nurse relationships.

When we take these principles into the conference room or the break room or wherever we interact with our fellow health care team members, we are given the opportunity to exercise the same emotional skill. The next sections will demonstrate how leaders and teams can integrate empathy into an effective nursing culture.

Outcomes of the Empathic Work Culture

Most people want to work for an organization that makes them feel safe and comfortable. This includes safety from physical harm and job loss, but it also includes protection from anxiety and fear. Increasing patient loads and responsibilities, not to mention spiraling technological advances and emphasis on controlling costs, are all factors that can lead to anxiety among nurses.

Organizations that emphasize empathy in their culture will naturally display a greater level of support for worker concerns and attention to worker safety than organizations that do not encourage empathy. In return, they will likely garner high company loyalty, low absenteeism, and, as a result, positive impact on their bottom line. When companies pay attention to threats or anxiety-producing situations within the workplace, they are taking the first step toward identification and resolution of emotional situations that could easily spiral out of control. In addition, organizations can create a corporate culture that uses emotions to build teamwork and trust and that assists employees in constructively channeling emotions to facilitate rather than impede work (Helge, 2001).

Creating a Team Culture That Responds Effectively to Change

In the past ten years, nursing has changed dramatically because of improved technology, demographic factors such as the increasing number of Generation X nurses in the workforce, and varying service delivery systems. Nursing needs to respond to change by becoming a more holistic practice that combines care with, among other things, technological savvy, skill in dealing with people, and an understanding of health care models (Higgins, 2003). Additionally, well-rounded practice includes relationship-centered care as well as relationship-centered practice.

Nursing teams must focus on relationships as they practice because relationships have become increasingly critical to working in health care. It is far more difficult today than it was perhaps twenty years ago to operate in a vacuum when it comes to patient care. One reason is that due to financial pressures, quality improvement programs, and expectations of patients, patient care delivery has to constantly be improved, and one nurse cannot improve patient care alone. One of the best ways to facilitate relationships is by encouraging and practicing empathy. There are several actions that can be promulgated by leaders to promote empathy within their team (Arthur, Wall, and Halligan, 2003).

EMPHASIZE QUALITY. Few things make a nurse unhappier than feeling that the quality of the care he provides is compromised by cost control, staff shortages, or overwork. The essence of nursing is quality care, although quality is frequently compromised by organizations seeking to establish or maintain a successful bottom line. The team leader needs to assure nurses that quality is given utmost importance in any decisions that are made. As nurses in a self-directed team or advisory council make recommendations, they should be encouraged to emphasize quality in their recommendations, with specific emphasis on how quality of care affects everything from efficiency to, ultimately, cost. Not only does this emphasis on quality have implications for the organization and patient care, but it also recognizes and uses a strong emotional issue, not shortchanging patient care, to promote a good outcome. Leaders who pay attention to quality and promote quality care promote empathy by sending the message, "I value your concern for good patient care, because your desire to give quality care is one reason you practice nursing."

CLARIFY OBJECTIVES. "The apparent lack of respect for nursing in terms of what professional nurses actually do in hospitals has been detrimental to the nursing profession," according to Ray, Turkel, and Marino (2002, p. 2). These authors posit that trust and fairness have eroded under the pressure of constant change. There is no better time than the present to reestablish with nurses what their roles actually are, so that they, their leaders, and their colleagues understand their role. This role has come to include acting as decision maker, facilitator, and business manager. Nurses who have been in the profession for a long time have felt the brunt of the change in the profession, while those who are newly educated may not have received adequate training in their respective programs. The empathic team leader will recognize the potential benefits in bolstering the nursing team's understanding of the objectives of their practice and who they need to be in order to reach those objectives. The leader who clarifies objectives is saying to constituents, "I know who you are and what you are capable of. Here is an affirmation of what you and your profession represent." This message promotes empathy by recognizing the professional capabilities of the individual nurse and showing concern for her perception of how she is valued.

INTRODUCE INNOVATION. Unfortunately, many of the ideas and innovations for health care reform that have been introduced over the past decade, including managed care, managed competition, and integrated care, have fallen short of expectations. The health care industry continues to strive for solutions that will support the polarities of cost and quality (Ham, 2003). A team of nurses faces a similar challenge on a much smaller scale. "Improvement of the performance of health care depends first and foremost on making a difference to the experience of patients and service users, which in turn hinges on changing the day-to-day decisions of doctors, nurses, and other staff," posits Ham (2003, p. 1978). When clinicians are engaged in orchestrating innovation in the organization, they feel they are leading the process rather than being led blindly through yet another change. In hospitals and health care service organizations that are empathic in culture, the need for nurses to participate in such innovation is understood and acted upon. Team members receive the message, "we understand you need input into the direction of your practice."

PROVIDE CLEAR LEADERSHIP. In recent times, scholars and researchers have proposed characteristics of leaders who support innovation and creativity. To cope with the reality of change in health care, the culture of an organization must nurture innovative ways of addressing issues and problems (Andriopoulos, 2001). Clear leadership involves clear direction throughout this innovation process. Particular attention should be given to how innovation affects people, partnerships, processes, and products (Dahlgaard and Dahlgaard, 1999). People should be recognized for their value in creating innovation, and the partnerships necessary for innovation should be encouraged. The teams should be in charge of creating processes and products that reflect their capability and make them proud of who they are. Clear leadership sends the message, "I know you need supportive direction to exercise your capabilities to the fullest, especially when the territory is new."

SET THE TONE WITH HIGH-QUALITY MEETINGS. The quality of meetings within an organization will influence the quality of informal interactions. Meetings are formalized, structured sessions in which team members learn to communicate in ways that take the feelings and reactions of others into account. Most communication, however, takes place outside of formal settings. Communication may occur in the form of dialogue about a patient, education of a family member, or chatting with a colleague about the events of the day.

Besides being boot camp for effective team interactions, all meetings serve a specific purpose. Meetings are called for the purpose of focusing on one specific goal or group of objectives, whether it is to communicate departmental issues or to work on an innovation by collecting viewpoints. The team leader must set the groundwork for respectful meetings in which agendas are followed, feelings and concerns are acknowledged, and negative emotions are not allowed to fester and impede the work of the group. At times, managing emotion and taking time for empathy involves stepping back and stepping away from the agenda. Meetings replete with emotional content will take time, but this time should be allotted, even if an issue needs to be tabled until a separate session. It is not wise to rush a purposeful meeting whose impact will be felt for some time to come (Wall, Solum, and Sobol, 1992). The key is effectively acknowledging emotions related to issues and not allowing them to get out of hand, while staying on track with the purpose and objective of the meeting itself. Making sure the emotional content of meetings is acknowledged and addressed sends the message, "I understand you have important feelings that influence your decisions and your perception of the situation."

PROMOTE HIGH LEVELS OF PARTICIPATION THROUGH UNDERSTANDING AND EDUCATION. Understanding nurses' continual need for education and skill development is key in helping them participate fully in their roles and the role of their department or organization. The frustration that results when a nurse is not aware of or able to adapt to new situations can be debilitating. The team leader should never assume that the nursing staff is aware of a new drug, a new machine, or a new unit policy. Constant education is needed to introduce these advances.

Recall the last time that everyone seemed to know about something—except you. This is an extremely uncomfortable feeling, one that team leaders and team members are tasked with identifying and managing. Bridging a knowledge gap can be accomplished through formal certification programs or distance learning arrangements (Rick, Kearns, and Thompson, 2003). Education on an issue or new technology points out that everyone needs to learn something new, not just one lone nurse who feels she may have missed the boat. Encouraging education sends the message to team members that they are indeed in the same boat with many others who need to learn, that they are expected to learn, and that their desire to practice competently is recognized. Empathy is promoted in the message, "I understand that you have a need to know new information, which in turn will enhance your confidence in your ability. I respect and support your need to know and encourage you to seek education and professional development."

PROMOTE DIVERSITY. The value of diversity awareness in twenty-first century nursing cannot be overemphasized, and at its root is the core essence of empathy. We must understand the issues that can arise from our inherent cultural differences in order to succeed as a team. We must remember at all times that the individual is in the foreground and the culture from which she comes is merely background. This applies in both patient care and team interactions (Manderson, 1998; Phillips, 2003). Parvis (2003) reminds us that multiculturalism actually stimulates creativity in groups. The empathic team openly invites the flexibility that multiculturalism provides; it is a gift!

Assessing the Culture for its Driving Force

Organizational culture can be described in a number of valid ways. Vestal, Fralicx, and Spreier (1997) define four dominant cultures that are demonstrated in health care; this book will refer to them as driving forces behind culture, or the chief motivators for the organization. The organization must understand the driving forces behind its dominant culture so that it can understand how to appropriately promote empathy within the culture. Organizations, like people, respond to different motivators. Each of these driving forces can be molded in an empathic framework, as long as they are understood. Further, although particular factors that have been agreed on by strategists and upper management often drive the culture within an organization, the environment of the organization can also be driven from within at the team level.

THE CULTURAL DRIVING FORCE THAT MAKES THE BEST USE OF TECHNOLOGY. A culture that is focused on making sure that technology is used to its fullest advantage describes the traditional culture, rich with hierarchies and management structures. Government agencies and subsidiaries frequently subscribe to this culture. This, of course, is the most traditional driving force in most business; the need to be on the cutting edge has motivated business for decades.

When technology is the driving force in an organization, work may be very specialized in order to reap the maximum benefit from technical expertise. Consequently, within the technological culture, there is perhaps more potential for silos and individual differences than in any other type of culture. The leader within this organization may have a particular challenge in forming and managing teams. A specific challenge involves integrating shared leadership into the organization, which contrasts with the traditional "decision at the top" methods. In addition, because this cultural driver results in an emphasis on rules over creativity, there is not as much opportunity for the leader to encourage team thought and consensus about a desired change. Efforts to affect the culture in this type of organization will result either in a slightly modified version of the traditional hierarchy or a complete change to a less structured, less hierarchical culture. In order to effect this, senior management must be willing to align with those driving the change, and adequate support must be garnered from the ranks to put the changes into motion. The leader in this case must be alert to the insecurities and sensitivities of people comfortable with a structured, rigid system and help them manage their emotions as they react to the change. Taking steps to let colleagues know that their sensitivities and insecurities are acknowledged can immediately promote a framework of empathy upon which to build.

THE CULTURAL DRIVING FORCE THAT EMPHASIZES QUALITY, CUSTOMER SATISFACTION, AND SERVICE. As a more patient-centered approach to service delivery becomes desirable due to both marketing and best practice factors, many organizations that were once motivated by keeping up with and obeying all the rules are turning to the quality and satisfaction driver to define their mission. The disease management company that I am affiliated with is an example of a company driven by these motivators. At the end of the day, the important factor is whether patients received quality care and were satisfied, so staff and management alike must focus on the outcomes of their work. A growing number of health service organizations, including hospitals and HMOs, are motivated by the drive to provide quality service and customer satisfaction. This results in a closer look at the patient experience: exactly how do patients perceive the care they receive, and what would they like to see improved? The empathic organizational desire to understand patients' feelings can be applied to staff as well.

The leader in this type of organization, then, has the delicate responsibility of balancing the needs of the customer with the needs of the staff. As we have seen, there is the potential for conflict between patient satisfaction and staff satisfaction. To successfully strike this balance, the leader can use empathy to understand the primary motivation of each team member and to sustain the vision espoused by the organization.

To maintain high standards for quality of care and service, the leader also must promote change and continual improvement of process. Placing team members in charge of the change process, cross-functional training, and continuing education activities (Vestal, Fralicx, and Spreier, 1997) shows that the team is growing in knowledge and that the leader empathizes with each team member's need to advance and learn as an individual as well as to perform functions as part of the team.

THE CULTURAL DRIVING FORCE THAT EMPHASIZES BEING THE FASTEST AND THE BEST. Organizations with this culture seek to do things faster and better than anyone else in the market; speed is of utmost importance, and the culture literally becomes time-based. Organizations adopt this mentality because of perpetual change in the environment and the need to keep ahead of change. Best suited to this type of culture are individuals who have a high sense of urgency and who are adaptable, intensively creative, and decisive. Organizations motivated by these factors usually have flatter, leaner hierarchies than other types of organizations, and they often use cross-functional work groups (Vestal, Fralicx, and Spreier, 1997). When staying ahead of rapid change is the driving force in an organization, the leader must be empathic with the emotional impact that rapid changes have on each team member. In this instance, the empathic framework is of utmost importance. A paradigm of empathy will not slow the pace of change, but it will bolster those who are shaken by it. Empathy in this case is focused on keeping employees happy and less disgruntled by continual, rapid change. When an individual is not well suited to his cultural driver (for example, perhaps the individual has a low sense of urgency) the leader will need to use empathy to understand what motivates urgency in that individual and work with her to make urgency a defining aspect of her behavior at work.

THE CULTURE DRIVEN BY FLEXIBILITY AND ADAPTIVE THINKING. This culture emphasizes the value of networks, or virtual organizations, in an attempt to respond to the need for flexibility in response to constant change in the market. Perhaps no cultural driver typifies the workplace of the future better than the network culture described by Vestal, Fralicx, and Spreier (1997), in part because of integration of services and the need to go outside the organization for resources. Leaders in this type of organization must be flexible, effective at finding and using resources even outside the organization, and able to think "outside the box." The use of network structures, or virtual structures, where individuals in teams may be in different buildings or across the country, is growing in many industries, including health care. Maintaining a network of diverse and multifaceted divisions—for example, the home health division, the rehabilitation division, the acute care division, the clinic division, the insurer— requires the empathic skills of facilitation and negotiation, skills that require identification of emotions and the ability to use them to facilitate thought. In short, this culture is most likely to involve relationship building with the added challenge of depending on team members who are across the country and coming from a different perspective of the same organization. The empathic framework reinforces the need to identify and acknowledge the diversity that characterizes virtual teams.

Supporting the Culture Through Empathy, and Building Empathy Through the Culture

Whatever an organization's dominant cultural type or cultural driving force, empathy can be applied to transform that culture. If the organization's chief objective, for example, is staying ahead of everyone else in the industry, that motivator can be interpreted in the framework of empathy to assist team members in meeting corporate goals effectively. If the health care institution's main goal is to improve patient satisfaction, the same is true. It is not as much about what drives the organization as about how effectively it is carried out. Both are aspects of culture.

Here are some steps for developing an empathic culture within an organization:

○ Attend to the dynamics of the group, and provide constructive feedback on group process (Cox, 2002). Feedback will help group members become more aware of the effectiveness of their interactions with others while building empathic skills.

○ Promote emotional learning within the culture (Segal, 2002). Emotional intelligence should be emphasized, not shrouded. Team members should be aware that their emotional intelligence needs to improve (as everyone's does) and be aware that coaching is occurring.

○ Eliminate perfectionism and encourage expansion (Segal, 2002). The need to be in control of all aspects of one's job, including the human emotions of one's team members, typifies the leader or team member who has eliminated a potential pathway of learning from mistakes. Ideally, we all want to have some measure of control over our jobs and our constituents' behavior, especially when we are in supervisory roles, but the notion that we can control *everything* is faulty. No one knows everything about what drives and motivates people, and learning possibilities are endless. Empathy helps facilitate the skill of perceiving people's motivations by allowing them to make mistakes and move on.

o Recognize personally held beliefs and values (Martin, Yarbrough, and Alfred, 2003). Regardless of the driving force behind the organizational or departmental culture, personal values will affect thoughts, reactions, and actions. Recognition of these values, admitting that they exist, is a key element of empathy.

o Nurture a team-centered approach to culture and process development, one that keeps the team's needs and values in mind. Within the guidelines of organizational goals, teams should have input into the benefits, as well as the drawbacks, of current or proposed processes. They should then be able to exercise as much creativity as possible in planning for change. Here, again, the value of open communication cannot be overemphasized: appropriate relationships within the organization must be continually cultivated so that a well-developed plan can be carried out effectively (Duchene, 2002). The team-centered approach highlights the individual's value as a team member and the team's value as a unit, and it fosters empathy simply by saying, "I see potential in you all, both as individuals and as a team."

Summary

Culture greatly influences our actions. In fact, culture defines the very environment in which we work and live. Culture in business has been studied more in recent years as a factor influencing employee behavior and work outcomes.

Emotional factors play an important role in culture. Each individual's emotional aptitude contributes to the culture of the work environment. Although the primary driving forces behind an organization's cultural pattern are usually directed by top management, the cultural infrastructure can be built with or without consideration of emotional factors. When emotional factors are considered and capitalized on, empathy characterizes the culture.

Leaders and team members should focus on working with constituents empathically and using the tools of identifying, using, understanding, and managing emotions appropriately in order to mold an emotionally relevant work culture. The relationship-centered environment that results will positively affect outcomes and team effectiveness, which will ultimately translate to better patient care.

TEN CRITERIA FOR AN EMPATHIC WORK CULTURE

1. Team collegiality is present, making for smoother team interactions.
2. Negative emotions are recognized and managed.
3. The team exhibits shared visions and goals.
4. There is an emphasis on quality in team interactions and products.
5. The team functions under clear objectives.
6. The team is equipped for participation through understanding and education.
7. There is a pervasive spirit of innovation.
8. Meetings are purposeful, and their respectful environment defines the environment of informal team interactions.
9. Leadership is clear and expectations are understood.
10. Diversity is understood and promoted within the team.

11

REBUILDING AND UPENDING THE HIERARCHICAL PYRAMID

IT SEEMS THAT improvement-minded individuals will never stop telling us how to fix things or make them better, even if those things do not seem to be altogether broken. As we discovered through a brief study of the life and work of Florence Nightingale, health care has come a long way and despite its challenges has emerged as a relatively respected set of professions with standards unrivaled by many other fields. Many of us would like to think we work for "good" organizations—hospitals or offices that care about patients, take quality seriously, and employ competent staff.

What Will Make Good Even Better?

Florence Nightingale had great insight into the future of nursing and of nursing leadership. One of the original nurse leaders, she began her *Notes on Nursing* text with the following philosophical principle:

> All disease, at some period or other of its course, is more or less a reparative process, not necessarily accompanied with suffering: an effort of nature to remedy a process of poisoning or of decay, which has taken place weeks, months, sometimes years beforehand, unnoticed, the termination of disease being then, while the antecedent process was going on, determined.
>
> If we accept this as a general principle, we shall be immediately met with anecdotes and instances to prove the contrary. Just so, if we were

to take, as a principle—all the climates of the earth are meant to be made habitable for man, by the efforts of man—the objection would be immediately raised—Will the top of Mount Blanc ever be made habitable? Our answer would be, it will be many thousands of years before we have reached the bottom of Mount Blanc in making the earth healthy. Wait until we have reached the bottom before we discuss the top [Nightingale, (1860) 1969, p. 7].

Nurses and physicians have been striving for decades to make health care as a professional arena healthy in terms of its systems, processes, and leadership. In making nursing leadership what it is today, the field has encountered much change, some intentional and some unintentional. Many organizations are frustrated that the visionary leadership at the top and the swarms of workers at the bottom do not automatically connect and share the same vision, goals, or plans. They put it into the hands of middle executives and frontline supervisors to make sure the job gets done in accord with the defined standards, and hope in so doing that the organization will profit, maintain above-standard quality, or simply become the best-rated in the business, according to what the driving force behind that organization's culture happens to be. For decades, this has worked sufficiently, but it can work better. The answer lies in reaching the bottom before we discuss the top.

The Group-Oriented Organization

Organizations, including health care providers, have made a noticeable shift over the years toward a group mentality, but there is still much work to do. Being clustered into groups with a defined purpose and producing effective outcomes through effective teamwork are vastly different accomplishments. "We may talk about the value of teamwork with our children," Wellins, Byham, and Wilson (1991) point out, "but much of the real world they see is oriented toward the individual. . . . When work begins, performance systems continue to reward individual accomplishments" (p. 5). Wellins and his colleagues go on to provide an interesting historical perspective about why the somewhat romanticized "Go, team" concept has been so difficult to infuse into business. During the time of Frederick Taylor, who was known as the father of modern industrial engineering, it was thought that highly specialized workers would be best left to focus on doing their highly specialized tasks, and that the planning, direction, and decision making should be left to someone who could control activities from the top (McConnell, 1998; Wellins, Byham, and

Wilson, 1991). Individuals who had been accustomed to independently producing a commodity or working with a couple of others to provide a service were forced by industrialization to surrender their autonomy in order to survive in a machine-based, volume-oriented industrial world. Worker empowerment was sacrificed, and the production workers, who were seen as the bottom echelon of the organization, lost their ability to direct the organization. The hierarchical pyramid was born.

Efforts to change this hierarchical structure in organizations continue, and research continues to provide evidence that it is important for leaders to listen to the people who do the work. Ronald Reagan consistently requested feedback from constituents (Strock, 1998). Authors and scholars such as Yukl (1998), Katzenbach and Smith (1993), and Fisher (1993) have clearly defined teamwork and the attributes of successful teams in their writings. Chiavenato (2001) says, "The rigid organizational hierarchy with its monolithic chain of command is giving way to integrated team networks based on autonomy and flexibility. . . . Emphasis on permanence, tradition and the past is giving way to creativity and innovation in the search for new solutions, new processes, and new products and services" (p. 18). Many of these efforts have been well accepted and applied in business.

The Learning-Achieving Cycle Upended: Learning Precedes Performance in Teams

Two major arenas in which group efforts will affect organizations are learning and performance. However, the order in which they should occur may come as a surprise.

LEARNING IN GROUPS. Group learning ability is described by Yukl (1998) as a predictor of team effectiveness. In other words, how well team members learn together indicates how well they can perform together. Goleman, Boyatzis, and McKee (2002) describes a process called action learning, which involves enabling participants or teams to draw on real-life challenges in order to learn and, secondarily, to achieve outcomes.

As individuals, our personality and worldview affect how and why we learn. Some people learn for the sake of learning; others learn because it will effect a change in their status; and still others crave the interactive social knowledge they can attain from the very process of learning (Chase, 1998). In the world most familiar to us, we go to school to learn, then we go out in the working world to achieve outcomes, and some element of learning is inherent in everything we do. The concept of group learning puts us back in "school" on a permanent basis and aligns learning with our chief objectives, placing learning before the secondary objective of actually accomplishing something.

What if work were really like that? Suppose we each walked onto our hospital unit or into our clinic or office suite and were told by our supervisors, "Today, everything you do will be for the purpose of learning. It does not matter what happens, as long as you learn something from it." Many of us would question that supervisor's mental status or even whether we were registering our own surroundings correctly. In most cases, our learning experiences at work come because we are doing something we should do better, but we certainly do not try to make mistakes just so we can learn. There are some things we do not want to learn the hard way, such as why it is wrong to give an overdose of a medication or why aberrant heart rhythms or complaints of increasing pain should not be ignored.

Team learning, fortunately, is quite different, for it allows more margin for error than does individual experimentation outside medically established boundaries. Teams have a directive to learn when they are working together to effect change in process, improve quality, or affect practice. They have to learn *first* in order to achieve these goals, just as we had to learn first in order to become competent nurses.

Yukl (1998) defines two primary steps to ensure team learning. The first is to review what went wrong and what went right after major activities. The focus of these review meetings should be constructive problem solving and not placing blame. In addition, the leader or the facilitator can use these opportunities to make relational assessments (for example, how well the team worked together and what emotional dynamics were noted) as well as performance assessments (for example, how smoothly the entire process went and what wrong turns could be corrected next time).

Another important factor in team learning is the ability of members to understand one another. In the process of learning, team members must be able to dialogue to discover their feelings and motivations on a particular issue. In this type of learning, understanding is just as much about feelings as it is about the best way to approach a task. The consequences of making assumptions without acknowledging feelings include possible excessive advocacy of a position, in which claims are exaggerated, opinions are presented as fact, and supporting evidence is incomplete. The emotional element helps explain our feelings for a particular position in a way that mere facts cannot. In addition, when a team member makes little effort to understand the feelings of others on the team who feel differently about an issue, so much effort may be applied to pushing through a particular position that it may be easiest for those in disagreement if they keep their mouths closed (Yukl, 1998), although it may not be better for the team in the long run.

Again, emotional ability as defined by Mayer, Salovey, and Caruso (2000, 2002) enters the game. It should be apparent that in both of Yukl's steps to group learning, emotional competence in leaders and team members is highly relevant. Yet exercise of emotional skill is more difficult than simply focusing on the task and the facts surrounding the issues. Goleman, Boyatzis, and McKee (2002) go on to say that when teams are working and learning together, "(they) must work on the projects, not individuals, and the teams need support throughout the duration of the project in creating a healthy climate, maintaining functional norms and emotional intelligence, dealing with conflict, focusing on learning rather than achievement, and so on" (p. 237). Specifically, the emotional intelligence component can and should include identifying the feelings that are present, knowing how those feelings are affecting the thoughts and contributions of team members, understanding where those feelings and thoughts can lead, and facilitating appropriate use of the emotions to reach a professional and well-grounded decision (Mayer, Salovey, and Caruso, 2000, 2002).

PERFORMANCE IN GROUPS. While teams are learning, their secondary role is to achieve outcomes. What conditions are necessary to foster strong performance by health care teams?

First, the organization itself needs to have a strong performance ethic. Most organizations that do not have such an ethic have difficulty commending their fate to teams. As a result, teams are not given the opportunity to perform in any arena that materially affects the organization as a whole (Katzenbach and Smith, 1993). Teams may be placed in charge of details that have little influence on the organization or kept busy with managing mundane matters. While day-to-day matters must always be addressed, they should not be the sole charge of teams. Teams, like individuals, need to feel that their work matters. Also, teams that are in a position to perform should be challenged to perform well, because stellar performance and successful accomplishment of objectives mean that the organization also performs well.

Second, effective team performance requires a culture of discipline. Culture, among other things, defines the "rules of the game" for getting along and performing well in an organization (Rondeau and Wagar, 1999). Collins (2001a) aptly states that while every company has a culture, and some have discipline, very few have a culture of discipline. A culture of discipline includes emotional discipline and conflict resolution discipline as much as it includes progress-oriented and objective-oriented discipline. When teams create and breathe within a culture of discipline, the need for hierarchy melts away. In other words, the culture of discipline becomes the paradigm within which innovative thought and action are managed, so there is no need for constant manipulation from the top.

A culture of discipline also contributes to learning by providing a structure for learning cycles within the organization or team. A discipline has its own organizational pyramid: at the top is the unique point of view of the discipline itself; the next level is based in tradition surrounding the discipline; the next is the procedures and strategies behind the discipline; and at the base are the tools and methods used to carry out the discipline. Although this pyramid is used primarily to define academic disciplines, it can also be applied to organizational disciplines, including quality improvement and process change (Aron, Dittus, and Rosenthal, 2002). There must be traditions, strategies, and tools in working through any situation or problem, capped by the unique points of view of the team members.

The third prerequisite for excellent team performance is a meeting of the minds about goals, procedures, and roles (Wall, Solum, and Sobol, 1992). A team, like an individual, will be unable to perform effectively if there is confusion about any of these. Imagine that you are a new manager and it is your first day on the job. How capable would you be of a stellar performance as a manager if you had no idea what unit you were assigned to, what time you were to start, and whom you were working with? This is a greatly simplified example, and as leaders, we hope that we will never be faced with that situation; however, teams face this dilemma all the time, albeit in a much subtler form. Indeed, it is possible for a team to sit in a room for hours, discuss a topic, and still not be clear on who is supposed to be doing what. Much of this not knowing is the result of conflict involving feelings and emotions surrounding the task. For example, one person may feel strongly about an initiative and want to assume a leadership role but be unsupported by others who are not as excited about what they see as the desired outcome. If that nurse flings herself into driving that initiative without obtaining and using emotional feedback of the group, the project will likely stall while others discuss alternate agendas. These alternate agendas are likely to be replete with individual desires and hopes, each with its own leader and each with its own desired outcome. Before long, everyone is confused, and someone has to step in and facilitate conflict resolution. Although conflict resolution skills are desirable in leadership, this type of conflict can be avoided altogether by establishing clear goals (not necessarily measures to meet those goals), roles (who will facilitate the team discussions), and procedures (guidelines for forming opinions, discussing views, and summarizing meeting content, preferably with attention to the emotional components of these transactions).

Multidisciplinary, Multiskilled Organizations

Teams must first learn and then perform. This concept is contiguous with the notion that organizations, especially those in health care, need to be multidisciplinary and multiskilled. When we emerged from nursing school and were rewarded with our first job, many of us were surprised to learn just how dependent we were on one another. IV teams, lab personnel, X-ray technicians, physical therapists, supply clerks, cashiers, dietary specialists, social workers, chaplains all made it possible or at least easier to do our job. In addition, nurses with more experience, more skills, and certain certifications were called on to do certain things for us that we were not yet prepared to do or at least to teach us what we needed to know. We soon had a small taste of two things we needed: cross empowerment and one another.

THE NEED TO CROSS-EMPOWER. The disease management organization with which I am affiliated had a clear impediment to efficient nursing service: nurses were spending hours on the telephone and on the Internet searching for social and personal resources for patients, something that nursing school had scarcely trained them to do. Because many of them knew very little about where to find support groups, respite care, or free equipment, they were struggling to find these through complicated networks and regional resource banks. When the organization hired social workers to assume this function, the nurses' burden was relieved, and patients received much more rapid response to their needs. However, as response to patients' needs improved, the value of the disease management services became more apparent to patients, who then used the services even more. As a result, they tapped into the resource identification function much more frequently, and they expected their nurses to help them quickly. Through collaboration with the social workers, nurses learned to access a database whose information can start a patient in the right direction, even if more thorough research must still be done by the social worker. This improvement in service represents a visible patient satisfaction initiative for the organization.

Because of the complexity of health care, nursing will probably always be nursing, dietary will always be dietary, and physical therapy will most likely always be physical therapy, although practice within those specific roles may grow and develop. In other words, nurses cannot be expected to practice like physical therapists or make completely informed dietary decisions in their day-to-day practice. However, nurses can and should be expected to understand the principles behind physical therapy, nutritional guidelines behind the food selections a dietician makes for certain patients, and even how to get a patient started in the right direction toward filling out forms to receive government aid. When learning tasks, skills, or knowledge expands the effectiveness of a nurse's role, it becomes more than cross training, it becomes cross empowerment. In other words, the nurse is not trained to step in and do the physical therapist's or dietician's job, but she is able to provide more effective patient care because she is connected through knowledge to the abilities of other disciplines. Likewise, physical therapists and dieticians who understand the disease process and the rationale behind some nursing interventions are equally empowered to reinforce the patient's plan of care.

Cross empowerment becomes increasingly important as people need more knowledge to do their jobs. We can no longer operate in silos: this is the crux of the team concept. Whether in a patient room or a board room, the nurse or nurse leader performs more effectively if she has knowledge shared mutually with her colleagues.

Knowledge sharing can occur through formal research or through a casual conversation in the hallway. Whatever the mechanism, knowledge sharing is becoming an essential, rather than a luxury, in nursing practice (Dixon, 2001).

The concept of cross empowerment can be applied in leadership as well. Leaders should cross-empower those who are not officially branded as leaders, and vice versa. Not everyone on the team can be a manager, but team members should at least understand some of the complexities that go into managerial decision making, so that they support the efforts of the manager rather than counteract them. Indeed, vision sharing and gaining agreement on the need to change (Kim and Mauborgne, 2003) are forms of cross empowerment; the leader shares, fundamentally, the prospect of betterment with team members and allows them to become a part of the solution. Related forms of cross empowerment include simply making known what goals and values one espouses (Reichheld, 2001) and promoting decision making by teams or, at least, team input into decisions (Charan, 2001).

On the other hand, leaders should be cross empowered by team members. Often, a manager will be caught up in the work involved in management and fail to recognize what the unit clerk or the staff nurse is doing each day. Some managers would be at a great loss if they needed to perform any staff member's job! Managers and leaders should have an idea of what staff members' work involves, even if it is not operational knowledge.

Cross empowerment, in summary, does three things. First, it allows everyone to understand where others' skills and abilities lie and how to work with everyone else to accomplish major goals. Second, it allows everyone, including leaders, to pass their core values and understandings to the collective knowledge bank of the team, so that decisions and actions can be taken collaboratively. Finally, and most important, it teaches us how much we need one another.

THE NEED FOR ONE ANOTHER. In multidisciplinary organizations, each person's unique skills and knowledge are essential. Team members are extremely interdependent; they need one another and thus need to cultivate effective relationships among themselves in order to leverage their talents for success. Interpersonal intelligence is described by Hatch (1997) in part as the ability to develop and sustain relationships with others. This is a skill that becomes apparent in early childhood, as children learn in preschool and even earlier to interact peacefully with one another, to negotiate, to befriend, and to lead.

As adults, we need to have this same type of interpersonal skill in our team interactions. In short, teamwork requires that we not do all of our thinking, feeling, and concluding on our own. Over time, we rely on the support and encouragement of the group as we share our individual thoughts and feelings. The result is a cumulative intelligence, facilitated by lowering of emotional barriers (Ryback, 1998).

The leader should keep this in mind and relay it to the team continually. We need one another; we need one another's thoughts, feelings, and opinions. The huge organization or even the small department is too large to be run effectively without collective input. That is because the huge organization or the small department is a collection of thoughts, feelings, and opinions, quite possibly well represented by everyone in the room. The thoughts, feelings, and opinions of others are *not* barriers to moving ahead. They fill in the gaps of what someone thinks is a perfect plan. They tie the knot on something that is just shy of a masterpiece. It does not matter how many thoughts, feelings, or opinions there are; we need them all.

In laying the emotional groundwork for an effective team process, the leader should encourage free flow of ideas, encourage dialogue that facilitates questions and answers (Yukl, 1998), and discourage criticism and the laying of blame. Often we forget how much we need one another, especially when we are confident in our own abilities and sure that we have the right answer to the problem. The leader should not allow a decision to happen in a group setting without first ascertaining that the opinions of all have had a chance to be heard.

In addition, it should be made perfectly clear, even when events are progressing at breakneck speed, how important it is to rely on one another. There are some who fear that asking for help or getting a second opinion is a sign of low intelligence or poor ability, but exactly the opposite is true. The norm, not the exception, should be collaboration and consultation when faced with a difficult situation. This is not a sign of weakness but rather a sign of fortitude in the area of relational behavior.

Building the Pyramid from the Bottom Up

We have established that the framework of an organization needs to be a culture of learning, growing, and performing teams that are both interdependent and empowered. Let us begin to ascend the organizational pyramid from its foundation, and see where it takes us.

Constructing the Pyramid

These days, *hierarchy* is almost a dirty word, its mention engendering visions of strict governance, bureaucracy, and harsh rules. If you happen to be low in the hierarchy, you have very little input into anything, and someone above you in the hierarchy can trump you at a moment's notice, simply by virtue of their position.

Pyramid is another word that stimulates thought about what it is like to be at the top and what it is like to be at the bottom. Most of us have seen and probably a few of us been a part of a human pyramid formed during a cheerleading routine. Those on the bottom must bear the most weight, but those on top have the most responsibility to balance and keep from falling. If the person on top falls, he or she could not only sustain significant personal injury but also injure someone else on the way down and take the pleasing symmetry of the formation with it. The whole point of forming a pyramid is to show off how wonderfully it can stay together, not how clumsily it can fall down.

We saw earlier in the chapter that since the advent of the industrial age, business structures have typically been constructed like pyramids, with fewer members functioning at each level of ascent. The workers and frontline supervisors are at the bottom; middle management is, naturally, somewhere in the middle, directing the supervisors; and the pinnacle is reserved for those in the executive offices, who reportedly make the most influential decisions for the organization. The workers (the bottom row) carry the weight of the entire organization, support the managers, and make sure that they do not shift enough to cause those at the top to lose their balance. The middle people must not only stand on what the workers are doing but also bear the weight of upper management on their shoulders while relying almost exclusively for their own balance on those below. Those at the top must constantly guard their steps, stretching their arms upward and smiling positively while secretly wanting to grab something below to hold on to. Those at the top risk the most exposure should they topple down, perhaps taking a few middle people with them. Top-down leadership makes perfect sense—until one stops to evaluate the weight and pressure on the individual workers, and the far-removed executive's dependency on processes about which he may have little practical knowledge.

A new type of pyramid is emerging for this increasingly technological age, a pyramid that is supported by the front line, stabilized by leadership, and topped off by a well-rounded, well-balanced, and fine-tuned group process. It is intended not to replace but to enhance the naturally occurring hierarchies in business by emphasizing group effectiveness and the power of the front line. Here is how it can be built.

THE FOUNDATION: THE FRONT LINE. We will begin by again thinking of the frontline workers as the foundation, or base, of the new pyramid. However, we will begin by thinking of the front line differently than we ever have before: we will think of the frontline workers in terms of their emotional abilities, thoughts, and feelings, not in terms of their productive skills.

One thing that human pyramid builders must be constantly aware of is a level surface. You would not want to build a pyramid on a sloping surface, nor would you want to have varying heights in the foundation. The inhabitants of the bottom row must have their backs level, or the people in the next row cannot appropriately balance on them.

For the same analogous reason, emotional ability on the front line should be level. One of the most arduous tasks of the leader is getting everyone on the same page emotionally. That means, among other things, assessing for emotional ability and assessing the use of emotional skills in team and group interactions. It means that when emotions are strong and team members are aggressive, some calming down may need to occur, and when someone would rather lie flat on the floor than support the team through the rendering of a thought, that must be dealt with also. If these situations aren't dealt with, the foundation will turn out to be a very bumpy surface that is entirely nonconducive to pyramid building.

Foundations for the future of nursing practice are also emerging in other areas of medical practice. Each nurse must have a vision of what the changing medical arena will look like in the areas of technology, genomics, pharmacology, and biotherapeutics (Porter-O'Grady, 2003). It is not enough to simply acknowledge our colleagues in other fields. We must align our backs with theirs, too.

THE CENTER BEAMS: MANAGEMENT AND LEADERSHIP. In the center of the traditional organizational hierarchy has always been management. Management typically has two roles: paying attention to the needs of the front line while satisfying the demands of upper management (McConnell, 1999). In our new pyramid, that is still essentially the case. However, *management* and *leadership* replace *managers* and *leaders* as these middle beams. The structure is determined not by how many bosses there are but by how good the leadership is.

These leaders, who ideally are supported by a level, emotionally solid foundation of nursing and multidisciplinary teams and are secure with the stable framework of a solid, group-oriented, interdependent, and empowering culture, are also doing a good deal of the support work themselves, although they are pulling upward rather than pushing downward. Whereas the function of management in the past was to bear down on employees to make sure they did a good job, the function of management in the new pyramid is to pull up and make sure there is stabilization by providing sturdy beams of support. In doing so, they ask questions rather than give answers, support team members rather than expect support, and seek depth of understanding rather than superficial agreement (Montgomery, 2003).

Good leadership provides support in a variety of ways. First, leadership erects the beam of trust—the beam that is never known to sway or topple over and is anchored firmly to the framework of empowering culture. Team members can grasp it and are reassured by it. Health care structures are changing whether we want them to or not; the options are to change with them effectively or to be changed by them ineffectively. Without trust, it becomes hard to work together as a team, especially when there is uncertainty as to what is happening in the rapidly changing environment (Laschinger, Finegan, and Shamian, 2001; Spath, 2003).

Second, effective leadership acts as a "signpost reader" (Porter-O'Grady, 2003, p. 59) for the team members and as such puts up the girder of forward thinking. While it is an asset for all team members to be forward-thinking, this skill especially becomes leaders, who have a specific responsibility to understand, anticipate, and manage change. The leader has to be on the lookout in order to advise the team. At their higher level, leaders have access to more knowledge; therefore, it is their duty to anchor this beam so that team members who grip it are properly aligned to do their work and direct their processes. To do otherwise would be like navigating without telling the driver where to turn, even though you very well understand what the map is telling you.

Third, effective leadership in the new pyramid is committed to making sure the right people are in the pyramid. The support beam of appropriate talent has perhaps never been more important than it is today. Team members, the foundation, hold on to this beam because they understand that the right talent leads to the right decisions and ultimately the right outcomes. Talent in today's dynamic workplace includes far more than ability: it involves the passion and the capacity to commit to the organization and whatever changes it needs to undergo to make it successful (Bradford and Sutton, 2003). For nurses, this means being committed to bettering patient care in the context of nursing practice and the individual unit or environment in which the nurse practices.

Leaders actually assume a followership role as they provide support for the team. They back up the team rather than pull from the front (Montgomery, 2002, 2003). They practice the essential art of listening in order to understand and identify team issues and emotions. They also concentrate on their own feelings, practicing self-reflection and self-regulation. In addition, they realize that the team's feelings and emotions as well as their own may be diverse, and they appreciate and promote that diversity (Montgomery, 2002).

THE PINNACLE: TEAM PROCESS. The new pyramid is clearly built of concepts rather than of people who happen to be in certain positions. The old way has valued position for far too long and as a result has negated the input and skill of many talented individuals. Perhaps most appropriate for this new pyramid structure is that at its top, where upper management would ordinarily reside, is the process of the team itself.

The process by which the team, unit, or organization functions is the part that results in visible outcomes. If the process comes tumbling down, it might take with it some of the supporting factors, but it will be rebuilt by continual learning and improvement of the supporting factors. The fall of a process is not nearly as dramatic, nor as traumatic, as the fall of an executive under the traditional hierarchy. The upper-level executive, as well as the organization, may or may not recover; the old hierarchy's basis in position, rather than learning and empowerment, has made it vulnerable to this potential. This is not to say that the executive level or other levels of management should not be involved in team processes; it is merely saying that the team's process should drive everyone's involvement. There will probably always be an upper level of management, and the goal is not to exclude them from the business. The goal is to enable all members of the organization to maximize their contributions through the new team structure.

Having said that, there are several necessary elements that will help form the capstone of the new pyramid. The team needs to rely heavily on its process to direct its culture and its vision.

First, the team process must guard against lack of vision, resistance to change, and pessimism (Silversin and Kornacki, 2003). These concepts have been stressed throughout this book, but they are worth mentioning again here. These three elements can kill enthusiasm and forward momentum more quickly than even lack of resources or funds. When the leader uses emotional skill, he can not only identify these detrimental qualities, but can understand their influence quickly and move to work with constituents to manage them.

Second, the process should emphasize knowledge and communication. One should only rarely be in a position to make decisions off the cuff or without sufficient supporting knowledge. Just as multiple sources of knowledge are needed for clinical skill at the bedside (Rycroft-Malone, Harvey, Kitson, McCormack, Seers, and Titchen, 2002), so they are in working with colleagues to reach decisions that affect the group. McKinley and others (1999) described a quality improvement team that evolved into a high-performance, self-directed team. They did this by operating in an informal, open environment; allowing balanced participation among members; and allowing and even encouraging disagreement. Consequently, the team members learned from one another and even looked forward to meetings. Properly facilitated, meetings should be enjoyed, not dreaded or seen as drudgery.

Third, and perhaps most important, the process should emphasize a core purpose and strategy, coupled with execution. Some business leaders emphasize execution over strategy, although both are important (Beckham, 2003). Strategy without execution is meaningless, and execution without strategy is purposeless. Teams must enlist and use both.

Structural Refinement of the New Pyramid

You may recall from other texts about changing organizational structures that the flatter, less hierarchical structures are coming to be better thought of than the taller ones with more levels of management. Flatter organizations are said to promote better communication and information flow, not to mention efficiency in making decisions and coordinating activities. (McConnell, 1998; Barnhart, 1997). I believe this as well, and it is this very point that leads us to structural refinement of the pyramid we have just built. How this is done is very important, because sudden flattening of an organizational structure that took years to build can be painful as well as frightening for everyone involved (McConnell, 1998).

How, then, can we make the pyramid better, more functional, and more conducive to an emotionally healthy organizational structure? The answer exists in considering, not the hierarchical positions themselves, but rather the functions and capabilities of everyone in the organization as we build and balance our new pyramid.

STRUCTURAL REFINEMENT A: BEGIN WITH A SHORTER REPLICA OF THE OLD PYRAMID. In the new pyramid, managers and leaders will necessarily become more responsive to the customer and the front line. No longer will the height of a traditional position-related pyramid serve to shield those on top from those nearer the ground. There will still be distinct staff and management functions, but the distance between these functions will become shorter. The uppermost functions of management will come closer to the middle level functions, so that there is more collaboration between the two and a greater attempt by upper management to understand each functional area of the organization. Likewise, the middle and supervisory functions will come closer to the functions of the front line, and the two will augment and support one another. As a result, all the elements of the new pyramid—the foundation (front line functions), the structural beams (leader functions), and the capstone (upper management functions) will naturally become closer together. The laws of physics tell us that shortening anything lowers its center of gravity and reduces the potential for it to be knocked off balance. Almost anything that is teetering high in the air is susceptible to a bad fall. The closer upper management is to the front line in function, the less likely it is to topple.

Teamwise, this shortening of all organizational functions brings the support and stability of the management process closer to the day-to-day work of the team members who make up the foundation. Not only does this create more tightness and closeness, but it also reduces the distance needed to travel to whatever is needed to reach the goal. Theoretically, communication within this structure is more direct, happens more quickly, and is less subject to misinterpretation or distortion (Rushmer, 2000).

In everyday life, we can think of tightening every connection in the pyramid in this way. Tighter team members are more attuned to one another's emotions, feelings, and interactions. When leaders are closer to their team members from the emotional perspective—that is, when they assist team members in recognizing and understanding, then managing, their emotions—team members are more likely to learn and respond in emotionally appropriate ways. The leaders are not close from a governing standpoint; they are close from a support standpoint. Their chief function is to provide support for the team. As such, they are more responsive to the team and the customer. They are one of the team themselves, with an added support function. Their "shortness" allows them to have their ear closer to the ground.

STRUCTURAL REFINEMENT B: EXPAND THE BASE OF THE PYRAMID. Remember that we are building a new pyramid from the ground up, not disbanding the pyramid we already have. We will use that one later. Right now, we are using elements of the old pyramid to build our new one.

Now, keeping the picture of the flattening pyramid in your mind, imagine the base of it being stretched out, as though the entire structure were made of rubber. What happens? Naturally, the pyramid will get even flatter. Flattening the hierarchy typically refers to reducing the number of levels of management and allowing more decision making at the frontline level. While this strategy is widespread and well known, in the context of our new pyramid it also means making teams more responsible and accountable for outcomes. If we think of influence as spreading over an area, it is obvious that the potential for the greatest influence lies at the foundation, which covers the greatest area of any part of the pyramid.

Stretching out the foundation means several things. It means giving teams the empowerment and accountability that frontline workers need to do their jobs and expand their roles, and it means giving more people the opportunity to participate. In shared leadership models, it is appropriate for different staff members to have the opportunity to rotate on and off committees at intervals. Not only do such committee members have the opportunity to learn while serving, but they also carry away with them a perspective that can influence their daily practice and interactions with others. Thus, what used to be "my job" becomes "our work" (Rushmer, 2000, p. 2244).

In addition, stretching out the foundation involves expanding the abilities of team members. This is also supported through an environment of empowerment and learning, the framework of the new pyramid. Therefore, by establishing the framework, the pyramid is able to sustain the expanded foundation.

Supporting the Pyramid from the Top Up

It is here that we begin to explore the upending of the pyramid. Although the theoretical structure of the new pyramid is very much based in relational concepts and not as much in position, it still resembles a traditional hierarchy, which has frontline workers (or team members) at the bottom. The purpose of building the new pyramid was not to make the hierarchy go away but to provide a new structure on which the organization (and its management and staff) can base its actions. Teams can be very good for integrating structure and process through all levels of the organization, even though positional levels can and should remain (Katzenbach and Smith, 1993). However, while gravity requires that many things be built from the bottom up, once completed, these structures can be lifted and balanced in such a way that they function as the engineer intended.

Balancing the Pyramid

The new pyramid, once built, can be balanced from the top up. What we have created in the new pyramid is *potential*: a concept of relationships and more interdependent functioning that brings management and frontline functions closer together. *Once* the team is established and performing effectively, it can be quite capable of effecting positive, influential decisions in an organization. To understand the counterintuitive concept of balancing from the top up, try to imagine the mature team-based pyramid flipped upside down onto its point and balancing solidly on its capstone. This pyramid requires three things: a sturdy point (top) on which to stand and pivot, some kind of mechanism to make sure that balance is maintained, and a broad, smooth, and stable surface, a kind of tabletop on which the organization can base its visions, plans, and goals.

THE PIVOT POINT: INTERACTIONS AND RELATIONSHIPS AMONG TEAMS IN THE ORGANIZATION. Whatever is balancing this new structure needs to be practically incapable of crumbling. The corners of crackers and of cardboard boxes are their most vulnerable parts, the most likely to be crushed by weight and the most likely to chip off when there is a disruption of any kind. That should not happen to the mature team pyramid. The top corner of the pyramid needs to be the sturdy element that can support its entire structure. When we upend the pyramid and balance it this way, the supporting end is made up of the interactions and relationships among teams. This is because in the new pyramid, everything pivots on one thing: how well the organization (including management and staff) communicates and interacts. In fact, management, especially upper management, which still resides in this capstone in the traditional pyramid, has the utmost responsibility to ensure that appropriate communication is maintained.

The importance of effective communication has been stressed throughout this book. It is so essential, that LaFasto and Larson (2001) say explicitly, "the fundamental guideline must be: *Use every means at your disposal to ensure that goals and priorities are clear. Leave nothing to chance. Communicate repeatedly in a variety of media. And when you think you're done, do it again*" (p. 185).

Interactive skills are not something with which every staff member, no matter what their level in the traditional "hierarchy," will come naturally equipped. These skills include conflict management, meeting leadership, negotiation, and the ability to influence others (Wellins, Byham, and Wilson, 1991). It is interesting to note that each skill has very much to do with emotional acuity. So important are these skills that supplemental training may be required if they are not present. Team leaders need to be especially careful that their message is heard consistently, and their message should include everything relevant (Fisher, 1993). Team members should be encouraged to do the same.

Often team interactions at all levels of the organization are hindered by distractions, excessive talkers, or team members who are hesitant to bring their views to the table. The use of circle communication technique can help mitigate some of these issues by requiring team members to focus on the speaker and concentrate on his communication. In circle communication, each person has the opportunity to speak, and other team members listen intently to that person's contribution. By doing this, team members practice active listening, conscious self-monitoring, and intentional speaking. Each person involved maintains a sense of individuality while contributing to the group consensus. Circle communication greatly contributes to shared leadership and avoids emphasizing one person over another. It is best used in situations where consensus is needed. It emerges from the common trait of humanity and breaks barriers created by position or perceived power. Circle communication is well worth practicing because it encourages different ways of being and knowing (Michaels, 2002).

THE CENTRAL BALANCING MECHANISM: CHARACTER BUILDING AND FEEDBACK FROM LEADERSHIP. While our theoretical pyramid balances, it cannot do so on good communication alone. Physiologically, our sense of balance is controlled by neurological functions involving the inner ear and cerebellum of the brain. Balance is a delicate phenomenon; it takes very little to throw off our sense of balance—for example, stepping on a small object on our way across a room or parking lot can do it. Cats and squirrels are equipped to balance in high, narrow places by using the fine-tuned movement of their tails. Humans tend to use their arms to do the same thing: notice a circus tightrope walker and his instinctive reaction to a near fall. Controlling balance is the result of an internal mechanism that alerts us when we are off balance. There should always be some mechanism for ensuring balance in teams as well.

To be effectively balanced in their process and interactions, teams need leadership feedback and evaluation. About evaluation and the nature of being human, the Danish philosopher Kierkegaard said that life must be lived moving forward, even though it is better understood looking backward. We must understand that people do not always behave predictably; often they behave differently when emotions, laziness, or uncertainty get in the way (Badaracco, 2002). Leaders should be prepared for this and need to be constantly vigilant in order to balance these factors with predictable ones. When someone lets his or her emotions get in the way of good judgment, it is an evaluative point that the leader should take up with that team member. This may strengthen character, or it may keep the same thing from happening again.

More than evaluation and feedback, teams need character development. Character evolves continually, just as emotional intelligence does. Building character involves recognizing where standards and values come from (family, faith, or perhaps both); promoting and demonstrating openness to change ideas and behaviors when presented with new evidence; moral accountability; and the ability to recognize destructive habits (Kowalski and Yoder-Wise, 2003).

To keep teams balanced and on track, evaluation is essential. However, the emphasis of team evaluations should be on nonfinancial performance measures such as customer satisfaction and benefit. Caution should be exercised here. Often, this is an area in which leadership falls short, because the measures have nothing to do with the company strategy, the measures are concocted and not scientifically based, the performance targets are out of line with financial goals, or they are measured incorrectly. To implement sound nonfinancial performance measures, leaders should determine which factors have an impact on the ultimate performance of the organization and continually measure and refine these factors (Ittner and Larcker, 2003). Rewards, in addition, can be nonfinancial and built into the goals of good performance (Hagland, 1995).

In addition, leaders should not neglect time for meeting with teams. The pressure of dealing with scarce resources often tests a leader's own character. In health care, it is often leaders who must infuse quality and improve work environments for nurses, resulting in a complex balancing act (Brunke, 2001) for the leader. Leadership must not get so involved in projects and management meetings, however, that they neglect having value-added meetings with front-line staff. Paying more attention in this area furthers the opportunity for two-way evaluation and feedback and emphasizes the support that teams are receiving from leadership.

THE SMOOTH SURFACE: OUTCOMES AND REFLECTIONS FROM THE FRONT LINE. The entire rationale for upending the new pyramid is to put the front line's contributions, conceptually, where they belong: at the top. Being at the top, however, adds responsibility and accountability. When the front line's contributions are critical to the organization's success, it naturally follows that the front line should take their contributions seriously and make concerted efforts to produce quality outcomes that will benefit the organization as a whole. Picture the top surface as a table-top or shelf: something that you would set something else on. As a review, the surface formed by the contributions of the front line is balanced by effective leadership and lifted up by pivotal communications within the organization, beginning at the management level. For the upended new pyramid to be effective, the organization itself must stand on the contributions and efforts of the front line, which are supported by, rather than merely supporting, management.

The entire "new pyramid" scenario is conceptual in nature. Nothing happens to the upper management or the middle management, and front line teams do not suddenly rule the organization without any guidance or authority from those in higher positions. In this ideal concept, however, teams whose outputs are literally driving the organization's mission fulfillment have attained the visibility and authority they need to get the job done. They have the respect of upper management, the support of leadership, and the respect of other teams and groups within the organization.

However, these are not the natural tendencies of today's organization. The proportionately largest group of health care professionals, nurses still typically receive low levels of organizational support (Laschinger, 1996). The changing work environment and job stress no doubt contribute to this phenomenon (Ndiwane, 2000). Nevertheless, it has never been more important to place nurses in a position of organizational influence than it is now, because changes in what is required of clinicians hit the front line before they hit anyone else. Who better to influence an adjustment to prepare for these changes than those who will have to deal with them?

Kutzscher, Sabiston, Laschinger, and Nish (1997) compared workplace satisfaction and empowerment among 170 employees working in hospital accreditation teams with 185 employees not working on teams. The results showed that involvement through teams affects employees' perceptions of access to power and ultimately job satisfaction. Collaboration with managers has been associated with job satisfaction and access to information associated with lower job stress (Almost and Laschinger, 2002).

Frontline significance in organizational leadership, however, does more for employees than enhance job satisfaction, and more for the organization than provide happy employees. We will now explore what can happen when frontline employees and teams participate where it really counts within the organization.

TOP-UP COMPETENCIES. Assuming that the team is supported and balanced, its contributions cover a wide, level expanse that can serve as a well-supported surface for moving ahead. Let us now explore some of the competencies that are built through a top-up approach to team functions.

Shared Leadership. Shared leadership is the primary manifestation of placing frontline workers at the top. The ability to share in the reality of making the organization, department, or unit run smoothly is based on the core principles of partnership, accountability, equity, and ownership (Ulrich, 2003). The shared leadership of all team members and the cross-organizational shared leadership of all teams provides the context for sustaining excellence within the organization (Ulrich, 2003).

Allowing Initiative. In traditional nursing education, there has been a disconnect between the humanistic, holistic aspects of patient care and the high level of technical knowledge and skill required by the profession. Specifically, there is a conflict between enabling to perform a role and empowerment to influence practice: nurses in the traditional educational structure have been entrenched in a hierarchy that unwittingly prevents them from being empowered to direct their own practice. After all, we are rightly taught to follow doctors' orders, stay within the bounds of Nurse Practice Acts, and sometimes communicate and justify professional judgment calls to the patient record as well as to the physician. Having inherited these well-educated nurses who are well aware of their professional boundaries, nurse leaders must constantly guard against their own need for control, which can rob teams even further of an empowering environment in which they could otherwise thrive (Espeland and Shanta, 2001; Laurent, 2000). The empowerment inherent in the mature team process and structure is what allows team members to actually achieve business results (Montebello, 1994). Whatever business they are in, be it primary care, tertiary care, or insurance, nurses have the capacity to affect results much more than they have been allowed to in the past. The team structure provides the perfect demonstration ground for their skills.

Anticipating the Next Need. Like good leaders, effective teams are known to anticipate the needs of the future, and the very existence of effective teams can foster an innovative climate. It has been noted that innovative organizations are supportive not only of innovation and creativity but also of the independent functioning of their members (Scott and Bruce, 1994) and, by extension, their teams. Innovation is defined as positive change that occurs when specialized knowledge is applied to a perceived problem (Gilmartin, 1998). It is a great accomplishment, indeed, for an organization to be able to present a problem to a team whose proven process and inter-action skills can bring forth a successful resolution to that problem. Having teams that are the top lookout for opportunities to change provides an additional level of maturity for the organization, because management need not always be the driving force behind needed improvements. In other words, teams that have reached this level are able to foresee and act on impending issues long before they become problematic.

Influencing Leadership. One challenge that faces all industries, including nursing, is that the workforce is changing. The younger members of the workforce have different expectations of employment than did their parents. For example, as few as two generations ago, a person joined a company's workforce and planned to stay there for a long time, perhaps for her lifetime. Most gave their skills and abilities to their organization so that in return their organization would provide them with a salary and some measure of security after retirement. Many of these of arrangements would be considered today as dead-end jobs: doing the same thing day after day with minimal personal or professional growth attached.

Today people seek not only financial security from their job but also opportunity. Many entering the workforce today do not see themselves doing the same job twenty or even ten years from now. Additionally, employment opportunities are increasingly diverse, and skilled individuals have choices. Nurses can work in a variety of different areas; they are usually not confined to the hospital for their entire career. Nurses seek personal and professional development as part of their job, so mentorship and leadership are doubly important. Teams that represent a cross-generational spectrum have the ability to influence leadership from the perspective of what leadership needs to become in order to adapt to the changing work-force (Wieck, Prydun, and Walsh, 2002). Managers and leaders must be tuned in and responsive to what teams need from them, just as teams should be open and responsive to feedback from leadership. Leadership is tasked with mobilizing the staff (Gokenbach, 2003) or creating teams that will engender staff mobilization.

Thriving, Dynamic Work Patterns and Successful Practice. A couple of emerging patterns and structures in the health care environment deserve men-tion here. First, business units that focus on specific functions can be estab-lished within departments and organizations in order to fulfill specific goals. Often teams are formed to address the business aspects, such as education and operations, that ultimately provide much of the support for management and the organization (Pinkerton, 2003). This structure not only allows the front line to participate more intimately in the primary functions of the orga-nization, it also underscores the importance of a company's mission by scaling it to the department level. For example, although the Disease Management Company with which I am affiliated has implemented an orga-nizationwide quality program, nurses within the clinical operations depart-ment manage quality within their own area by participating in different committees at the staff and management levels. Their initiatives and progress benefit their areas while ultimately feeding the organization's quality program.

A second emerging pattern is the consultant role of nursing. That is, nurses can and should become expert in their specific field and spend time developing other nurses (Higgins, 2003). The upended new pyramid is a perfect breeding ground for this nurse role in that it provides the empow-erment, education, and attention to process necessary for such a role. Nurse experts who have devoted time, research, and attention to changes and advances in one particular field are a valuable resource for patients, families, other team members, and organizational leadership.

The mature, well-balanced team structure can be a springboard for these and several other areas of advanced practice, many of which have yet to be discovered. By putting its best face to the world, the team will cause the organization to flourish in ways previously untapped and currently undiscovered.

Summary

We have come to think of business in terms of a traditional hierarchy of position in which upper management, middle management, and frontline workers form a pyramid. While it is unlikely that management will or even should dissolve into a distant memory, a new kind of hierarchy is needed, one that places frontline workers at the foundation, leadership as the supportive beams, and team process at the top, all with empowerment, education, performance expectation, and interdependency as the environmental framework. Once this initial pyramid is constructed, it grows shorter and flatter, with leadership and the front line coming closer to each other, and wider, with a greater expanse of accountability on the front line.

Establishing effectiveness within teams, once they are built, requires that the structure figuratively be set on its head, resulting in a top-up perception. The pivotal point on which the entire team balances is its ability to interact and communicate effectively. Leadership provides the mechanism and measures for balance. Frontline workers are responsible for outcomes that most affect business and organizational success, so they provide the smooth surface from which organizational processes are driven. Supported by such a solid structure, the organization is thus poised to make an effective contribution to the future of health care, with all the innovations, change, and empowerment it will entail.

TEN CRITERIA FOR THE NEW ORGANIZATIONAL PYRAMID

1. Teams' primary function is to learn, both emotionally and practically.
2. Teams' secondary function is to perform and produce results based on learning.
3. Team members are cross empowered, which means that they grow in their understanding of what other team members are doing and need from them.
4. Team members recognize and draw on their need for one another.
5. The abilities and characteristics of the front line make up the foundation of the pyramid.
6. Leadership and management provide the supportive beams of trust, appropriate talent, and observing signs of things to come.
7. Team process is the capstone of the pyramid and pervades the organization.
8. Team communication and interaction are stable and refined enough so that the pyramid, if inverted, could be entirely based on that one aspect.
9. Leadership balances the inverted pyramid through character development, feedback, and evaluation.
10. The maturity and balance of the new structure provides a suitable platform for decisions and actions that affect the business as a whole.

12

THE FUTURE OF EMOTIONAL INTELLIGENCE FOR NURSING LEADERSHIP

IT PROBABLY COMES AS no surprise that the last chapter of this book is about the future. As nurses, we are always thinking of the future; for example, we have goals and plans for the patients under our care. Everything we do ultimately influences our future, and most of us live with that in mind.

Why Think About the Future of Nursing Leadership Now?

The preceding chapters provide insight into the crucial role that emotional intelligence plays in leadership, specifically nursing leadership. Often, a reader may absorb or contemplate material in all its detail, all the while wondering what the crux of the matter really is; in other words, why is it all so important? For this book, here is the answer to that question: in the future, effective nursing leadership will become increasingly dependent on the development and use of emotional skills. In this final chapter, the specifics behind this belief will be demonstrated, as well as how emotional skill will come increasingly into play as we inaugurate the twenty-first century.

The Increasing Demands of Leadership Require a Courageous Stance

Some leadership mantras have become classic; *visionary thinking, strategy, communication skills,* and *teamwork* are all familiar terms to leaders who have read or studied management styles or principles, so it should come as no surprise that this book has championed all of these principles and more. One of the chief objectives of this book, one that sets it apart from other books of its kind, has been to point out the inseparably emotional side of these principles. I have demonstrated how carving out and integrating this additional layer of intelligence, which has varying levels and abilities, enhances effective leadership. Unlike cognitive intelligence, emotional skill requires the individual to integrate qualities that may be held as personal or even sacred—for example, self-awareness or feelings attached to a specific event or item. For that reason, applying emotional skill may often take more courage than the application of other skills or abilities.

If we were to be entirely honest, we would admit that anything worth having or worth investing in requires some measure of courage. For example, as leaders, we are often called on to believe implicitly in a decision, even if we are not certain of the outcome. The lack of the "courage of our convictions," as it is so often called, actually smacks of bad leadership and the inability to truly decide, no matter how many literal or actual decisions one may make or communicate on a daily basis. While it is important to maintain flexibility, it is equally important, if not more so, to maintain an air of assuredness. Sometimes, however, that air of assuredness takes a great deal of courage and self-discipline.

Leaders will need to fill critical roles in the future: change manager, master strategist, relationship builder, and talent developer. Among other skills, these roles will require that leaders develop organizational and personal communication skills, strategic thinking ability, and the ability to develop talent (Giganti, 2003b). In the future, courage will become much more important, and it will go beyond merely believing in one's own stance. It will be needed more and more in those leadership principles that we are all extremely familiar with. Because of increased focus on teams, more interdependent roles, an abundance of technological and ethical issues, and the need to change more rapidly, emotional involvement will be required to make our leadership work. The nurse leader will also need courage to often step out of her comfort zone and make changes proactively, all the time monitoring and helping bolster the emotions of constituents.

Additionally, emotional knowledge must be applied because of who we are leading: an increasingly diverse workforce perhaps more keen than ever before to their feelings and emotions. We must know how to help them identify exactly what these emotions are and how to effectively use, understand, and manage them.

Increased Diversity Requires an Honest Look at Oneself and Others

"We don't look so much at what or where people have studied but rather at their drive, initiative, cultural sensitivity, and readiness to see the world as their oyster," says CEO Stephen Green (Green, Hassan, Immelt, Marks, and Meiland, 2003, p. 40). Truly, sensitivity to diversity will typify the effective nurse leader of the future. The increasing diversity of the U.S. population alone is enough to convince us that we must accept and celebrate diversity.

The value of diversity will need to be promoted in the organization of the future. Diverse team members may evaluate team communications from varying perspectives, but reinforcing stereotypes only hinders team communication. Suggested approaches to increasing diversity awareness and the value teams place on diversity include evaluation of the community's and the organization's ethnic and racial composition; assessing the level of diversity in higher management; and involving minorities in mentoring activities that will poise them to advance in their careers (Mateo and Smith, 2001).

Not only is the workforce culturally diverse, but it is also generationally diverse. As of 2002, two-thirds of the nursing force was over age forty, and 40 to 60 per cent of those nurses were expected to retire within fifteen years (Cordeniz, 2002, p. 237). Nurses born between 1963 and 1977 are making up more and more of the workforce, and they have different expectations than their predecessors as to what makes up an acceptable work environment. To maintain the loyalty of this new generation of nurses, leaders should realize that many of these individuals are more loyal to themselves than to their company (in other words, they do not typically begin a job hoping that they will remain with the same organization for twenty to thirty years); that they expect and demand training and learning as part of their job; and that they are looking for a job that allows them to have time and energy for a personal life (Billingsley, 2000). Nurse leaders will need to be aware of these factors as Generation X nurses stream into the vacancies created by retiring nurses.

Increased Knowledge Must Be Applied

In the words of Florence Nightingale, men of thought and men of action should be indistinguishable from one another (Jacobs, 2001). As nurses and as leaders, we are exposed to an increasing wealth of information and knowledge. This knowledge places us in a position and even invokes an obligation to apply it in our daily practice. Our predecessors in nursing leadership had neither the technology nor the leadership theory that we have today.

Specific to knowledge of emotional intelligence, we are living and practicing in an environment that is increasingly attuned to the emotional competencies needed to excel in leadership. Emotional intelligence has been identified as a competency of star performers by leaders and authors in many disciplines (Strickland, 2000; Goleman, 1998a, 1998b). This text has emphasized emotional intelligence and the fact that it can be learned, developed, and applied in leadership situations. Further, emotional intelligence skills enhance the leadership abilities of those in positions of formal or informal leadership.

The female-dominated nursing field is often thought to be characterized by qualities that are frequently associated with femininity: caring, nurturing, and relationship-centered behavior. High levels of emotional intelligence are said to contribute to the softer business results of cooperation and increased employee satisfaction (Strickland, 2000). All nurses, male and female alike, would benefit from learning emotional skills and translating them into their work environments.

Equipping the Nurse Leader with Emotional Courage for Nursing Leadership in the Twenty-First Century

This book has provided a discussion of emotional intelligence as it relates to nursing leadership in a very systematic way, discussing the emotional capabilities of nurse leaders from four perspectives: understanding the elements of emotional intelligence; intelligently creating, sharing a vision, and setting an example; intelligent transfer of information; and changing the culture of nursing and the organization. The nurse leader who is best positioned for the future will possess emotional acuity and will demonstrate unprecedented leadership courage.

Courage can be described as part of an individual's disposition and can be manifested morally, physically, or even emotionally (Clancy, 2003). Courage can seem to be depleted by intervening factors such as setbacks and disappointments. It must, however, be consistently applied in order to maintain beliefs and convictions; leaders who do not hold true to their convictions may compromise care and the development of staff. In times of crisis, this ability takes the form of the mind-over-matter approach. More specifically, however, we as leaders need to renew and refresh our courage at times by tuning into what we are feeling, acknowledging it, understanding where it is leading us, and managing it. Managing feelings of despair or discouragement may include seeking support from a trusted colleague or listing possibilities related to the current situation. In any case, we must maintain our courage if we are to lead.

This courage does require emotional skill. The abilities to identify, use, understand, and manage emotion will uphold the courageous nurse leader in unparalleled ways. Let us explore those ways as we discuss some of the leader capabilities that will be so important in the future.

Identifying Emotions

The ability to identify emotions (Mayer, Salovey, and Caruso, 2000, 2002) has been cited as a fundamental and foundational skill throughout this book. In preparing for the future, nurse leaders can apply this skill to three courageous acts: honoring oneself, being self-aware, and leading through the needs of the group.

SELF-MANAGEMENT AND THE COURAGE TO HONOR ONESELF. "To the extent that we can be emotionally honest . . . we find our voice, we become real," say Cooper and Sawaf (1997, p. 7). "Without experiencing potent feelings—which can be powerful catalysts for change—we'd never be forced to take a good, clear look at who we are."

Indeed, taking a good, clear look at who one is can be a powerful yet intimidating experience. This good, clear look forces the observer, the self alone, to assess that which motivates, excites, terrifies, and saddens it— and it causes the self to understand how it reacts to these emotions. Even more important, emotional honesty allows others to appreciate these aspects of the individual without the trouble of a façade, an excuse, or an explanation.

There is a delicate balance involved here. Many people plausibly believe that too much emotional honesty is detrimental to business and political relationships. No one in their right mind or at least with any sense of propriety, they reason, would let themselves be seen sweating in the face of everyday adversity or blissfully overjoyed at a small success. On the other hand, too much masquerading equates to emotional dishonesty and can be damaging to relationships.

Self-management can bridge the gap between too much and too little honesty. While self-management involves the avoidance of tantrums and meltdowns, it also involves, more subtly, the finesse to present what makes a person real in a productive, acceptable way. Those who live the principle of emotional management as if it implies beating emotions into submission may well come across as stoics who display no feeling. Those who are dedicated to developing their emotions to their fullest potential are practicing self-management to its most productive extent, and they are able to use their emotional honesty to establish positive relationships in the workplace.

In the future of nursing leadership, this self-management will involve a new type of courage: the courage to honor oneself. While that may seem paradoxical (after all, shouldn't honoring oneself be one of the easiest things to do?), honoring oneself is a skill that often needs to be developed. Caregiving dominates the health care professional's day, and the care is rarely reciprocated. Strength is more or less expected; calmness is construed as professionalism; and questionable character traits are fodder for intense speculation. At home at the end of the day, the health care professional is left to tend her self. If that self is to be honored, courage is required to change the focus of the day. Even more courage is required to exude the same honoring of the self at work.

Knowing and honoring oneself is foundational. Yet many bypass that foundation when building their career. They build a career on criteria, projections, optimism, pessimism, hopes, dreams, expectations, rigor, routine—anything but a true knowledge of self and an acceptance and consideration of who that self is. However, any other foundation hinders effective leadership. When it comes to the part of leadership that is driven by the self, one may reach for someone or something else to sustain one's motivation, but ultimately, the self is all one has.

Pagonis (2001) points out that knowing oneself is the first essential step in effective leadership. If something comes naturally (such as humor, public speaking, or charisma), by all means, know it, value it, and use it. If something does not come naturally or is more difficult, Pagonis recommends spending less time trying to use it. The ability to say, "I am better at x than I am at y" takes honesty with and honoring of the self. This implies not only an acknowledgment of personal worth but also an appreciation of it. The leader who masters this skill has a much easier time accepting those working under his guidance. Because I have a nose and ears, I am less likely to be curious about the mysterious lumps and squiggles on the faces of just about everyone else I meet. Because I understand who I am and that I have complexities, strengths, and weaknesses, I am not surprised when weaknesses and strengths typify nearly every other human being I come across. Also, if I am adept at acknowledging and managing these, I am in a much better position to help others do the same.

When the self is acknowledged and appreciated, emotional honesty, with oneself and with others, becomes much more realistic. Many people are afraid to reveal their feelings because they are afraid their feelings will not be understood or accepted. These individuals would rather create rational explanations for their actions, lack of action, or delayed commitment. Emotional honesty, tempered with self-management and self-awareness, involves being true and real, not hiding or avoiding or performing acrobatics to skirt the issue. Saying "There have been unexpected delays (or we underestimated the timeline), and we need more time to finish the project" is more emotionally honest than declaring "two additional weeks will allow us to enhance the quality of the ultimate product." Explaining "I am not comfortable with that decision from an ethical standpoint" is more honest than expounding on how another decision would make more sense financially. It all comes down to being real, and these days, that takes courage.

GOOD BUSINESS SENSE AND THE COURAGE TO BE SELF-AWARE. The perception that one has of oneself affects one's motivation, thought processes, emotional reactions, and behaviors (Bandura, 1977; Kelly, 2002). When we understand and accept where we are, we are more inclined to accept where others are and to be there with them. As painful as this process may be, it is essential, and it takes courage. Caring, a virtue that is claimed by nursing as a core value, is actually downplayed in the workplace as making one too vulnerable (Sherwood, 2003). I believe that a primary paradigm shift is occurring, from a primary focus on business acumen to a blended focus combining business ability with self-awareness and awareness of what makes others successful (including a caring spirit) within themselves and their organization.

EFFECTIVE GUIDANCE AND THE COURAGE TO LEAD THROUGH THE NEEDS OF THE GROUP. In the future, the focus of leadership will shift to those who are being led and away from the leader himself. Emotional aptitude will be key for navigating this transition and moving forward in the bold new era of participative health care leadership. At any given time, a leader may find himself in a servant role, a facilitator role, or a collaborator role. That is what it means to lead through the needs of the group, which involves validating the emotions of both staff and management (Staring and Taylor, 1997).

Imagine a young boy scout troop on an overnight outing. The scoutmasters who lead the adventure suit up, pack up, and maybe hike for a great distance in order to provide an unforgettable experience for a covey of giggling, adventurous boys. Everything is designed with the scouts in mind: what they should eat, what they will learn, what they will see, whether they will be safe. The focus is on those being led.

This model of leadership is being infused into our organizations. First, the troop members (the workforce) are the beneficiaries of our leadership, not us. They, not we, are the organization. They, not we, are in a position to reap the rewards of the successful organization they help to create. The education, nourishment, and safety that comes from our leadership is all for their benefit.

Second, leading for the leader's own personal edification is akin to the scoutmaster sleeping in an air-conditioned shelter, complete with cable television, while the troop sleeps under the stars. It does not make sense, and it does not look good. We sleep under the stars, too—with the crickets and the passing showers. That is effective and credible leadership.

Using Emotion to Facilitate Thought

Mayer, Salovey, and Caruso's (2000, 2002) concept of emotional facilitation has been cited throughout the text. Our thoughts and actions, unfortunately, are often thought to be hindered by our emotions, when in fact they can be facilitated by them in a positive way. Using emotions to facilitate our thoughts appropriately can result in the courage to listen and to address conflict as it arises.

COMMUNICATION AND THE COURAGE TO LISTEN. Listening does more than give us information; it sometimes gives us information that we would rather not know. There is a certain amount of information that we receive, and although much of it depends on the sender and the message itself, a great deal of it also depends on what we as the recipient allow to enter. We tend to filter and categorize information without even realizing it, and what we pay attention to matters just as much as what the message is and how the sender sent it.

Often, listening to ugly things requires a certain amount of action on our part, which is why effective listening involves somewhat of a risk and a commitment. If we do not give credence to the ugly and the unpleasant, we have less of a personally felt obligation to change it. Many experienced managers realize that poor listening skills will ultimately catch up with them; anything they are hearing from the ranks but ignoring will probably snowball if not addressed early. Some managers prefer to focus solely on successes and not address these little annoyances. These may be less experienced managers trying to put their best foot forward, but they may also be seasoned managers who are just accustomed to constantly putting out fires when the flames are lapping outside their office door. Neither has developed the courage to really listen.

Listening allows us to effectively participate in emotionally honest transactions. If the sender of the message is being emotionally honest, we need to hear that honesty in a way that does not translate the message into something different without first seeking to clarify what was meant by the sender. Consider the example given in the earlier section on honoring oneself. "We need more time to finish the project" could be interpreted in several different ways, from "these people are just lazy and didn't stay on top of their plan" to "I don't think they know what they are doing; they're just stalling." What the statement could really mean is this: "We need more time to finish the project. There were unexpected obstacles, which have been very frustrating. We appreciate the importance of a deadline and regret that it was not met. We are coming to you as our leader because we trust that you will understand and possibly even give feedback as to what we can do to more quickly overcome some of these obstacles." Rather than blowing the statement off as another excuse or request for delay, the courageous listener can help the sender to elaborate on what is honestly going on. In this case, the listening involves some dialogue and possibly some problem solving. This kind of courageous listening, using effective communication tools and attitudes (Kowalski and Yoder-Wise, 2003), will typify effective leadership in the future.

INTERPERSONAL SKILLS AND THE COURAGE TO ADDRESS CONFLICT. Job applicants frequently characterize themselves as having good interpersonal skills. For years, having excellent interpersonal skills has been a criterion for working in any job dealing with people.

Now imagine an interviewee who says, "I have to be honest with you. My interpersonal skills are not the best. I am actually very difficult to get along with. I don't work well with others, and I go around picking fights at every opportunity. I am technically qualified for this job; if I am hired, I will request an office as far away from my coworkers as possible so that I can give you my best work."

Of course, that fictional applicant had better hope that his skills are superior to anyone else's on the planet and that the fate of the entire world hinges on what he does for a living. Although the foregoing example is extreme, it is not unrealistic. There are indeed individuals working in facilities, offices, and clinics right now whose interpersonal skills are far from well developed. Most of us can name one or two whom we have worked with in the past. Interpersonal skills are something that most of us would like to say we have but that actually exist in varying degrees.

Interpersonal skills involve emotional ability to a great degree; think of how identification, facilitation, understanding, and management of emotions (those of both oneself and others) play into our overall ability to work with and deal with people. A culture that is focused on the needs of people makes work and practice more meaningful for employees (Sherwood, 2003). One interpersonal skill that will become increasingly valuable and needed in the future is conflict management.

Conflict management, without a doubt, takes a great deal of courage. It often separates those who are interpersonally skilled from those who are less so, because it requires active listening, problem solving, and keeping one's cool, all at the same time. People are comfortable with conflict management to varying degrees. Those who practice it and embrace its importance will contribute greatly to their success in nursing leadership in the future. The bottom line is this: conflict is on the increase—whether from external stressors, internal motivating factors, cultural differences, ethical dilemmas, or a shortage of staff. Conflict is, essentially, the reason that management is needed. Effective nurse leaders will be more and more conflict-savvy in the future.

Understanding Emotions

To be able to understand emotions and how they progress from one to the other is a high-level emotional skill, according to Mayer, Salovey, and Caruso (2000, 2002). Mastery of this skill can help leaders evaluate emotions and their prospective impact on both present and future situations. Nurse leaders will increasingly need the skill of understanding emotions, as well as the courage to understand the environment and to solve problems collaboratively. This will be true, in part, because of the growing complexity of nursing, the increasingly collaborative nature of the field, and the ethical, fiscal, and purely human decisions that will continue to face nurses in the years to come.

ENVIRONMENTAL ASSESSMENT AND THE COURAGE TO UNDERSTAND. In the story of Noah and the great flood, after the rain had stopped, Noah sent out a dove to assess the environment. He wanted to find out whether the water had receded below the level of the treetops, and he determined this by whether the dove returned with anything in its beak. The first findings were discouraging. The bird came back without anything. Later, when the water had receded, the dove brought back an olive leaf (Genesis 8:8–12). It is a simple story, but it illustrates a very important principle: you must know how high the waters are before you step out into them. If they are higher than your head, using a boat rather than wading is a good idea. If they are ten feet higher than yesterday, you get a pretty good idea of what is happening as well.

Assessing the environment takes courage. Chances are that we do not want to know that there is not a tree in sight. However, not knowing can contribute to backsliding or even demise of a career.

One thing is certain: the environment is constantly changing. *Who Moved My Cheese?* is a tale of two smart mice and two reluctant, almost somnolent human beings who notice that their world is changing at noticeably different rates. The characters who anticipate and keep up with the change get far ahead of those who do not. In fact, they are able to eat to their hearts' content while the slackers starve, search, and scratch their heads. This simple story paints a perfect picture of the health care environment. The cheese will move, and we must move with it—and it is much easier to move with it if we know where it is moving (Johnson, 1998).

Watching the environment is an arduous, sometimes rather mundane task but nevertheless a necessary one. Regulations, standards, and even legal actions can cause a complete shift in priorities in a health care organization or even the entire industry. (Consider the recent impact of the Health Insurance Portability and Accountability Act (HIPAA) on nearly all aspects of health care.) Being ahead of the game requires skill, and understanding what is out there requires courage. Motivating the organization to understand what is coming and act on it with the sense of urgency felt by the leader takes even more courage. Kotter (1996) remarks that the biggest mistake made by leaders who sense that change is needed is plunging ahead without making sure that others understand the urgency.

Being proactive because of anticipated shifts in the environment requires far more courage than reacting to actual shifts or even reacting to a crisis. When we react, usually we have no choice. It is usually imperative that we react (even if it is by inaction), and we are expected to do something. Our response and what we are responding to is usually quite visible and understood. In contrast, we do not have to be proactive. Reaction is controlled partially by the situation we are reacting to; proactive actions are controlled by those taking the actions. Proactive action takes courage, and in many cases, this approach may mean stirring up urgencies that others are not ready for.

Every nurse is responsible for shaping the type of environment that promotes satisfaction and excellence (Sherwood, 2003). We must determine where the floodwaters are. The need to be far ahead of the game will typify leadership in the future.

STRATEGIC LEADERSHIP AND THE COURAGE TO SOLVE PROBLEMS COLLABORATIVELY.

Yukl (1998) outlines several steps for formulating a strategy. Long-term objectives or priorities must be determined, and strengths and weaknesses must be assessed. Then core abilities (technical expertise, application skills) should be recognized and evaluated. Because there may be a current strategy in place, the leader must evaluate whether incremental change in the current plan or a completely new plan is needed. So that there are no surprises, the likely outcomes of the new strategy should be evaluated. Yukl is also careful to point out that strategies should be formulated in conjunction with other executives; crucial decisions should not be made alone.

One of the nice things about a new strategy is that it looks good on paper, and often the paper is a clean sheet. In other words, planning can be done all day and no obstacles will surface, no matter how unrealistic the plan. If obstacles appear likely, the strategy has a plan for dealing with them. When the plan begins to be executed, however, the obstacles arise, and we had better be able to solve problems. Problem solving also takes courage and must be done collaboratively.

"If you're not involving people in planning and problem solving and in the execution of their responsibilities," say Kouzes and Posner, "you're underutilizing the skills and resources in your organization" (1995, p. 175). Why in the world would we want to do that? Underutilization of resources is more tangible when we are talking about MRI machines or desk space and much less so when we are referring to the skills of people. The amount of attention given to underutilization will probably increase in the future as the value of human resources and of intellectual ability continue to soar.

When people participate in organizational leadership, they share in implementing the vision for the organization. They should also participate in the strategy and problem solving required to refine the vision. When obstacles occur, the strategy may change drastically or slightly. Therefore, strategic leadership is a fluid, dynamic, and ongoing process that goes far beyond initial planning. Kouzes and Posner go so far as to say that 90 percent of the organization's workforce should be involved in problem solving and planning.

We should never underestimate the capabilities of those working with us. When we are placed in a position of leadership, it is not always because we are capable of doing the work better than anyone else. Rather, it is often because we are trusted to facilitate getting the work done by those who do it best. Leadership requires a shift in skill away from doing the work and toward an entirely different focus on the effective use of resources. The human nature of our most important resources adds a new level of accountability. We must collaborate and help those on our team to be successful, because they have the answers and we have stewardship of the wealth that they bring to the table.

Managing Emotions

Managing emotions is the highest of all emotional skills and as such requires the most advanced emotional learning (Mayer, Salovey, and Caruso, 2000, 2002). Managing emotions involves the ability to moderate and influence emotions in oneself and in others, skills that are needed to successfully lead through the courageous acts of creating, sharing a vision, and setting an example that others not only want to follow but will follow well.

GOOD THINKING AND THE COURAGE TO CREATE. In their book *The Knowing-Doing Gap,* Pfeffer and Sutton (2000) refer to "the pressure for consistency" as a psychological force that can easily hinder good, creative thinking (p. 73). People generally seek to appear consistent rather than confused or hypocritical, they say. In addition, it may be more efficient to be consistent and not stumble into the pitfalls of change. Also, when people do not quite know what to do, they may imitate others who are similar or follow historical precedents (Pfeffer and Sutton, 2000). The problem with consistency and relying on memory to dictate current direction is fairly easy to realize. If change begets change, then old solutions won't fit new problems, right? Yet the old psychological forces often have a tight grip.

Good thinking involves what we are accustomed to: learning from our mistakes and our history and understanding the competition or what others like us are doing. But it also involves something that we may not be as accustomed to: understanding the present, anticipating the future, and creating around them both. This takes courage, because it usually involves doing what no one has ever done before or at least taking a new spin on what was done earlier. But leaders must find ways to buck the trends against creativity in order to have a creative vision for the future. In addition, leaders need courage in order to bring about changes that may be difficult (Samuel, 2003).

Chapter Four was devoted to the emotional skills required in leaders who create. Perhaps one of the most courageous acts involved in creating is challenging the present norm. The leader must not only create an environment that is ripe for change but also change people's mind-sets, realizing that resistance is possible and even probable. Once the environment is right, the leader must engender in followers a spirit of participation and willingness to challenge the norm that will transcend the present in order to manifest the vision of the future. This involves risk and attention to new ideas but also the willingness to prevent failures from discouraging creativity.

A LOOK FORWARD AND THE COURAGE TO SHARE THE VISION WITH OTHERS. Wall, Solum, and Sobol (1992) give this insightful look into visionary leadership: "Your decision to become a visionary leader must come from your heart. Empirically, there is ample evidence from enlightened companies that empowering employees and building a participative work environment will yield substantial productivity gains. But the new paradigm is based on the understanding that, while profits are our end goal, they are not our most powerful leadership focus. . . . The irony of the role of the visionary leader is that they must be a servant to those they lead. The paradox is that they can lead only by giving their power away" (p. 226–227).

Wall, Solum, and Sobol conclude by calling visionary leadership a courageous act that requires stamina. A critical ingredient in successful leadership is ensuring that an organization's vision and mission ultimately become reality (Spitzer, 2003). Truly, courage is involved in both the sharing of the vision and the sharing of the leadership. Visionary leadership goes beyond simply making people see. It involves letting people participate, make decisions, have accountability, and lead their contributions forward.

In basic genetics lessons, most health professionals learn about the phenomenon of mitosis. Cells divide, and each new cell is a representative of the original. A well-executed vision is much like this. As the vision is shared, each participant becomes representative of the vision. They live it and act on it. The leader gives the vision to those she is leading so that they can carry out the work. It becomes theirs, and they treat it as such. A vision and leadership in implementing it can be effectively shared in a multitude of ways. The leader must define the challenges clearly, understand feelings and expectations, and help constituents manage them so that their focus on the vision is clear. Additionally, the leader must be able to temper and align the vision not only with the ideal but with organizational realities—resources, policies, and culture—and teach constituents to do the same (Vestal, 2003).

Participative leadership allows the leader to bridge the gap between needing to lead and needing to foster success in those being led. Leaders who know themselves and their strengths are better equipped to see those of their constituents, as I noted earlier. Also, leaders who are willing to trust their constituents—strengths, weaknesses, and all—with the execution of a well-formulated vision will be courageously contributing to the growth of themselves, their colleagues, and the organization.

MOTIVATION AND THE COURAGE TO SET AN EXAMPLE. Kouzes and Posner (1995) cite research on leader credibility, asserting that credibility is undoubtedly the foundation of leadership. When asked what typifies a credible leader, respondents answered in rather elementary phrases: "They walk the talk," "They practice what they preach," and, most frequently, "They do what they say they will do." To do this, the researchers continue, three things must happen. The leader must clarify her own values and those of others, must gain unity around shared values, and must be vigilant as to how the values are being lived—by herself as well as others. Setting an example requires being up front with oneself and others as to feelings and beliefs, perceived obstacles, and goals. Motivation in and of itself is not a bad thing—in fact, it is a very good thing—but it is not the only thing. Because leaders do not operate in a vacuum, motivation is at best the equivalent of a stimulating, inspirational dream that occurs night after night.

Therefore, with setting an example, the focus is not so much on the leaders but on the team members. What kind of example do they need? They need an example that is not only articulated but also followed by us. That takes courage and the ability to facilitate experiences that empower nurses (Campbell, 2003). This implies living the vision, not just speaking of it. The motivation flows into us and should exit us as example. That should be motivation enough for our constituents.

Summary

Emotionally intelligent leadership will typify the health care organization of the future. The ability to embrace change, to make decisions that support and allow for environmental influences, and to lead through the needs of others will require the emotional knowledge, facilitation, understanding, and management that are hallmarks of emotionally skilled managers.

There will be leaders that are less skilled than others, just as there are leaders less prepared in business acumen and emotional skill today. Those who hone their skills now will be more prepared for the future. The readers of this book, because they will make up a part of this future leadership, are encouraged to take advantage of the opportunity now to learn about, understand, and manage the emotional part that makes them who they are.

Preparing for the future is important because of the increasing demands of leadership; the need to understand, accept, and promote cultural and generational diversity; and the sheer amount of knowledge available. Facing the twenty-first century of nursing, with its anticipated changes, will require courage on the part of the nurse leader that can be passed on to teams and organizations. This courage will be augmented by attention to and development of emotional competencies within teams and the field of nursing itself.

TEN CRITERIA FOR THE COURAGEOUS TWENTY-FIRST CENTURY NURSE LEADER

1. The courageous nurse leader first has the courage to know and to honor himself or herself.

2. The courageous nurse leader supports good business decisions with self-awareness.

3. The courageous nurse leader leads through the needs of the group.

4. The courageous nurse leader listens, even though it might mean hearing things that he or she may not want to hear.

5. The courageous nurse leader addresses conflict with resolve and with the understanding that conflict actually betters the team and the organization.

6. The courageous nurse leader assesses the environment for future and current implications for the profession.

7. The courageous nurse leader solves problems collaboratively.

8. The courageous nurse leader creates through thinking that envisions the need for change.

9. The courageous nurse leader is able to have a vision of the ideal and to share it with others.

10. The courageous nurse leader sets an example for the organization and motivates teams to accomplish great purposes through their own actions.

REFERENCES

Adams, K. E., Cohen, M. H., Eisenberg, D., & Jonsen, A. R. (2002). Ethical considerations of complementary and alternative medicine therapies in conventional medical settings. *Annals of Internal Medicine, 137*(8), 660–664.

Aiken, L. H., Havens, D. S., & Sloane, D. M. (2000). The magnet nursing services recognition program: A comparison of two groups of magnet hospitals. *American Journal of Nursing, 100*(3), 26–36.

Alcock, B., Berter, E., Hawkins, J., Madsen, P., & McCall, M. (2002). Communication: What to say and when to say it. *AORN* [Association of Operating Room Nurses] *Journal, 76*(5), 875–878.

Almost, J., & Laschinger, H. (2002). Workplace empowerment, collaborative work relationships, and job strain in nurse practitioners. *Journal of the American Academy of Nurse Practitioners, 14*(9), 408–420.

Ambulance Work and Nursing—A Handbook on First Aid to the Injured with a Section on Nursing, Etc. (c. 1898). Chicago: W. T. Keener. Retrieved on March 11, 2004, from http://ENW.org/1895 Nursing.htm

American Nurses Association. (2001). *Code of Ethics for Nurses with Interpretive Statements.* Washington, DC: American Nurses Publishing.

Andriopoulos, C. (2001). Determinants of organizational creativity: A literature review. *Management Decision, 39*(10), 834–840.

Appel, S. (1995). Freud on civilization. *Human Relations, 48*(6), 625–646.

Aron, D., Dittus, R., & Rosenthal, G. (2002). Exploring the academic context for quality improvement: A scientific discipline in need of a career path. *Quality Management in Health Care, 10*(3), 65–70.

Arthur, H., Wall, D., & Halligan, A. (2003). Team resource management: A programme for troubled teams. *Clinical Governance, 8*(1), 86–91.

Ashforth, B. E., & Humphrey, R. H. (1993). Emotional labor in service roles: The influence of identity. *Academy of Management Review, 18*(1), 88–115.

Ashforth, B. E., & Humphrey, R. H. (1995). Emotions in the workforce: A reappraisal. *Human Relations, 48,* 97–125.

Ashley, J. A. (1997). Nursing power and healthcare reforms. In K. Wolf (Ed.), *Jo Ann Ashley: Selected readings* (pp. 103–120). New York: National League for Nursing.

Badaracco, J. (2002). *Leading quietly.* Boston: Harvard Business School Press.

Badaracco, J. L., Jr. (1997). *Defining moments.* Boston: Harvard Business School Press.

Bandura, A. (1977). *Social learning theory.* Englewood Cliffs, N.J.: Prentice-Hall.

Barden, C. (2003). Bold voices: Fearless and essential. *American Journal of Critical Care, 12*(5), 418–423.

Bardwick, J. M. (1996). Peacetime management and wartime leadership. In F. Hesselbein, M. Goldsmith, & R. Beckhard (Eds.), *The leader of the future.* San Francisco: Jossey-Bass.

Barker, L. L., Cegala, D. J., Kibler, R. J., & Wahlers, K. J. (1979). *Groups in process: An introduction to small group communication.* Englewood Cliffs, NJ: Prentice Hall.

Barnhart, T. (1997). Save the bureaucrats (while reinventing them). *Public Personnel Management, 26*(1), 7–14.

Bar-On, R. (2000). Emotional and social intelligence. In R. Bar-On & J. Parker (Eds.), *The handbook of emotional intelligence.* San Francisco: Jossey-Bass.

Barton, A. (1991). Conflict resolution by nurse managers. *Nursing Management, 22*(5), 83–85.

Beckham, D. (2003). Sustainable leadership. *Health Forum Journal, 46*(3), 43–44.

Beglinger, J. (2003). Transforming nursing. *Health Progress, 84*(4), 25–32.

Benner, P. (1984). *From novice to expert: Excellence and power in clinical nursing practice.* Menlo Park, CA: Addison-Wesley.

Bennett, M. (2003). Implementing new clinical guidelines: The manager as agent of change. *Nursing Management, 10*(7), 20–23.

Benton, D. (1999). Assertiveness, power and influence. *Nursing Standard, 13*(52), 48–53.

Berwick, D. (2003). Disseminating innovations in health care. *Journal of the American Medical Association, 289*(15), 1969–1975.

Billingsley, M. (2000). Satisfying Gen X: Can we do it? *Nursing Connection, 13*(1), 72–74.

Birrer, R. B. (2002). The physician leader in health care. *Health Progress, 83*(6), 27–30.

Blake, R. R., & McCanse, A. A. (1997). *Leadership dilemmas—grid solutions.* Houston: Gulf.

Blake, R. R., & Mouton, J. S. (1978). *The new managerial grid.* Houston: Gulf.

Boyatzis, R. E. (2001). How and why individuals are able to develop emotional intelligence. In C. Cherniss & D. Goleman (Eds.), *The emotionally intelligent workplace.* San Francisco: Jossey-Bass.

Bradford, B., & Sutton, M. (2003). From survival to success. *Nursing Administration Quarterly, 27*(2), 106–119.

Brazill, S. (2002). Let's get this show on the road: Primary health care. *SMA Newsbulletin, 4*(4), 2.

Broccolo, G. T. (2002). Integrating business and spirituality. *Health Progress 83*(3), 36–39, 67.

Bronstein, L. (2003). A model for interdisciplinary collaboration. *Social Work 48*(3), 297–306.

Brunke, L. (2001). Workplace issues remain a priority. *Nursing BC, 33*(5), 38.

Buckingham, M., & Clifton, D. O. (2001). *Now, discover your strengths.* New York: Free Press.

Byrne, M. (2002). The feelings nurses and patients/families experience when faced with the need to make bioethical decisions. *Association of Operating Room Nurses (AORN) Journal, 76*(1), 185.

Byrne, M., & Keefe, M. (2002). Building research competence in nursing through mentoring. *Journal of Nursing Scholarship, 34*(4), 391–396.

Cadman, C., & Brewer, J. (2001). Emotional intelligence: A vital prerequisite for recruitment in nursing. *Journal of Nursing Management, 9*(6), 321–324.

Campbell, S. (2003). Cultivating empowerment in nursing today for a strong profession tomorrow. *Journal of Nursing Education, 42*(9), 423–426.

Campbell, S., Roland, M., & Wilkin, D. (2001). Improving the quality of care through clinical governance. *British Medical Journal* (International Edition), *322*(7302), 1580–1582.

Chaffee, M., & Arthur, D. (2002). Failure: Lessons for health care leaders. *Nursing Economics, 20*(5), 225–231.

Chapman, L., & Howkins, E. (2003). Work-based learning: Making a difference in practice. *Nursing Standard, 17*(34), 39–42.

Charan, R. (2001). Conquering a culture of indecision. *Harvard Business Review, 79*(4), 74–82.

Chase, R. (1998). Knowledge navigators. *Information Outlook, 2*(9), 17–26.

Chen, P. Y., & Spector, P. E. (1992). Relationship of work stressors with aggression, withdrawal, theft and substance use: An exploratory study. *Journal of Occupational and Organizational Psychology, 65*(3), 177–184.

Chernin, P. (2002). Creative leadership: The strength of ideas, the power of the imagination. *Vital Speeches of the Day, 68*(8), 245–249.

Cherniss, C. (2000). Social and emotional competence in the workplace. In R. Bar-On & J.D.A. Parker (Eds.), *The handbook of emotional intelligence.* San Francisco: Jossey-Bass.

Cherniss, C. (2003). The business case for emotional intelligence. Available: www.eiconsortium.org.

Chesbrough, H. W., & Teece, D. J. (2002). Organizing for innovation: When is virtual virtuous? *Harvard Business Review, 80*(8), 127–135.

Chiavenato, I. (2001). Advances and challenges in human resource management in the new millennium. *Public Personnel Management, 30*(1), 17–26.

Christensen, C. M., & Raynor, M. E. (2003). Why hard-nosed executives should care about management theory. *Harvard Business Review, 81*(9), 66–74.

Church, E. B. (2003). Sensitivity to others. *Parent and Child, 11*(3), 72.

Citrin, J. (2002). *Zoom: How twelve exceptional companies are navigating the road to the next economy.* New York: Doubleday.

Clancy, T. R. (2003). Courage and today's nurse leader. *Nursing Administration Quarterly, 27*(2), 128–132.

Clarke, L. (2003). Nurse education: Why Socrates would disapprove. *Nursing Standard, 17*(52), 36–37.

Cline, D., Reilly, C., & Moore, J. (2003). What's behind RN turnover? *Nursing Management, 34*(10), 50–53.

Cohen, S. G., & Bailey, D. E. (1997). What makes teams work: Group effectiveness research from the shop floor to the executive suite. *Journal of Management, 23*(3), 239–290.

Colleagues remember talented leader. (2003). *Nursing Standard, 17*(30), 4.

Collins, J. (2001a). *Good to great.* New York: HarperCollins.

Collins, J. (2001b, Jan.). Level 5 leadership. *Harvard Business Review.*

Connolly, K. H. (2002). The new IQ. *Nursing Management, 33*(7), 17–18.

Cooper, R., & Sawaf, A. (1997). *Executive EQ: Emotional intelligence in leadership and organizations.* New York: Grosset Putnam.

Cordeniz, J. (2002). Recruitment, retention, and management of Generation X: A focus on nursing professionals. *Journal of Healthcare Management, 47*(4), 237–249.

Covey, S. R. (1990). *The seven habits of highly effective people: Powerful lessons in personal change.* New York: Simon & Schuster.

Covey, S. R. (1991). *Principle-centered leadership.* New York: Summit Books.

Covey, S. R., Merrill, A. R., & Merrill, R. R. (1994). *First things first.* New York: Simon & Schuster.

Cox, S. (2002). Emotional competence—the rest of the story. *Nursing Management, 33*(10), 64–66.

Cranton, P. (1996). *Professional development as transformative learning: New perspectives for teachers of adults.* San Francisco: Jossey-Bass.

Csikszentmihalyi, M. (1997). *Finding flow: The psychology of engagement with everyday life.* New York: HarperCollins.

Daddario, D. (2003). Mentorship: Taking medical-surgical nurses to new heights. *Med-Surg Matters, 12*(1), 16.

Dahlgaard, J., & Dahlgaard, S. (1999). Integrating business excellence and innovation management: Developing a culture for innovation, creativity and learning. *Total Quality Management, 10*(4/5), S465–S472.

Davidhizar, R., & Shearer, R. (2002). Taking charge by "letting go." *The Health Care Manager, 20*(3), 33–38.

de Beauport, E. (1996). *The three faces of mind.* Wheaton, IL: Theosophical Publishing House.

Dearborn, K. (2002). Studies in emotional intelligence redefine our approach to leadership development. *Public Personnel Management, 31*(4), 523–530.

DePaulo, B. M. (1992). Nonverbal behavior and self-presentation. *Psychological Bulletin, 111,* 203–243.

De Ville, K. A. (2001). The ethical and legal implications of handheld medical computers. *Journal of Legal Medicine, 22*(4), 447–466.

Dimond, E., Calzone, K., Davis, J., & Jenkins, J. (1998). The role of the nurse in cancer genetics. *Cancer Nursing, 21*(1), 57–75.

Dixon, N. (2001). What is true? Looking at the validity of shared knowledge. *Information Outlook, 5*(5), 32–34.

Dossey, B. (1996). Help your patient break free from . . . anxiety. *Nursing, 26*(10), 52–54.

Dossey, B. M. (2000). *Florence Nightingale: Mystic, visionary, healer.* Springhouse, PA: Springhouse Corporation.

Drucker, P. (2001). *The essential Drucker.* New York: HarperCollins.

Druskat, V. (2001). Building the emotional intelligence of groups. *Harvard Business Review, 79*(3), 80–90.

Druskat, V., & Wolff, S. (2001). Group emotional intelligence and its influence on group effectiveness. In C. Cherniss & D. Goleman (Eds.), *The emotionally intelligent workplace.* San Francisco: Jossey-Bass.

Duchene, P. (2002). Leadership's guiding light. *Nursing Management, 33*(9), 28–30.

Duff, C. (1999). *Learning from other women: How to benefit from the knowledge, wisdom and experience of female mentors.* New York: AMACOM.

Eaton, J., & Johnson, R. (2001). *Coaching Successfully.* London: Dorling Kindersley.

Edmondson, A., Bohmer, R., & Pisano, G. (2001). Speeding up team learning. *Harvard Business Review, 79*(9), 125–132.

Egan, G. (1994). *Working the shadow side.* San Francisco: Jossey-Bass.

Eisen, M. (2001). Peer-based professional development viewed through the lens of transformative learning. *Holistic Nursing Practice, 16*(1), 30–42.

Eisenstat, R., & Dixon, D. (2000). Building organizational fitness. *Health Forum Journal, 43*(4), 52–55.

Elfenbein, H. A., & Ambady, N. (2002). Predicting workplace outcomes from the ability to eavesdrop on feelings. *Journal of Applied Psychology, 87*(5), 963–971.

Epstein, R. M. (2003). Mindful practice in action: Part I. Technical competence, evidence-based medicine, and relationship-centered care. *Families, Systems and Health, 21*(1), 1–9.

Eskildsen, J., Dahlgaard, J., & Norgaard, A. (1999). The impact of creativity and learning on business excellence. *Total Quality Management, 10*(4/5), S523–S530.

Espeland, K., & Shanta, L. (2001). Empowering versus enabling in academia. *Journal of Nursing Education, 40*(8), 342–346.

Evans, S. A. (1991). Conflict resolution: A strategy for growth. *AACN Clinical Issues in Critical Care Nursing, 20*(2), 20A–24A.

Evashwick, C., & Ory, M. (2003). Organizational characteristics of successful innovative health care programs sustained over time. *Family and Community Health, 26*(3), 177–193.

Farnham, A., Faircloth, A., & Carvell, T. (1996). Are you smart enough to keep your job? *Fortune, 133*(1), 34–40.

Farson, R., & Keyes, R. (2002). The failure-tolerant leader. *Harvard Business Review, 80*(8), 64–71.

Feifer, C., Nocella, K., DeArtola, I., Rowden, S., & Morrison, S. (2003). Self-managing teams: A strategy for quality improvement. *Topics in Health Information Management, 24*(1), 21–28.

Feinstein, K. (2003). We can't reward what we can't perform: The primacy of learning to change systems. *Health Affairs,* Web Exclusives 2002, W118–W121.

Fernandez-Araoz, C. (2001). The challenge of hiring senior executives. In C. Cherniss & D. Goleman (Eds.), *The emotionally intelligent workplace.* San Francisco: Jossey-Bass.

Fewtrell, D., & O'Connor, K. (1995). *Clinical phenomenology and cognitive psychology.* New York: Routledge.

Fisher, K. (1993). *Leading self-directed work teams.* New York: McGraw-Hill.

Fisher, K. W., Shaver, P. R., & Carnochan, P. (1990). How emotions develop and how they organize development. *Cognition and Emotion, 4,* 81–127.

Fleeger, M. E. (1993). Assessing organization culture: A planning strategy. *Nursing Management, 24*(2), 39–41.

Flower, J. (2000). The uncomfortable and the unanswerable. *Health Forum Journal, 43*(3), 24–27.

Fontaine, D. (1998). Lessons from a mentor: A dance for two. *Journal of Cardiovascular Nursing, 12*(2), 29–32.

Freshman, B., & Rubino, L. (2002). Emotional intelligence: A core competency for health care administrators. *The Health Care Manager, 20*(4), 1–9.

Freud, S. (1935). *Autobiography.* New York: Norton.

Freud, S. (1960). *Origins and development of psychoanalysis.* New York: Regnery-Gateway.

Freud, S. (1972). *The history of the psychoanalytic movement* (4th ed.). New York: Collier. (Original work published 1914)

Fuller, G. (1990). *The supervisor's portable answer book.* Paramus, NJ: Prentice-Hall.

Gardner, D., & Cary, A. (1999). Collaboration, conflict, and power: Lessons for case managers. *Family and Community Health, 22*(3), 64–77.

Gardner, H. (1983). *Frames of mind* (rev. ed.). New York: Basic Books.

Gardner, J. W. (1990). *On Leadership.* New York: Free Press.

Garrison, A. (2003). Between a rock and a hard place. *Journal of the American Medical Association, 290*(9), 1217–1218.

Gebelein, S. H., Lee, D. G., Nelson-Neuhaus, K. J., & Sloan, E. B. (1999). *Successful executive's handbook.* Minneapolis, MN: Personnel Decisions International.

Giganti, E. (2003a). Developing leaders for 2010. *Health Progress, 84*(1), 11–12.

Giganti, E. (2003b). Mission and mentoring at St. Joseph Health System. *Health Progress, 84*(3), 8–9.

Gilmartin, M. (1998). The nursing organization and the transformation of health care delivery for the 21st century. *Nursing Administration Quarterly, 22*(2), 70–86.

Goertz, J. (2000). Creativity: A component for effective leadership in today's schools. *Roeper Review, 22*(3), 158–162.

Gokenbach, V. (2003). Infuse management with leadership. *Nursing Management, 34*(1), 8, 10.

Gold, E. R., & Caulfield, T. A. (2002). The moral tollbooth: A method that makes use of the patent system to address ethical concerns in biotechnology. *Lancet, 359*(9325), 2268–2270.

Goleman, D. (1995). *Emotional intelligence.* New York: Bantam Books.

Goleman, D. (1998a). What makes a leader? *Harvard Business Review, 76*(6), 93–104.

Goleman, D. (1998b). *Working with emotional intelligence.* New York: Bantam Books.

Goleman, D. (2000). Leadership that gets results. *Harvard Business Review, 78*(2), 78–90.

Goleman, D. (2003). *Destructive emotions: How can we overcome them? A scientific dialogue with the Dalai Lama.* New York: Bantam Books.

Goleman, D., Boyatzis, R., & McKee, A. (2002). *Primal leadership.* Boston: Harvard Business School Press.

Grandey, A. (2000). Emotional regulation in the workplace: A new way to conceptualize emotional labor. *Journal of Occupational Health Psychology,* 5(1), 95–110.

Grazier, K. L. (2003). Interview: Philip A. Newbold, FACHE, president and CEO, Memorial Hospital and Health System, South Bend, Indiana. *Journal of Healthcare Management,* 48(1), 2–5.

Green, S., Hassan, F., Immelt, J., Marks, M., & Meiland, D. (2003). In search of global leaders. *Harvard Business Review,* 81(8), 38–44.

Greenhalgh, P. (1994). *Emotional growth and learning.* New York: Routledge.

Greenspan, S. I. (1997). *The growth of the mind.* New York: Addison-Wesley.

Grossman, R. (2000). Emotions at work. *Health Forum Journal,* 43(5), 18–22.

Gustafson, B. (2003). Are you meeting customers' emotional needs? *Healthcare Financial Management,* 57(4), 44–48.

Haack, P., & Smith, M. V. (2000). Mentoring new music teachers. *Music Educator's Journal,* 87(3), 23–27.

Hagenow, N. (2001). Care executives: Organizational intelligence for these times. *Nursing Administration Quarterly,* 25(4), 30–35.

Hagland, M. (1995). Incent me. *Hospitals and Health Networks,* 69(17), 7.

Halm, M., & Penque, S. (1999). Spirit at work: Supporting patients and colleagues. *Dimensions of Critical Care Nursing,* 18(5), 34–39.

Ham, C. (2003). Improving the performance of health services: The role of clinical leadership. *Lancet,* 361(9373), 1978–1980.

Hanna, L. (1999). Lead the way. *Nursing Management,* 30(11), 36–39.

Hart, R. (1984). *Verbal style and the presidency.* San Diego: Academic Press.

Harvard Business Review. (2003). Emotional intelligence is still smart. *Harvard Business Review,* 81(4), 95.

Hatch, T. (1997). Friends, diplomats, and leaders in kindergarten: Interpersonal intelligence in play. In P. Salovey & D. Sluyter (Eds.), *Emotional development and emotional intelligence.* New York: Basic Books.

Haviland-Jones, J., Gebelt, J. L., & Stapley, J. C. (1997). The questions of development in emotion. In P. Salovey & D. Sluyter (Eds.), *Emotional development and emotional intelligence.* New York: Basic Books.

Hayward, S. F. (1997). *Churchill on leadership.* Rocklin, CA: Prima.

Helge, D. (2001). Turning workplace anger and anxiety into peak performance: Strategies for enhancing employee health and productivity. *AAOHN Journal,* 49(8), 399–408.

Higgins, A. (2003). Leadership and change: The developing role of the consultant nurse. *Nursing Management,* 10(1), 22–28.

Hirschhorn, L. (2002). Campaigning for change. *Harvard Business Review,* 80(7), 98–104.

Hochschild, A. R. (1983). *The managed heart: Commercialization of human feeling.* Berkeley: University of California Press.

Hoffmaster, B. (2003). Fear of feeling. *Hastings Center Report, 33*(1), 45–47.

Holloway, M. (2003). The mutable brain. *Scientific American, 289*(3), 78–85.

Hom, E. (2003). Coaching and mentoring new graduates entering perinatal nursing practice. *Journal of Perinatal and Neonatal Nursing, 17*(1), 35–49.

Hughes, S. (2002). Ethical theories and dilemmas. *British Journal of Perioperative Nursing, 12*(6), 211–217.

Humphrey, J. (1998). *Job stress.* Needham Heights, MA: Allyn & Bacon.

Hunsaker, P., & Alessandra, A. (1986). *The art of managing people.* New York: Simon & Schuster.

Hutton, D. (2003). Help for CEOs. *Health Forum Journal, 46*(3), 21–24.

Institute of Medicine. (2001). *Crossing the quality chasm: A new health system for the 21st century.* Washington, DC: National Academy Press.

Ittner, C., & Larcker, D. (2003). Coming up short on nonfinancial performance measurement. *Harvard Business Review, 81*(11), 88–95.

Jacobs, B. (2001). Respect for human dignity: A central phenomenon to philosophically unite nursing theory and practice through consilience of knowledge. *Advances in Nursing Science, 24*(1), 17–35.

James, H. (1963). *Psychology* (abridged ed.). New York: Fawcett.

Johnson, G., Scholes, K., & Sexty, R. W. (1989). *Exploring strategic management.* Englewood Cliffs, NJ: Prentice Hall.

Johnson, J. (2002). Six steps to ethical leadership in health care. *Patient Care Management, 18*(2), 1–9.

Johnson, S. (1998). *Who moved my cheese? An amazing way to deal with change in your work and in your life.* New York: Putnam.

Jones, M. (1997). UnConventional wisdom. *Psychology Today, 30*(5), 34–36.

Jones, M. A. (1992). Job conflict resolution styles of nurses. *Journal of Nursing Administration, 22*(11), 63.

Joshua-Amadi, M. (2002). Recruitment and retention: A study in motivation. *Nursing Management, 9*(8), 17–22.

Kanter, R. M. (2003). Thriving locally in the global economy. *Harvard Business Review, 81*(8), 119–127.

Katzenbach, J. R., & Smith, D. K. (1993). *The wisdom of teams.* Boston: Harvard Business School Press.

Kaye, K. (1994). *Workplace wars and how to end them.* New York: AMACOM.

Kelly, C. (2002). Investing in the future of nursing education: A cry for action. *Nursing Education Perspective, 23*(1), 24–29.

Kenny, N., Sargeant, J., & Allen, M. (2001). Lifelong learning in ethical practice: A challenge for continuing medical education. *Journal of Continuing Education in the Health Professions, 21*(1), 24–32.

Kerfoot, K. (1998). Leading change is leading creativity. *Pediatric Nursing, 24*(2), 180–181.

Kerfoot, K. (2002). Warming your heart: The energy solution. *Dermatology Nursing, 14*(3), 197–198.

Kim, W. C., & Mauborgne, R. (2003). Tipping point leadership. *Harvard Business Review, 81*(4), 60–69.

Kinsella, L. (2001). Truth telling in patient care. *Nursing, 31*(12), 52–55.

Kotter, J. P. (1996). *Leading change.* Boston: Harvard University Press.

Kotter, J. P., & Cohen, D. S. (2002). *The heart of change: Real-life stories of how people change their organizations.* Cambridge, MA: Harvard Business School Press.

Kouzes, J., & Posner, B. (1995). *The leadership challenge.* San Francisco: Jossey-Bass.

Kowalski, K., & Yoder-Wise, P. (2003, September/October). Five C's of leadership. *Nurse Leader,* pp. 26–31.

Kram, K. E., & Cherniss, C. (2001). Developing emotional competence through relationships at work. In C. Cherniss & D. Goleman (Eds.), *The emotionally intelligent workplace.* San Francisco: Jossey-Bass.

Kramer, R. M. (2002). When paranoia makes sense. *Harvard Business Review, 80*(7), 62–69.

Kubsch, S., Henniges, A., Lorenzoni, N., Eckardt, S., & Oleniczak, S. (2003). Factors influencing accruement of contact hours for nurses. *Journal of Continuing Education in Nursing, 34*(5), 204–212.

Kutzscher, L., Sabiston, J. A., Laschinger, H.K.S., & Nish, M. (1997). The effects of teamwork on staff perceptions of empowerment and job satisfaction. *Health Management Forum, 2*(10), 12–17.

Lachman, V. (1998). Care of the self for the nurse entrepreneur. *Nursing Administration Quarterly, 22*(2), 48–59.

LaFasto, F., & Larson, C. (2001). *When teams work best.* Thousand Oaks, CA: Sage.

Laschinger, H.K.S. (1996). A theoretical approach to studying work empowerment in nursing: A review of studies testing Kanter's theory of structural power in organizations. *Nursing Administration Quarterly, 20*(2), 25–42.

Laschinger, H., Finegan, J., & Shamian, J. (2001). The impact of workplace empowerment, organizational trust on staff nurses' work satisfaction and organizational commitment. *Health Care Management Review, 26*(3), 7–23.

Laurent, C. (2000). Control addicts: A 12-step program for nurse managers. *Nursing Forum, 35*(4), 15–22.

Lennox, R. D., & Wolfe, R. N. (1984). Revision of the self monitoring scale. *Journal of Personality and Social Psychology, 46*(6), 1349–1364.

Levey, S., Hill, J., & Greene, B. (2002). Leadership in health care and the leadership literature. *Journal of Ambulatory Care Management, 25*(2), 69–74.

Levinson, W., Gorawam-Bhat, R., & Lamb, J. (2000). A study of patient clues and physician responses in primary care and surgical settings. *Journal of the American Medical Association, 284*(8), 1021–1027.

Lippman, T. W. (2000). *Madeleine Albright and the new American diplomacy.* Boulder, CO: Westview Press.

Lundberg, T., & Tulczak, L. (1997). *Slash your workers' comp costs.* New York: American Management Association.

Maher, C. A. (1991). A systems approach to managing conflict. *Orthopedic Nursing, 10*(3), 35–44.

Malloch, K. (2002). Trusting organizations: Describing and measuring employee-to-employee relationships. *Nursing Administration Quarterly, 26*(3), 12–19.

Manderson, L. (1998). *Cultural diversity: A guide for health professionals.* Brisbane, Australia: Queensland Government.

Martin, C. (2002). The theory of critical thinking in nursing. *Nursing Education Perspectives, 23*(5), 243–247.

Martin, P., Yarbrough, S., & Alfred, D. (2003). Professional values held by baccalaureate and associate degree nursing students. *Journal of Nursing Scholarship, 35*(3), 291–296.

Marvel, K., Bailey, A., Pfaffly, C., Gunn, W., & Beckman, H. (2003). Relationship-centered administration: Transferring effective communication skills from the exam room to the conference room. *Journal of Healthcare Management, 48*(2), 112–124.

Mateo, M., & Smith, S. (2001). Workforce diversity: Challenges and strategies. *Journal of Multicultural Nursing and Health, 7*(2), 8–12.

Mayer, J. D., Caruso, D. R., & Salovey, P. (1999). Emotional intelligence meets traditional standards for an intelligence. *Intelligence, 27*(4), 267–298.

Mayer, J. D., & Salovey, P. (1993). The intelligence of emotional intelligence. *Intelligence, 17*(4), 433–442.

Mayer, J. D., & Salovey, P. (1994). Emotional intelligence and the construction and regulation of feelings. *Applied and Preventive Psychology, 4*, 197–208.

Mayer, J. D., & Salovey, P. (1997). What is emotional intelligence? In P. Salovey & D. J. Sluyter (Eds.), *Emotional development and emotional intelligence: Educational implications.* New York: Basic Books.

Mayer, J. D., Salovey, P., & Caruso, D. (1999). *MSCEIT research version 1.1* (3rd ed.). Unpublished test manual, University of New Hampshire, Durham, NH.

Mayer, J. D., Salovey, P., & Caruso, D. (2000). Emotional intelligence as zeit-geist, as personality, and as a mental ability. In R. Bar-On and J. Parker, *The handbook of emotional intelligence*. San Francisco: Jossey-Bass.

Mayer, J. D., Salovey, P., & Caruso, D. R. (2002). *MSCEIT user's manual*. North Tonawanda, NY: Multi Health Systems.

Mayer, J. D., Salovey, P., Caruso, D. R., & Sitarenios, G. (2001). Emotional intelligence as a standard intelligence. *Emotion, 1*(3), 232–242.

McCannon, M., & O'Neal, P. (2003). Results of a national survey indicating information technology skills needed by nurses at time of entry into the work force. *Journal of Nursing Education, 42*(8), 337–340.

McConnell, C. (1998). Fattened and flattened: The expansion and contraction of the modern organization. *Health Care Supervisor, 17*(1), 72–83.

McConnell, C. (1999). Balancing inside and outside: Preparing for tomorrow while fulfilling today's responsibilities. *Health Care Manager, 18*(2), 73–82.

McKinley, C., Parmer, D., Saint-Amand, R., Harbin, C., Roulston, J., Ellis, R., Buchanan, J., & Leonard, R. (1999). Performance improvement: The organization's quest. *Quality Management in Health Care, 7*(2), 50–59.

McLean, T. R. (2002). Cybersurgery: An assessment for enterprise liability. *Journal of Legal Medicine, 23*(2), 167–210.

McLeod, J. (1999). A narrative social constructionist approach to therapeutic empathy. *Counseling Psychology Quarterly, 12*(4), 377–394.

McNeil, B. J., Elfrink, V. L., Bickford, C. J., & Pierce, S. T. (2003). Nursing information technology knowledge, skills, and preparation of student nurses, nursing faculty, and clinicians: A U.S. survey. *Journal of Nursing Education, 42*(8), 341–349.

Mezirow, J. (1991). *Transformative dimensions of adult learning*. San Francisco: Jossey-Bass.

Mezirow, J., & Associates. (2000). *Learning as transformation: Critical perspectives on a theory in progress*. San Francisco: Jossey-Bass.

Michaels, C. (2002). Circle communication: An old form of communication useful for 21st century leadership. *Nursing Administration Quarterly, 26*(5), 1–10.

Miller, P. H. (1993). *Theories of developmental psychology* (3rd ed.). New York: Freeman.

Miller, S. A. (2003). Lessons in loving. *Parent and Child, 11*(3), 70.

Mintzer, B. (2003). The power of a vision: The nurse's journey through health care. *Urologic Nursing, 23*(1), 82–86.

Miskell, J. R., & Miskell, V. (1994). *Motivation at work*. Burr Ridge, IL: Irwin.

Mitroff, I., & Alpaslan, M. (2003). Preparing for evil. *Harvard Business Review, 81*(4), 109–115.

Montebello, A. (1994). *Work teams that work*. Minneapolis, MN: Best Sellers.

Montgomery, K. (2002). Leadership: An old topic with a new face—leading a coalition. *Patient Care Management, 17*(10), 10–12.

Montgomery, K. (2003). Becoming a follower: A new competency for the organizational leader. *Patient Care Management, 19*(2), 1–10.

Morris, J. A., & Feldman, D. C. (1996). The dimensions, antecedents, and consequences of emotional labor. *Academy of Management Review, 21*(4), 986–1010.

Morrison, P. (2000). Learning from other women: How to benefit from the knowledge, wisdom and experience of female mentors [Book review]. *Surgical Services Management, 6*(10), 73.

Moss, M. T. (2001). *Emotional determinants in health care executive management styles.* Unpublished doctoral dissertation, Medical University of South Carolina, Charleston, SC.

Moss, M. T., Rau, W., Craig, J., & Strack, G. (2000). *Characteristics of leaders.* Unpublished manuscript, Medical University of South Carolina, Charleston, SC.

Ndiwane, A. (2000). The effects of community, co-worker and organizational support to job satisfaction of nurses in Cameroon. *ABNF Journal, 11*(6), 145–149.

Neuwirth, Z. E. (1999). The silent anguish of the healers. *Newsweek, 134*(11), 79.

Nightingale, F. (1969). *Notes on nursing: What it is and what it is not.* New York: Dover. (Original work published 1860)

Nussbaum, M. (2001). *Upheavals of thought: The intelligence of emotions.* New York: Cambridge University Press.

Olesen, E. (1993). Twelve Steps to *Mastering the winds of change.* New York: MacMillan.

Olson, L. (2002). Ethical climate as the context for nurse retention. *Chart, 99*(6), 3–4.

O'Sullivan, M. J. (1999). Strategic learning in healthcare organizations. *Hospital Topics, 77*(3), 13–21.

Otto, D. A. (1999). Regulatory statutes and issues: Clinical accountability in perioperative settings. *AORN* [Association of Operating Room Nurses] *Journal, 70*(2), 241–252.

Owens, J., & Patton, J. (2003). Take a chance on nursing mentorships: Enhance leadership with this win-win strategy. *Nursing Education Perspectives, 24*(4), 198–204.

Pagonis, W. (2001). Leadership in a combat zone. *Harvard Business Review, 79*(11), 107–116.

Parvis, L. (2003). Diversity and effective leadership in multicultural workplaces. *Journal of Environmental Health, 65*(7), 37, 65.

Peddy, S. (1998). *The art of mentoring.* Houston: Bullion Books.

Perra, B. (2001). Leadership: The key to quality outcomes. *Journal of Nursing Care Quality, 15*(2), 68–73.

Pfeffer, J., & Sutton, R. I. (2000). *The knowing-doing gap.* Boston: Harvard Business School Press.

Pfeill, M. (2003). The skills-teaching myth in nurse education: From Florence Nightingale to Project 2000. *International History of Nursing Journal, 7*(3), 32–40.

Phillips, M. (2003). The challenge of cultural diversity. *Dermatology Nursing, 15*(4), 311, 338.

Pinkerton, S. (2003). Supporting the nurse manager to improve staff nurse retention. *Nursing Economics, 21*(1), 45–46.

Pitman, B. (2003). Leading for value. *Harvard Business Review, 81*(4), 41–47.

Place, M. (2002). A shared history of "doing what needs to be done." *Health Progress, 83*(4), 6, 54.

Poole, C. (2003). Developing empathy. *Parent and Child, 11*(3), 68–69.

Porter-O'Grady, T. (2003). Of hubris and hope: Transforming nursing for a new age. *Nursing Economics, 21*(2), 59–64.

Porter-O'Grady, T., & Afable, R. (2002). Reforming the health care structure. *Health Progress, 83*(1), 17–20.

Porter-O'Grady, T., Hawkins, M. A., & Parker, M. L. (1997). *Whole systems shared governance.* Gaithersburg, MD: Aspen.

Poste, G. (1997). Managing discontinuities in healthcare markets and technology: Creativity, cash and competition. *Vital Speeches of the Day, 63*(10), 309–313.

Press, C. (2001). Why strategies fail. *Health Forum Journal, 44*(2), 26–31.

Qubein, N. R. (1997). *How to be a great communicator in person, on paper, and on the podium.* New York: Wiley.

Raingruber, B. (2000). Being with feelings as a recognition practice: Developing clients' self-understanding. *Perspectives in Psychiatric Care, 36*(2), 41–50.

Rapaport, R. (1993). To build a winning team: An interview with head coach Bill Walsh. *Harvard Business Review, 71*(1), 110–120.

Rashotte, J., & Thomas, M. (2002). Incorporating educational theory into critical care orientation. *Journal of Continuing Education in Nursing, 33*(3), 131–137.

Ray, M. A., Turkel, M. C., & Marino, F. (2002). The transformative process for nursing in workforce redevelopment. *Nursing Administration Quarterly, 26*(2), 1–14.

Read, H., Fordham, M., Adler, G., & McGuire, W. (Eds.). (1971). *The collected works of C. G. Jung* (Vol. 6, Bollingen Series 20) (Rev. ed., R. Hull). Princeton, NJ: Princeton University Press.

Reichheld, F. (2001). Lead for loyalty. *Harvard Business Review, 79*(7), 76–84.

Reinick, C. (2002). Leadership's guiding light, part 2: Create a learning organization. *Nursing Management, 33*(10), 42–43.

Restall, G., Ripat, J., & Stern, M. (2003). A framework of strategies for client-centered practice. *Canadian Journal of Occupational Therapy, 70*(2), 103–112.

Rick, C., Kearns, M., & Thompson, N. (2003). The reality of virtual learning for nurses in the largest integrated health care system in the nation. *Nursing Administration Quarterly, 27*(1), 41–57.

Robbins, C., Bradley, E., Spicer, M., & Mecklenburg, G. (2001). Developing leadership in healthcare administration: A competency assessment tool/practitioner application. *Journal of Healthcare Management, 46*(3), 188–199.

Robbins, S., & Hunsaker, P. (1996). *Training in interpersonal skills* (2nd ed.). Upper Saddle River, NJ: Prentice Hall.

Roberts, R. D., Zeidner, M., & Matthews, G. (2001). Does emotional intelligence meet traditional standards as an intelligence? Some new data and conclusions. *Emotion, 1*(3), 196–231.

Roberts, W. (1987). *Leadership secrets of Attila the Hun.* New York: Warner Books.

Rondeau, K., & Wagar, T. (1999). Hospital choices in times of cutback: The role of the organizational culture. *Leadership in Health Services, 12*(3), xiv–xxii.

Ross, R. R., & Altmaier, E. M. (1994). *Intervention in occupational stress.* London: Sage.

Rugh, W. A. (1999). Past, present and future leadership. *Middle East Policy, 6*(4), 30–33.

Rushmer, R. (2000). What will it mean to have a flatter team-based NHS structure? *British Journal of Nursing, 9*(21), 2242–2248.

Ryback, D. (1998). *Putting emotional intelligence to work.* Boston: Butterworth-Heinemann.

Rycroft-Malone, J., Harvey, G., Kitson, A., McCormack, B., Seers, K., & Titchen, A. (2002). Getting evidence into practice: Ingredients for change. *Nursing Standard, 16*(37), 38–43.

Sabatier, K. (2002). The Institute for Johns Hopkins Nursing—a collaborative model for nursing practice and education. *Nursing Education Perspectives, 23*(4), 178–182.

Salovey, P., & Mayer, J. D. (1990). Emotional intelligence. *Imagination, Cognition, and Personality, 9,* 185–211.

Salovey, P., & Mayer, J. D. (1994). Some final thoughts about personality and intelligence. In R. J. Sternberg & P. Ruzgis (Eds.), *Personality and intelligence* (pp. 308–318). New York: Cambridge University Press.

Samuel, P. (2003). Lead the way. *Nursing Standard, 18*(1), 96.

Sauter, S., Murphy, L., Colligan, M., Swanson, N., Hurrell, J., Scharf, F. S., Grubb, P., Goldenhar, L., Alterman, T., Johnston, J., Hamilton, A., & Tisdale, J. (1999). Stress . . . at work (DHHS NIOSH Publication No. 99–101). Retrieved from http://www.cdc.gov/niosh/stresswk.html.

Savage, C. (2003). Nursing leadership: Oxymoron or powerful force? *AAACN Viewpoint, 25*(4), 1, 11–14.

Schreiber, R., & Bannister, E. (2003). Challenges of teaching in an emancipatory curriculum. *Journal of Nursing Education, 41*(1), 41–45.

Schutte, N., Malouff, J., Bobik, C., Coston, T., Greeson, C., Jedlicka, C., Rhodes, E., & Wendorf, G. (2001). Emotional intelligence and interpersonal relations. *Journal of Social Psychology, 141*(4), 523–536.

Scott, S., & Bruce, R. (1994). Determinants of innovative behavior: A path model of individual innovation in the workplace. *Academy of Management Journal, 37*(3), 580–608.

The secret skill of leaders. (2002). *U.S. News & World Report, 132*(1), 8.

Segal, J. (2002). Good leaders use "emotional intelligence." *Health Progress, 83*(3), 44–46, 66.

Sessa, V. I. (1998). Using conflict to improve effectiveness of nurse teams. *Orthopedic Nursing, 17*(3), 41–48.

Sherwood, G. (2003, September/October). Leadership for a healthy work environment: Caring for the human spirit. *Nurse Leader,* pp. 36–40.

Shultz, B. (2003). What makes a good leader? *AORN* [Association of Operating Room Nurses] *Journal, 78*(1), 9–11.

Sigma Theta Tau International (2001, July). *Facts on the nursing shortage.* Available: http://www.nursesource.org/facts_shortage.html. Accessed Nov. 2003.

Silversin, J., & Kornacki, M. J. (2003). Implementing change: From ideas to reality. *Family Practice Management, 10*(1), 57–62.

Simpson, R. L., & Keegan, A. J. (2002). How connected are you? Employing emotional intelligence in a high-tech world. *Nursing Administration Quarterly, 26*(2), 80–86.

Slater, J. (1999). That winning feeling. *Far Eastern Economic Review, 162*(39), 68.

Smith, C. A., & Lazarus, R. S. (1993). Appraisal components, core relational themes, and the emotions. *Cognition and Emotion, 7,* 233–269.

Smith, S., Tutor, R., & Phillips, M. (2001). Resolving conflict realistically in today's health care environment. *Journal of Psychosocial Nursing and Mental Health Services, 39*(11), 36–47.

Sokol, A. J., & Molzen, C. (2002). The changing standard of care in medicine: E-health, medical errors, and technology add new obstacles. *Journal of Legal Medicine, 23*(4), 449–490.

South, I. (1857). *Facts Relating to Hospital Nurses*. London, St. Thomas's Hospital.

Spath, P. (2003). Sharing the knowledge. *Health Forum Journal, 46*(2), 16–19, 47.

Spitzer, R. (2003, September/October). The magnetism of management. *Nurse Leader*, p. 4.

Staring, S. (1999). When in doubt, call in RIC: Respect, integrity and compassion. *Surgical Services Management, 5*(5), 25–27.

Staring, S., & Taylor, C. (1997). A guide to managing workforce transitions. *Nursing Management, 28*(12), 31–32.

Staw, B., Sutton, R., & Pelled, L. (1994). Employee positive emotions and favorable outcomes at the workplace. *Organization Science, 5*(1), 51–71.

Stayer, R. (1990). How I learned to let my workers lead. *Harvard Business Review, 68*(6), 66–69, 72–74, 80, 82–83.

Sternberg, R. J. (1985). *Beyond IQ*. New York: Cambridge University Press.

Sternberg, R. J., & Wagner, R. K. (1986). *Practical intelligence*. New York: Cambridge University Press.

Stonecipher, H. (1998). Innovation and creativity: From the light bulb to the jet engine and beyond. *Vital Speeches of the Day, 64*(12), 370–374.

Strickland, D. (2000). Emotional intelligence: The most potent factor in the success equation. *Journal of Nursing Administration, 30*(3), 112–117.

Strock, J. (1998). *Reagan on leadership: Executive lessons from the great communicator*. Rocklin, CA: Prima.

Sutton, R. (2001). The weird rules of creativity. *Harvard Business Review, 79*(8), 94–103.

Swann, W., Stein-Seroussi, A., McNulty, S. (1992). Outcasts in a white-lie society: The enigmatic worlds of people with negative self-conceptions. *Journal of Personality and Social Psychology, 62*(4), 618–624.

Tanner, C. (2003). Cultivating the nurse within. *Journal of Nursing Education, 42*(7), 287–288.

Taylor, R. (2003). Leadership is a learned skill. *Family Practice Management, 10*(9), 43–48.

Tesser, A., & Rosen, S. (1975). The reluctance to transmit bad news. *Advances in Experimental Social Psychology, 8*, 193–232.

Tichy, N., & Charan, R. (1995, March-April). The CEO as coach: An interview with AlliedSignal's Lawrence A. Bossidy. *Harvard Business Review, 73*(2), 69–78.

Truby, B. (2000). Conflict management and resolution. *Surgical Services Management, 6*(6), 21–25.

Turkle, S. (2003). Technology and human vulnerability. *Harvard Business Review, 81*(9), 43–51.

Turski, G. W. (1994). *Toward a rationality of emotions*. Athens, OH: Ohio University Press.

Tyler, J. L. (2003). Core competencies: A simplified look at a complicated issue. *Healthcare Financial Management, 57*(5), 90–94.

Ulrich, B. (2003). Leader to watch: Tim Porter-O'Grady, EdD, PhD, RN, FAAN. *Nurse Leader, 1*(5), 20–25.

Ulrich, D. (1996). Credibility x Capability. In F. Hesselbein, M. Goldsmith, & R. Beckhard (Eds.), *The Leader of the Future.* San Francisco, Jossey-Bass.

Upenieks, V. V. (2003). The interrelationship of organizational characteristics of magnet hospitals, nursing leadership, and nursing job satisfaction. *The Health Care Manager, 22*(2), 83–98.

Useem, M. (2001a). The leadership lessons of Mount Everest. *Harvard Business Review, 79*(9), 51–58.

Useem, M. (2001b). A manager for all seasons. *Fortune, 143*(9), 66–72.

Vanman, E. J., & Miller, N. (1993). Applications of emotion theory and research to stereotyping and intergroup relations. In D. M. Mackie & D. L. Hamilton (Eds.), *Affect, cognition, and stereotyping* (pp. 213–238). San Diego, CA: Harcourt Brace Jovanovich.

Vargo, J. (1997). Teaching weaves the brain's neuron connections. In P. Salovey & D. J. Sluyter (Eds.), *Emotional development and emotional intelligence: Educational implications.* New York: Basic Books.

Verdejo, T. (2002). Mentoring: A model method. *Nursing Management, 33*(8), 15–16.

Vestal, K. (2003, Sept./Oct.). The change-dazed manager. *Nurse Leader,* 6–7.

Vestal, K., Fralicx, R., & Spreier, S. (1997). Organizational culture: The critical link between strategy and results. *Hospital and Health Services Administration, 42*(3), 339–365.

Vinten, G. (1992). Thriving in chaos: The route to management survival. *Management Decision, 30*(8), 22–28.

Vitello-Cicciu, J. M. (2002). Exploring emotional intelligence: Implications for nursing leaders. *Journal of Nursing Administration, 32*(4), 203–210.

Waldroop, J., & Butler, T. (1996). The executive as coach. *Harvard Business Review, 74*(6), 111–117.

Wall, B., Solum, R., & Sobol, M. (1992). *The visionary leader.* Rocklin, CA: Prima.

Watson, J. (2000). Leading via caring-healing: The fourfold way toward transformative leadership. *Nursing Administration Quarterly, 25*(1), 1–6.

Weisinger, H. (1998). *Emotional intelligence at work.* San Francisco: Jossey-Bass.

Wellins, R., Byham, W., & Wilson, J. (1991). *Empowered teams: Creating self-directed work groups that improve quality, productivity, and participation.* San Francisco: Jossey-Bass.

Wesorick, B. (2002). 21st century leadership challenge: Creating and sustaining healthy, healing work cultures and integrated service at the point of care. *Nursing Administration Quarterly, 26*(5), 18–32.

West, C. (1854). *How to Nurse Sick Children.* London: Longman, Brown, Green and Landmans.

Wheatley, M. J., & Kellner-Rodgers, M. (1996). *A simpler way.* San Francisco: Berrett-Koehler.

Wieck, K., Prydun, M., & Walsh, T. (2002). What the emerging workforce wants in its leaders. *Journal of Nursing Scholarship, 34*(3), 283–288.

Woodham Smith, C. (1951). *Florence Nightingale, 1820–1910.* New York: McGraw-Hill.

Wright, A. (2002). Precepting in 2002. *Journal of Continuing Education in Nursing, 33*(3), 138–141.

Young, A., & Perrewe, R. (2000). The exchange relationship between mentors and protégés: The development of a framework. *Human Resource Management Review, 10*(2), 177–209.

Yukl, G. (1998). *Leadership in organizations* (4th ed.). Upper Saddle River, NJ: Prentice Hall.

Zeidner, M., Matthews, G., & Roberts, R. D. (2001). Slow down, you move too fast: Emotional intelligence remains an "elusive" intelligence. *Emotion, 1*(3), 265–275.

Zimmerman, B. J., & Phillips, C. Y. (2000). Affective learning: Stimulus to critical thinking and caring practice. *Journal of Nursing Education, 39*(9), 422–425.

NAME INDEX

A

Adams, K. E., 39
Adler, G., 199, 205n1
Afable, R., 26, 27, 160
Aiken, L. H., 7
Albright, M., 114–115
Alcock, B., 123
Alessandra, A., 189, 190, 192, 204
Alfred, D., 164, 236
Allen, M., 135
Almost, J., 258
Alpaslan, M., 20
Altmaier, E. M., 154
Ambady, N., 15, 146, 147
Andriopoulos, C., 71, 230
Appel, S., 48
Aron, D., 243
Arthur, D., 17, 124, 158
Arthur, H., 71, 229
Ashforth, B. E., 14, 15, 145
Ashley, J. A., 169
Attila, 112

B

Badaracco, J., 44, 73, 128, 130, 256
Bailey, A., 16, 150, 151
Bailey, D. E., 137
Bandura, A., 268
Bannister, E., 165
Barden, C., 105
Bardwick, J. M., 7
Barker, L. L., 142
Barnhart, T., 252
Bar-On, R., 133, 175
Barton, A., 193, 196, 197

Beckham, D., 16, 94, 101, 251
Beckman, H., 16, 150, 151
Beglinger, J., 167, 171, 220
Benner, P., 175
Bennett, M., 137
Benton, D., 153
Berger, S., 115–116
Berter, E., 123
Berwick, D., 86, 106
Bickford, C. J., 26, 30
Billingsley, M., 264
Birrer, R. B., 5, 45, 156
Blake, R. R., 5, 45
Bohmer, R., 147, 149
Boyatzis, R. E., 126, 147, 197, 240, 242
Bradford, B., 71, 250
Bradley, E., 45
Brazill, S., 120
Breuer, 48
Brewer, J., 31
Broccolo, G. T., 128
Bronstein, L., 113
Bruce, R., 78, 259
Brunke, L., 257
Buckingham, M., 146–147
Butler, T., 174
Byham, W., 239, 255
Byrne, M., 27, 169

C

Cadman, C., 31
Calzone, K., 5, 39
Campbell, S., 135, 169, 177, 276
Carnochan, P., 12

SUBJECT INDEX

A

Abnormal accidents, 20

Acceptance, desire for, 75

Accommodation response, 196, 197, 199, 201

Accomplishment: of leading change, 70; sense of, providing, 220

Accountability: delegating, 199; fostering, 137; increased, 65; individual and mutual, 142; key, 173; for mistakes, accepting, 124; new level of, 273; for outcomes, 253, 257; for patients, 17; preserving, 157; ultimate, 90

Achievement: outcomes, 240, 242; sense of, providing, 220

Acknowledgement: versus agreement, 203; of challenges, 107–108; of contributions, 155; of ideas and arguments, 124; of opinions, 151; of polarities, 223; of self, 267; of work, 8, 48, 49, 89

Action: balanced with reflection, 171; call to, example of defining, 108–109; change in, and behavior, 166; and emotion, relationship between, understanding, 179; enduring, 44; extending vision sharing into, 181; proactive, versus reaction, 272; providing framework for, 49; tied to vision, 105; willingness to take, 46, 226–227. *See also* Leadership actions

Action learning, 240

Action plans, 178, 210–211

Actions, everyday. *See* Behavior

Active listening: applying, 202–203; practicing, 255; skills required for, 189, 190–192

Adapting to change, 93

Adaptive thinking, driven by, 234

Adoption of technology, 24–25

Affiliative leaders, 196, 197

Agendas, alternate, problem with, 243

Aggression response, 196, 199

Aggressive reactive behavior, 153

Agreement, acknowledgment versus, 203

Air travel, advent of, 158–159

Alignment: with colleagues in other fields, 249; of culture with philosophies of empathic care, 227–236; with results, leadership actions and, 46; of vision with the ideal and reality, 275. *See also* Belief-behavior alignment

All-forgiving leader, 225

Alliances, building, 153–154

Alternate agendas, problem with, 243

Ambassadors, acting as, 156–158

Ambulance Work and Nursing, 4

American Hospital Association, 24

American Nurses Association, 28

Analysis, use of, 43, 56, 108; for conflict resolution, 187, 193–200, 208–209

Annual evaluations, 133–134

Annual feedback, 134

Anxiety disorders, 219

Anxiety-producing situations. *See* Stressors

R